PHYSICAL FITNESS ASSESSMENT

Principles, Practice and Application

Prepared under the aegis of the
International Committee for Physical Fitness Research

Past president L. Larson
President   L. Novak
Vice-president R. J. Shephard
Secretary   T. Ishiko

with the support of a grant from Recreation Canada.

Physical Fitness Assessment

PRINCIPLES, PRACTICE AND APPLICATION

Edited By

ROY J. SHEPHARD

Department of Preventive Medicine and Biostatistics
University of Toronto
Toronto, Ontario, Canada

and

HUGUES LAVALLÉE

Department of Health Sciences
University of Québec
Trois-Rivières, Québec, Canada

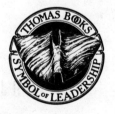

CHARLES C THOMAS • PUBLISHER
Springfield • Illinois • U.S.A.

Published and Distributed Throughout the World by
CHARLES C THOMAS · PUBLISHER
Bannerstone House
301-327 East Lawrence Avenue, Springfield, Illinois, U.S.A.

© *1978, by* CHARLES C THOMAS·PUBLISHER
ISBN 0-398-03701-9
Library of Congress Catalog Card Number; 77-24900

Library of Congress Cataloging in Publication Data
Main entry under title:

Physical fitness assessment.

Proceedings of a conference held at the University of Québec at Trois-Rivières,
prepared under the aegis of the International Committee for Physical Fitness Research.
  Includes index.
  1. Physical fitness—Congresses. 2. Physical fitness—Testing—Congresses.
3. Physical education and training—Congresses. I. Shephard, Roy J. II. Lavallée,
Hugues. III. International Committee for Physical Fitness Research. [DNLM: 1.
Physical fitness—Congresses. 2. Sport medicine—Congresses. 3. School health—
Congresses. 4. Community health services—Congresses. 5. Physical education and
training—Congresses. QT255 P579 1976]
GV205.P5   613.7   77-24900
ISBN 0-398-03701-9

*With THOMAS BOOKS careful attention is given to all details of
manufacturing and design. It is the Publisher's desire to present books that are
satisfactory as to their physical qualities and artistic possibilities and
appropriate for their particular use. THOMAS BOOKS will be true to those
laws of quality that assure a good name and good will.*

Printed in the United States of America
M-3

CONTRIBUTORS

O. Bar-Or
Department of Research and Sports Medicine
Wingate Institute for Physical Education and Sports
Wingate, Israel

C. Beaucage
Department of Health Sciences
Université du Québec à Trois-Rivières
Trois-Rivières, Québec, Canada

D. M. Berkson
Department of Community Health and Preventive Medicine
Northwestern University Medical School
Chicago, Illinois, U.S.A.

G. Beunen
Departement Lichamelijke Opvoeding
Katholieke Universiteit Leuven
Leuven, Belgium

S. R. Brown
Department of Kinesiology
Simon Fraser University
Burnaby, British Columbia, Canada

J. E. L. Carter
Department of Physical Education
San Diego State University
San Diego, California, U.S.A.

D. Chakrabarti
Department of Physiology
Calcutta University College of Science and Technology
Calcutta, India

B. J. Crepin
Department of Physical Recreation and Athletics
Carleton University
Ottawa, Ontario, Canada

v

G. R. Cumming
Department of Cardiology
Children's Hospital
Winnipeg, Manitoba, Canada

T. K. Cureton
University of Illinois
Urbana, Illinois, U.S.A.

C. T. M. Davies
MRC Environmental Physiology Unit
London School of Hygiene and Tropical Medicine
London, England

R. Dotan
Department of Research and Sports Medicine
Wingate Institute for Physical Education and Sports
Wingate, Israel

R. A. Faulkner
Department of Kinesiology
Simon Fraser University
Burnaby, British Columbia, Canada

H. Fujimatsu
Department of Exercise Physiology
School of Physical Education
Chukyo University
Aichi, Japan

T. Fukunaga
Department of Exercise Physiology
School of Physical Education
Chukyo University
Aichi, Japan

M. Hebbelinck
Institute of Physical Education
Free University
Brussels, Belgium

H. Heck
Institute for Sports Medicine and Circulation Research
German Sports University
Cologne, West Germany

K. Hirata
Chukyo University
Aichi, Japan

W. Hollmann
Institute for Sports Medicine and Circulation Research
German Sports University
Cologne, West Germany

I. B. Iliev
Department of Functional Diagnosis
Sport-medical Dispensary
Plovid, Bulgaria

O. Inbar
Department of Research and Sports Medicine
Wingate Institute for Physical Education and Sports
Wingate, Israel

T. Ishiko
Department of Physical Fitness
Juntendo University
Chiba, Japan

J. C. Jéquier
Department of Health Sciences
Université du Québec à Trois-Rivières
Trois-Rivières, Québec, Canada

P. L. Jooste
Industrial Hygiene Division
Chamber of Mines of South Africa
Johannesburg, Republic of South Africa

M. R. Kar
Department of Physiology
Calcutta University College of Science and Technology
Calcutta, India

T. Kavanagh
Toronto Rehabilitation Centre
Toronto, Ontario, Canada

V. Klissouras
Physiology Department and Physical Education Department
McGill University
Montreal, Quebec, Canada

M. Kobayashi
Department of Exercise Physiology
School of Physical Education
Chukyo University
Aichi, Japan

R. LaBarre
Department of Health Sciences
Université du Québec à Trois-Rivières
Trois-Rivières, Québec, Canada

B. Lake
Sydney, Australia

R. R. J. Lauzon
Fitness Consultant
Recreation Canada
Ottawa, Ontario, Canada

H. Lavallée
Department of Health Sciences
Université du Québec à Trois-Rivières
Trois-Rivières, Québec, Canada

A. Mader
Institute for Sports Medicine and Circulation Research
German Sports University
Cologne, West Germany

A. Magazanik
Heller Institute of Medical Research
Sheba Medical Center
Tel-Hashomer, Israel

A. Matsuo
Department of Exercise Physiology
School of Physical Education
Chukyo University
Aichi, Japan

A. Meroz
Heller Institute of Medical Research
Sheba Medical Center
Tel-Hashomer, Israel

P. K. Nag
Department of Physiology
Calcutta University College of Science and Technology
Calcutta, India

M. Ostyn
Departement Lichamelijke Opvoeding
Katholieke Universiteit Leuven
Leuven, Belgium

J. Pařízková
Research Institute FTVS
Charles University
Prague, Czechoslovakia

J. Pauwels
Departement Lichamelijke Opvoeding
Katholieke Universiteit Leuven
Leuven, Belgium

C. W. Poole
Department of Physical Recreation and Athletics
Carleton University
Ottawa, Ontario, Canada

M. K. Rajic
Department of Health Sciences
Université du Québec à Trois-Rivières
Trois-Rivières, Québec, Canada

R. L. Rasmussen
Department of Physical Education
St. Francis Xavier University
Antigonish, Nova Scotia, Canada

G. G. Ray
Department of Physiology
Calcutta University College of Science and Technology
Calcutta, India

D. B. Read
Industrial Hygiene Division
Chamber of Mines of South Africa
Johannesburg, Republic of South Africa

R. Reisenauer
Research Institute of Endocrinology
Prague, Czechoslovakia

R. Renson
Departement Lichamelijke Opvoeding
Katholieke Universiteit Leuven
Leuven, Belgium

N. J. Rick
Department of Physical Recreation and Athletics
Carleton University
Ottawa, Ontario, Canada

W. D. Ross
Department of Kinesiology
Simon Fraser University
Burnaby, British Columbia, Canada

R. Rost
Institute for Sports Medicine and Circulation Research
German Sports University
Cologne, West Germany

H. Ruskin
Department of Physical Education
Hebrew University
Jerusalem, Israel

S. G. Savov
Sport-Medical Dispensary
Plovdiv, Bulgaria

R. N. Sen
Department of Physiology
Calcutta University College of Science and Technology
Calcutta, India

Y. Shapiro
Heller Institute of Medical Research
Sheba Medical Center
Tel-Hashomer, Israel

Y. Sheonfeld
Heller Institute of Medical Research
Sheba Medical Center
Tel-Hashomer, Israel

R. J. Shephard
Department of Preventive Medicine and Biostatistics
University of Toronto
Toronto, Ontario, Canada

E. Shvartz
Heller Institute of Medical Research
Sheba Medical Center
Tel-Hashomer, Israel

W. E. Sime
Department of Kinesiology/Health Studies
University of Waterloo
Waterloo, Ontario, Canada

J. Simons
Departement Lichamelijke Opvoeding
Katholieke Universiteit Leuven
Leuven, Belgium

Š. Šprynarová
Research Institute of the Faculty of Physical Education and Sports
Prague, Czechoslovakia

J. Stamler
Department of Community Health and Preventive Medicine
Northwestern University Medical School
Chicago, Illinois, U.S.A.

N. B. Strydom
Industrial Hygiene Division
Chamber of Mines of South Africa
Johannesburg, Republic of South Africa

P. Swalus
Departement Lichamelijke Opvoeding
Katholieke Universiteit Leuven
Leuven, Belgium

J. Taylor
Department of Kinesiology
Simon Fraser University
Burnaby, British Columbia, Canada

B. Vanden Eynde
Departement Lichamelijke Opvoeding
Katholieke Universiteit Leuven
Leuven, Belgium

D. Van Gerven
Departement Lichamelijke Opvoeding
Katholieke Universiteit Leuven
Leuven, Belgium

I. T. Whipple
Department of Community Health and Preventive Medicine
Northwestern University Medical School
Chicago, Illinois, U.S.A.

D. Zwiren
Department of Research and Sports Medicine
Wingate Institute for Physical Education and Sports
Wingate, Israel

FOREWORD

THE OCCASION OF THE Montreal Olympic Games brought to Canada a vast number of internationally known experts in the fields of physical activity and human performance. The International Committee for Physical Fitness Research (I.C.P.F.R.) decided to profit from this serendipitous gathering of intellect by organizing a conference on the principles, practice, and application of physical fitness assessment, and the edited proceedings of the meeting provided the basis for the present volume.

Some international conferences make poor reading. This is not due to a lack of expertise on the part of the contributors, but reflects rather the difficulty that many foreigners and even North Americans find in effective use of the English language. The present editors have taken considerable liberties with the texts of some manuscripts; they hope that in so doing they have conserved the authors' intentions, while making their ideas much more accessible to the reader.

The I.C.P.F.R. gathering was hosted and supported financially by the Health Sciences Department of the French-speaking University of Québec at Trois-Rivières, Canada. Happily for Anglophone readers, the hosts graciously consented to conduct the entire meeting in English. The papers covered a wide range of very practical topics for those concerned with fitness testing, assessment of athletic performance, improvement of school programs of physical education, and the promotion of community health. Specific topics included a comparison of various international proposals for the standardization of fitness testing; a detailed consideration of body build, inheritance, test repetition, and environment as factors modifying test results; application of test procedures to the evaluation of existing and experimental programs of physical education; use of fitness tests in the assessment of athletes at various levels of competition; and the place of fitness testing in primary, secondary, and tertiary medical care. This varied material should have appeal to an equally diverse audience—physical educators, exercise physiologists, sports physicians, and many others concerned with schoolchildren, athletes, and the promotion of health within the community.

ROY J. SHEPHARD
HUGUES LAVALLÉE

CONTENTS

Chapter *Page*

Opening Remarks 3

**Section One: VARIABLES AFFECTING FITNESS
TESTING** 5

1. MERITS OF VARIOUS STANDARD TEST PROTOCOLS—A
   COMPARISON BETWEEN I.C.P.F.R., W.H.O., I.B.P, AND
   OTHER GROUPS
   T. Ishiko 7
2. BODY SIZE AND THE ASSESSMENT OF PHYSICAL PERFORMANCE
   G. R. Cumming 18
3. BODY DIMENSIONS AND PHYSIOLOGICAL INDICATORS OF
   PHYSICAL FITNESS DURING ADOLESCENCE
   Š. Šprynarová and R. Reisenauer 32
4. BODY WEIGHT AND ITS RELATIONSHIP TO PERFORMANCE ON
   THE BICYCLE ERGOMETER AND TREADMILL
   D. Van Gerven, M. Ostyn, and B. Vanden Eynde 39
5. KINANTHROPOMETRY, TERMINOLOGY AND LANDMARKS
   W. D. Ross, S. R. Brown, M. Hebbelinck,
   and R. A. Faulkner 44
6. RACIAL DIFFERENCES IN FUNCTIONAL CAPACITY
   V. Klissouras 51
7. HEIGHT-WEIGHT COMPARISON OF CANADIAN
   SCHOOLCHILDREN
   M. K. Rajic, H. Lavallée, R. J. Shephard, J. C. Jéquier,
   R. Labarre, and C. Beaucage 60
8. LEARNING AND HABITUATION AS FACTORS AFFECTING FITNESS
   TESTING
   C. T. M. Davies 75
9. SEASONAL VARIATIONS OF C.A.H.P.E.R. PERFORMANCE TESTS
   J. C. Jéquier, R. Labarre, R. J. Shephard, H. Lavallée,
   C. Beaucage, and M. Rajic 85

10. ENVIRONMENTAL VARIABLES AFFECTING FITNESS TESTING
    N. B. Strydom 94
11. AN ASSESSMENT OF EXERCISE AND HEAT ORTHOSTATISM
    E. Shvartz, A. Meroz, A. Magazanik, Y. Sheonfeld,
    and Y. Shapiro 102

Section 2: FITNESS TESTING AND THE PREDICTION OF
ATHLETIC PERFORMANCE   111

12. THE PREDICTION OF ATHLETIC PERFORMANCE BY
    LABORATORY AND FIELD TESTS—AN OVERVIEW
    R. J. Shephard 113
13. RELATIONSHIPS AMONG ANAEROBIC CAPACITY, SPRINT AND
    MIDDLE DISTANCE RUNNING OF SCHOOLCHILDREN
    O. Bar-Or and O. Inbar 142
14. OXYGEN DEBT AND INTEGRATED EMG DURING SPRINT
    RUNNING
    T. Fukunaga, M. Kobayashi, A. Matsuo, H. Fujimatsu ... 148
15. THE INFLUENCE OF ENDURANCE TRAINING ON ROWING
    PERFORMANCE
    P. L. Jooste, D. B. Read, and N. B. Strydom 156
16. THE A.A.H.P.E.R. NATIONAL YOUTH FITNESS TEST:
    RESEARCHED, SLIGHTLY REVISED, AND REPUBLISHED, 1976
    T. K. Cureton 163
17. MAXIMAL AEROBIC POWER IN GIRLS AND BOYS AGED 9 TO 16
    YEARS WHO PARTICIPATE REGULARLY IN SPORT
    I. B. Iliev 172
18. PREDICTION OF ATHLETIC PERFORMANCE IN SWIMMERS AND
    RUNNERS BY MEASURES OF LACTIC ACID AFTER EXERCISE
    AT THE SPORTS GROUND
    A. Mader, H. Heck, and W. Hollmann 177

Section 3: FITNESS TESTING IN THE ASSESSMENT OF
SCHOOL PHYSICAL EDUCATION PROGRAMS   179

19. FITNESS TESTING IN ASSESSING SCHOOL PHYSICAL
    EDUCATION PROGRAMS
    J. Simons 181
20. SEASONAL DIFFERENCES IN AEROBIC POWER

R. J. Shephard, H. Lavallée, J. C. Jéquier, R. LaBarre, M. Rajic, and C. Beaucage 194

21. THE RELATIONSHIP BETWEEN SOMATIC DEVELOPMENT AND MOTOR ABILITY, AND THE THROWING VELOCITY IN HANDBALL FOR SECONDARY SCHOOL STUDENTS
J. Pauwels 211

22. PHYSICAL FITNESS AND SKELETAL MATURITY IN GIRLS AND BOYS 11 YEARS OF AGE
S. G. Savov 222

23. MOTOR PERFORMANCE AS RELATED TO CHRONOLOGICAL AGE AND MATURATION
G. BEUNEN, M. Ostyn, R. Renson, J. Simons, and D. Van Gerven 229

24. THE IMPACT OF ECOLOGICAL FACTORS AND PHYSICAL ACTIVITY ON THE SOMATIC AND MOTOR DEVELOPMENT OF PRESCHOOL CHILDREN
J. Pařízková.. 238

25. SOCIAL DIFFERENTIATION OF PHYSICAL FITNESS OF PREADOLESCENT BELGIAN BOYS
R. Renson, G. Beunen, M. Ostyn, J. Simons, P. Swalus, and D. Van Gerven 248

26. ANTHROPOMETRIC AND PHOTOSCOPIC SOMATOTYPING OF CHILDREN
W. D. Ross, J. E. L. Carter, R. L. Rasmussen, J. Taylor .. 257

27. CHANGES IN THE BODY TYPE OF JAPANESE PUPILS FROM 1955 TO 1975
K. Hirata 263

28. PHYSICAL PERFORMANCE OF SCHOOL CHILDREN IN ISRAEL
H. Ruskin 273

29. PHYSICAL FITNESS IN YOUNG BENGALESE MALE STUDENTS
R. N. Sen, M. R. Kar, and D. Chakrabarti 321

Section Four: FITNESS TESTING IN PROGRAMS OF COMMUNITY HEALTH 327

30. THE CANADIAN HOME FITNESS TEST IN THE HEALTH ENVIRONMENT

R. R. J. Lauzon 329

31. ON THE STAGE DURATION FOR A PROGRESSIVE EXERCISE TEST
    PROTOCOL
    R. J. Shephard and T. Kavanagh 335

32. FACTORS AFFECTING AN EXERCISE TOLERANCE TEST
    B. Lake 345

33. CORRELATIONS AMONG AEROBIC FITNESS TESTS AND $\dot{V}O_2$
    MAX IN MEN WHO VARY IN AEROBIC POWER
    O. Bar-Or, D. Zwiren, and R. Dotan 356

34. EVALUATION OF WORK CAPACITY IN "HEALTHY" OLDER
    PEOPLE AND PATIENTS WITH CORONARY HEART DISEASE
    R. Rost and W. Hollmann 363

35. PROLONGED EFFECTS OF A CAUTIOUS EXERCISE PRESCRIPTION
    C. W. Poole, B. J. Crepin, and N. J. Rick 367

36. VARIABILITY OF HEART RATE, BLOOD PRESSURE, AND
    RATE-PRESSURE PRODUCT DURING BICYCLE ERGOMETER
    EXERCISE IN MIDDLE-AGED MEN
    W. E. Sime, I. T. Whipple, J. Stamler, D. M. Berkson ... 377

37. RELATIONSHIP BETWEEN SEGMENTAL AND WHOLE BODY
    WEIGHTS OF SOME INDIAN SUBJECTS
    R. N. Sen, G. G. Ray, and P. K. Nag 384

PHYSICAL FITNESS ASSESSMENT
Principles, Practice and Application

OPENING REMARKS

M. Le Recteur,
Dr. Lavallée,
Invités Distingués.
Mesdames et Messieurs.

C'est avec un grand plaisir que je voudrais adresser mes mots de bienvenue au Québec, Province Olympique, et à Trois-Rivières, siège de cette réunion du Comité International de recherche sur la capacité physique.

Nous avons encore en mémoire la dernière réunion qui a eu lieu à Jérusalem, sous la présidence bienveillante du Dr. Hillel Ruskin et nous sommes tous peinés que des circonstances imprévues l'empêchent d'être présent à notre réunion d'aujourd'hui. Heureusement, son collègue Dr. Bar-Or a accepté de présenter son communiqué. Personnellement, j'ai gardé beaucoup de souvenirs agréables d'Israel, particulièrement le certificat que j'ai reçu pour la course la plus vite entre notre hôtel et la salle de conférence!

Au dernier Congrès, les participants ont eu beaucoup d'ennuis à cause de difficultés dans le transport aérien; quelques participants Orientaux, même notre distingué Secrétaire, n'ont pu réaliser leurs projets de voyage. La semaine dernière, nous avons souffert également de grèves aux aéroports canadiens, mais heureusement tout s'est réglé avant notre réunion.

J'espère que nos discussions permettront d'étudier plus à fond tous les problèmes complexes de mesure de la capacité physique, particulièrement l'application des méthodes standardisées aux comparaisons internationales. De cette façon, nous pourrons vérifier s'il y a vraiment une différence entre les Suédois et les Canadiens; ce qui constitue une étape préliminaire pour toutes les considérations sérieuses de l'activité physique et la santé publique. J'espère aussi que vous trouverez

3

beaucoup de plaisir à rencontrer vos amis des réunions précédentes et à savourer l'ambiance de la vie Québécoise. S'il y a quelque chose que je puisse faire pour augmenter le confort et le plaisir de votre séjour parmi nous, je vous prierais de me le demander ou de vous adresser au secrétariat.

Maintenant, je voudrais remercier sincèrement Monsieur Boulet et Dr. Lavallée qui ont soutenu et vaincu tous les problèmes pratiques de cette réunion, et de déclarer le congrès officiellement ouvert.

Roy J. Shephard

Section One

VARIABLES AFFECTING FITNESS TESTING

Chapter 1

MERITS OF VARIOUS STANDARD TEST PROTOCOLS—A COMPARISON BETWEEN I.C.P.F.R., W.H.O., I.B.P., AND OTHER GROUPS

T. Ishiko

Abstract

The International Committee for Physical Fitness Research (I.C.P.F.R.), the International Biological Programme (I.B.P.), and the World Health Organization (W.H.O.) have all published standard protocols for physical fitness testing. Procedures of the former two bodies have much general similarity in terms of examining comprehensive physical fitness, while the latter group considers only physiological measurements obtained during exercise. Such standard protocols are useful for researchers who wish to obtain information pertaining to the physical fitness of a given population in comparison with others or to determine longitudinal trends of fitness within a specific region. The author is concerned that a slight discrepancy between tests, such as the pattern of loading in an exercise test or the formula for calculating body fat from body density, could invalidate comparisons and lead to false conclusions. The validity of the standard protocols is a future problem; it has yet to be seen whether valuable information will be produced by using these tests.

D UE TO A RECENT world-wide concern about national levels of physical fitness, fitness tests have been devised in many countries. Internationally authorized bodies, including I.C.P.F.R., I.B.P., and W.H.O., have published standard protocols for physical fitness testing in an attempt to clarify the relative physical fitness of various populations and the relationship of such fitness to life-style. Substantial coincidence of the test items may be detected, as would be anticipated from the

7

common concepts used by the working groups engaged in the construction of these physical fitness tests. However, there are also significant differences, due to the differing viewpoints of these various bodies.

Test composition of I.C.P.F.R., I.B.P., and W.H.O.

I.C.P.F.R. was established in 1964 in order to develop a standardized international fitness test battery. After ten years of discussion, this was published in 1974.[1] The I.C.P.F.R. tests include four clear-cut elements: medical examination; physiological measurements and indices; measures of physique and body composition; and basic physical performance tests. Additionally, a standardized form for the recording of personal data was proposed. This classification provides a good model for those who wish a comprehensive understanding of physical fitness tests.

The International Biological Programme was organized from a much wider perspective. The tests are described in various I.B.P. handbooks of which Handbook No. 9 details field tests on human biology.[3] Therefore, physical fitness tests are included in this volume. It has eight chapters: A. growth and physique; B. genetic constitution; C. work capacity and pulmonary function; D. climatic tolerance; E. nutritional studies; F. medical and metabolic studies; G. demographic assessment and related sociocultural factors; and H. environmental description. Correspondence of the I.B.P. and I.C.P.F.R. tests can be seen in chapter C and, to a lesser extent, in chapter F. The W.H.O. considers only physiological measurements during exercise in its technical report No. 388.[4]

Medical examination

The I.C.P.F.R. medical examination test is a prerequisite to stress testing. It consists of three parts: Form A (medical history), Form B (physical examination), and Form C (laboratory data). Forms A and B are mandatory, except for the section concerning examination of the reproductive system. Form C is optional, with the exception of urinalysis. An important characteristic of the I.C.P.F.R. medical examination form is that it requests the physician performing the examination to specify clearly whether a given subject may or may not participate in stressful fitness tests.

The I.B.P. medical examination is aimed primarily at yielding information on the health of a community. It consists of a personal examination and laboratory investigations (Table 1-I). The I.B.P. and the I.C.P.F.R. forms are almost identical in content and have a nearly identical system of coding. However, no part of the I.B.P. examination is indicated as mandatory or optional. The I.B.P. form includes many additional clinical items relating to regional infectious diseases such as yaws, leprosy, and trypanosomiasis, which I.C.P.F.R. lacks. These diseases are of interest in the study of human biology, as part of the I.B.P. project, but are not a primary concern of I.C.P.F.R. participants. There is apparently no obligation for a physician of I.B.P. to give a subject permission to participate in the physiological tests. A comparison of I.C.P.F.R. and I.B.P. medical examinations is shown in Table 1-I.

TABLE 1-I

A COMPARISON OF THE MEDICAL EXAMINATIONS RECOMMENDED BY ICPFR AND IBP

Item	*ICPFR*	*IBP*
Aim of medical examination	Prerequisite to stressful testing of an individual	Medical status of the community
Medical history	Many items with family history	Only yaws and chest illness, without family history
Physical Examination	Many items	Many items with investigations relating to many regional infectious diseases
Laboratory data	VC, FEV Blood ECG	Stool Sputum Blood

Physiological tests

The I.C.P.F.R. physiological tests are limited to standard laboratory exercise, the main aim being to obtain a value for maximal oxygen intake, either directly or indirectly. The modes of exercise described by I.C.P.F.R. include the treadmill, bicycle ergometer, and stepping ergometer. I.B.P. physiological tests (Table 1-II) include both exercise and resting measurements. The former comprise indirect and direct measurements of $\dot{V}_{O_2}$ max and estimates of anaerobic power, while the latter include forced expiratory volume and vital capacity. The treadmill is omitted from the apparatus recommended by I.B.P., since it is inappropriate for field use. But it is strange that running up a staircase, not always available in the field, has been selected as a measurement of anaerobic power. The W.H.O. describes exercise tests only, the treadmill, bicycle ergometer, and stepping ergometer being employed as in the I.C.P.F.R. recommendations. The variables measured in the W.H.O. tests are somewhat different from those of I.B.P. and I.C.P.F.R.; they include various indices of cardiovascular function such as heart rate, blood pressure, ECG, $\dot{Q}$, and $\dot{V}_{O_2}$.

TABLE 1-II

A COMPARISON OF PHYSIOLOGICAL TESTS RECOMMENDED BY ICPFR AND IBP

Measures	ICPFR	IBP	WHO
	Direct $\dot{V}_{O_2}$ max	Direct $\dot{V}_{O_2}$ max	
	Indirect $\dot{V}_{O_2}$ max	Indirect $\dot{V}_{O_2}$ max	
		Anaerobic Power	
		FEV	
		VC	
			Heart Rate
			Blood Pressure
			ECG
			$\dot{Q}$
			$\dot{V}_{O_2}$
Apparatus	Treadmill		Treadmill
	Bicycle ergometer	Bicycle ergometer	Bicycle ergometer
	Stepping ergometer	Stepping ergometer	Stepping ergometer
		Staircase	

The common measurement between I.C.P.F.R., I.B.P., and W.H.O. is, therefore, the $\dot{V}O_2$ max. The characteristic of the I.C.P.F.R. measurement of $\dot{V}O_2$ max is that the load is increased in a stepwise fashion. The same increment of load (Mets) is adopted irrespective of the apparatus used: the treadmill grade is increased by 2.5 percent, keeping a constant speed of walking (80 m/min); in the case of the bicycle ergometer, the initial load is 1 watt per kilogram of body weight, and this load is augmented by ⅓ watt per kg of body weight; in a stepping ergometer test, 33 lifts per minute are performed on an adjustable bench, starting at 4.5 cm and increasing the height by 4.5 cm every two minutes.

In the I.B.P. measurement of $\dot{V}O_2$ max, an indirect measurement is made in order to obtain a rough idea of the subject's $\dot{V}O_2$ max. Thereafter, a formal maximal test is performed. If the bicycle ergometer is used, the initial load is set at approximately 70 percent of the subject's $\dot{V}O_2$ max. The required work is next increased to the expected $\dot{V}O_2$ max, as predicted from the indirect measurements. The setting is further increased in steps of 200 kg-m/min until the subject is exhausted. The maximum step test is performed on an eighteen-inch bench in the same manner as in the bicycle test (an initial load approximately 70 percent of $\dot{V}O_2$ max, with an increase in the rate of working every two minutes until exhaustion). The increase of work load is accomplished by increasing the stepping speed, while maintaining a fixed bench height.

The W.H.O. protocol describes bicycle, treadmill, and stepping apparatus but does not recommend procedures; instead, it discusses each approach critically, pointing out its merits and demerits. As a result, W.H.O. concludes that the best apparatus for universal exercise testing is an upright bicycle ergometer, exercise being performed at several increasing work loads, each lasting at least four minutes without intervening rest pauses.

In order to compare the I.C.P.F.R. and I.B.P. tests of $\dot{V}O_2$ max, the author measured the actual $\dot{V}O_2$ max of five male subjects (Tables 1-III and 1-IV). The I.B.P. and I.C.P.F.R. propose an almost identical criterion for the attainment of $\dot{V}O_2$

max; the former protocol requires three measurements of $\dot{V}O_2$ coincident within 5 percent, while the latter requires two coincident measurements. Applying such criteria to the experimental data, the I.B.P. requirement was not invariably satisfied; however, it was met in nine of ten cases when using the bicycling and stepping tests of I.C.P.F.R. Possible reasons for the discrepancy between the two protocols were (1) the increase in work load with the I.B.P. test was so rapid that there was not enough time to reach a levelling-off of $\dot{V}O_2$ and (2) the I.B.P. criterion of three coincident measurements was too severe. In order to test the first explanation, the time to exhaustion was noted (Table 1-IV). With the I.B.P. protocol, the test duration was shorter than ten minutes in six of ten cases. In the bicycling exercise, no subject was able to exercise for more than seven minutes. With regard to the second explanation, the duration of levelling-off must exceed six minutes to yield three coincident $\dot{V}O_2$ measurements, since

TABLE 1-III

COMPARISON OF $\dot{V}O_2$ MAX (ML/MIN) OBTAINED BY IBP AND ICPFR
PROTOCOLS.

	IBP				ICPFR			
	Indirect		Direct		Direct			
Subject	bicycle	step	bicycle	step	bicycle	step	Treadmill	
							(1)	(2)
A	2938	3140	2366*	2777*	2800	2844	2941*	3071
B	3703	3228	3129*	3429*	3243	3098	3554*	3824
C	3616	3572	3333*	3503*	3716	3690	3929*	3752
D	2582	2589	2693*	2857*	2786*	2891	3119*	3020
E	3169	3099	2862*	2729*	2807	2897		3080
X	3202	3126	2877	3059	3070	3084	3386	3349
SD	±419.0	±315.8	±336.6	±335.6	±366.1	±315.4	±384.8	±359.4

*leveling-off was not attained.

(1) Values obtained with constant walking speed 100 m/min and 2 percent increase of slope every minute (Superstandard test).

(2) Values obtained by constant walking speed 100 m/min with 2.5 percent increase of slope every two minutes (Superstandard speed with standard slope).

TABLE 1-IV
COMPARISON OF TIMES TO EXHAUSTION FOR IBP AND ICPFR TESTS OF
MAXIMUM OXYGEN UPTAKE.

	IBP		ICPFR			
Subject	Bicycle	Step	Bicycle	Step	Treadmill	
					(1)	(2)
A	4'12"0	9'51"7	17'31"2	21'46"2	12'46"8	18'54"7
B	4'56"4	14'45"0	15'00"0	23'26"5	14'49"4	20'22"7
C	5'20"2	20'00"0	16'40"0	23'57"0	11'45"0	19'16"9
D	7'00"0	13'50"5	16'00"0	18'00"0	12'14"4	18'00"0
E	3'44"0	14'30"0	15'51"5	18'18"5		18'26"2
X	5'02"4	14'35"4	16'12"5	21'05"6	12'53"9	19'00"0
SD	±1'07"6	±3'13"9	±50"6	±2'30"5	±1'10"2	±48"8

measurements are made every two minutes. It may not be easy
to endure such a period of exhausting work. If the same
criterion were to be applied to the W.H.O. method, which
recommends four minutes of exercise at each work load,* the
duration of levelling-off would be more than twelve minutes,
which is definitely impracticable. On the contrary, most subjects
met the I.C.P.F.R. criterion during both bicycling and stepping
tests. However, the criterion was not satisfied with the
I.C.P.F.R. treadmill test unless there was a gradual increase of
work load.

From these experiments, it was concluded that the I.B.P. test
demanded a too rapid increase of work load and applied a too
severe criterion for attainment of an oxygen plateau. The
I.C.P.F.R. bicycling and stepping tests were appropriate,
however, while the I.C.P.F.R. treadmill test was also appropriate when workloads were applied gradually.

Physique and Body Composition

An assessment of body build is essential not only when
examining physical fitness, but also as a background to

---

*The W.H.O. four-minute per stage test was intended primarily for submaximum
effort.—Eds.

measurements of work capacity and physical performance. I.C.P.F.R. and I.B.P. each describe many anthropometric measurements (Table 1-V). The items common to the I.C.P.F.R. and I.B.P. protocols are weight, height, sitting height, certain diameters (biacromial, bicristal, biepicondylar), chest circumference, and three skinfold thicknesses (triceps, subscapular, suprailiac). There are some differences of test items between the I.C.P.F.R. and I.B.P., probably an expression of differing opinions among researchers engaged in such tests (Table 1-V). The determination of body fat by the underwater weighing method is described by both I.C.P.F.R. and I.B.P., but the recommended equation for calculating body fat is somewhat different (see also Table 1-VI).—

I.C.P.F.R.: % Fat = 4.570/density − 4.142
I.B.P.: % Fat = 4.95/density − 4.5

Relative to I.B.P., the I.C.P.F.R. technique underestimates fat in the obese person, but overestimates it in the lean person. Radiographic measurement of the thigh is described in the I.B.P. protocol but is lacking in I.C.P.F.R. Sophisticated measurements such as total body water and total body potassium are described in I.C.P.F.R. while they are lacking in I.B.P., since such procedures are not easily used as field tests. Maturation is described under anthropometry in I.C.P.F.R., while it is found under growth and physique in the I.B.P. protocol.

Performance Tests (including dynamometry)

The I.C.P.F.R., I.B.P., and Japanese Physical Fitness Tests[2] are compared in Table 1-VII. The I.C.P.F.R. performance test consists of eight items measured in metric units, but it lacks the Harvard step test and a ball throw; the former test does not measure physical performance and the latter is inappropriate, since throwing performance is much influenced by sociocultural patterns of physical activity. The I.B.P. performance items comprise the A.A.H.P.E.R. (American Alliance for Health, Physical Education and Recreation) fitness test battery and the Harvard step test; distances are expressed in yards.

TABLE 1-V
COMPARISON OF MEASURES OF PHYSIQUE AND BODY COMPOSITION
RECOMMENDED BY ICPFR AND IBP

	ICPFR	*IBP*
Anthropometry	Weight	Weight
	Height:	Height:
	standing, acromiale, radiale, dactylion, trochanterion, tibial, sitting, suprasternal when seated	standing sitting
		Length: total arm length
	Diameter: biacromial, bicristal, biepicondylar humerus,	Diameter: biacromial, biiliac, bicondylar humerus, wrist, chest (transverse, anterio-posterior)
	Circumference: chest, upper arm(contracted, relaxed) thigh	Circumference: chest
	Skinfold: Biceps, triceps, subscapular suprailiac, thigh (medial and lateral)	Skinfold: triceps, subscapular suprailiac
Body Composition	Underwater weighing Total body water Total body potassium	Underwater weighing X ray of the thigh
Maturation	Puberty rating pubic hair (both sexes) genital development (males) breast development (females) Skeletal age	A2. Puberty rating pubic hair (both sexes) genital development (males) breast development (females) A4. Skeletal age
Somatotyping		A3. Photogrammetry

TABLE 1-VI
COMPARISON OF BODY FAT CALCULATED WITH I.C.P.F.R. AND I.B.P. EQUATIONS.

Subject	Density	ICPFR	Body Fat % IBP	Difference
Very Obese	1.00	42.8	45.0	−2.2
Very Lean	1.08	8.9	8.3	0.6

TABLE 1-VII

COMPARISON OF PERFORMANCE TESTS INCLUDING DYNAMOMETRY AS RECOMMENDED BY I.C.P.F.R., I.B.P. AND JAPANESE TEST.

Item	I.C.P.F.R.	I.B.P.	Japanese Test	
			A. Fitness Diagnostic Test	B. Motor Performance Test
Endurance		Harvard step test	Modified Harvard test	
Jumping power	Standing broad jump	Standing broad jump	Standing vertical jump	Running broad jump
Speed	50-m sprint	50-yd sprint		50-m sprint
Chinning	Pull-ups (males) Flexed arm hang (females)	Pull-ups (males) Modified pull-ups (females)		Pull-ups (males) Modified pull-ups (females)
Agility	Shuttle run (10-m)	Shuttle run (10-yd)	Side-steps (20-sec)	
Abdominal strength	Sit-ups (30-sec)	Sit-ups (1-min)		
Distance run	2000 or 1000 m (males) 1500 or 800 m (females) 600 m (children)	600-yd run		1500m (males) 1000m (females)
Dynamometry	Grip	Grip Back Pull and Push Leg extension Trunk flexion Soft ball throw	Grip Back	
Throwing power				Handball throw
Flexibility	Trunk forward flexion		Trunk forward flexion Trunk backward extension	

Dynamometry is listed as a separate item in I.B.P. The I.B.P. protocol lacks flexibility measurements.

Japan has two youth fitness tests, a fitness diagnostic test and a motor performance test. The former is aimed at measuring basic general fitness, the latter at measuring athletic fitness. If items from both tests are combined, they cover almost all phases of the performance tests recommended by both I.C.P.F.R. and I.B.P. Results of the Japanese youth tests are issued every year by the Japanese Ministry of Education.

Conclusion

Standardized fitness tests are indispensable for the comparison of data obtained from various parts of the world. Such requirements are partly fulfilled by the guidebooks published in recent years, but a clear understanding of similarities and differences between these guidebooks is of grave importance for research workers who must deal with international and interorganizational data. The validity and reliability of the tests are not yet completely established for populations of various regions. Moreover, the results presented thus far are insufficient. Existing studies should be repeated and new populations should be examined in the future.

References

1. Larson, L. A. (Ed.): *Fitness, Health and Work Capacity. International Standards for Assessment.* MacMillan Publishing Co., New York, 1974.
2. Ministry of Education in Japan: *Survey of Japanese Physical Fitness,* 1964.
3. Weiner, J. S. and Lourie, J. A. (Ed.): *Human Biology. A Guide to Field Methods.* I.B.P. Handbook No. 9, London, 1969.
4. W.H.O.: *Exercise Tests in Relation to Cardiovascular Function.* Wld Hlth Org Techn Rep Ser 388, Geneva, 1968.

Chapter 2

BODY SIZE AND THE ASSESSMENT OF PHYSICAL PERFORMANCE

G. R. CUMMING

Abstract

Size is an important variable influencing the oxygen cost of standardized submaximal exercise tests. Body weight increases the oxygen requirement of stepping and of bicycle ergometry at the same kg-m work load. When walking, the oxygen consumed (ml/kg-min) is less for a heavy person than for someone who is lighter. Extra height reduces the oxygen cost of both treadmill walking and of bicycle ergometer work. The extra oxygen cost of graded treadmill walking does not seem to be related to body weight. There is insufficient data concerning the oxygen cost of treadmill walking and running in children; reported values range from the same as adults, to 10 to 20 percent greater. The treadmill speed at which the oxygen cost of running becomes less than that of walking may vary in subjects of differing size. While there is theoretical merit in relating the maximal oxygen uptake to height (in m²), in practice units of ml/kg-min are likely to be used. When studying children from 6 to 16 years of age, the correlation of aerobic power to weight and height is so great that any other body dimension or functional capacity related to body size will appear to be a valuable predictor of $\dot{V}o_2$ (max). It is preferable that studies of $\dot{V}o_2$ (max) predictions be confined to a narrow age group. Body size is often a better predictor of performance in physical tests than laboratory tests.

BODY DIMENSIONS ARE of obvious importance in the selection of athletic careers, such as basketball or American football, and the findings of Tanner on the 1960 Olympians are well known.[1] The author will not discuss further the relationship between body dimensions and elite athletic performance, but wishes to review two areas—the relationship of body size to the prediction of oxygen uptake in laboratory tests, and some

18

aspects of physical performances of children in relationship to body dimensions.

Stepping and Cycling

It is usually assumed that the oxygen cost of stepping is directly related to body weight, and that the O_2 cost of cycling is independent of body size. Cotes reviewed the effect of body weight on the energy expenditures involved in stepping, cycling, and treadmill walking and found that heavier persons used more oxygen to do the same amount of work.[2] In the stepping test, the load was constant (350 kg-m/min), yet a man of 80 kg required about 10 percent more oxygen than a man of 60 kg. Presumably a large part of the extra energy was lost in acceleration and deceleration of body parts with each step.*

A similar relationship was found when cycling on the laboratory ergometer. At a load of 450 kpm/min, a person who was 10 kg heavier required about 6 percent more oxygen. The oxygen cost of cycling on the laboratory ergometer is usually held to be independent of body weight. However, Cotes suggested that it cost more to move heavier legs—and the differences were not insignificant.

In extremely obese subjects (averaging 62 percent over-weight) I. Åstrand et al.[3] found that the efficiency of bicycle ergometer work was reduced. When performing 300 kpm of external work, obese women required an additional 200 ml of oxygen and obese men 180 ml more oxygen—differences of 24 and 20 percent from results for average sized persons. Unfortunately, the oxygen consumed at heavy work loads was not sufficiently explored.

These examples illustrate the problem of assuming that the oxygen cost of some forms of submaximal exercise tests are independent of, or linearly related to, body weight.

Wyndham and his colleagues[4, 5] have made extensive study of weight, height, and exercise $\dot{V}o_2$ relationships in miners.

---

*Since many of the oxygen consumption data discussed are *gross* values, a part of the increased oxygen usage of the heavy person may refleet a greater resting energy expenditure rather than a difference in the efficiency of working.—Eds.

Their data was summarized in 1971. They selected four groups of men, tall and light, short and light, tall and heavy, and short and heavy. The mean $\dot{V}o_2$ max of each group was about 42 ml/kg-min. The $\dot{V}o_2$ requirement for bicycle ergometer work (three loads) was greater in the heavier men and smaller in the taller men. Even when working on the bicycle ergometer, it paid to be tall and lean. Similar results were observed for walking and for walking pushing a mine car—$\dot{V}o_2$ was higher in heavier persons and lower in taller persons. While weight accounted for 70 percent of the variability in $\dot{V}o_2$, height accounted for 4 percent and could not be neglected completely. The Johannesburg workers have also found a higher $\dot{V}o_2$ max in ml/kg body weight in heavier mining recruits. This is the reverse of what others have reported; nutritional factors or other peculiarities of the Bantu may be involved.

Walking and Running

The classical review of human energy expenditure by Passmore and Durnin[6] noted differences in the oxygen cost of walking (ml/kg-min) with body weight; for example, a light person (36.4 kg) required 21 percent more oxygen than a person of 72.8 kg. A 91.2 kg person walking at the same speed required only 3 percent less oxygen than the 72.8 kg person. The coefficient of variation for the metabolic cost of walking was given as 15 percent, with size factors accounting for some of the interindividual differences.

Workman and Armstrong[7] showed that the number of steps taken per minute at a given speed of treadmill walking depended on body weight, the relationship being sufficiently constant to allow a prediction of the rate of stepping from height. These authors also found that the $\dot{V}o_2$ per step divided by body weight had a consistent mathematical relationship to walking speed, allowing them to prepare a nomogram[8] to estimate the oxygen cost of level walking. Jankowski et al.[9] have demonstrated the validity of this nomogram for coronary patients. The data in Table 2-I is derived from the Workman-Armstrong nomogram. It shows the predicted $\dot{V}o_2$ (ml/kg-min) for four theoretical subjects. Weight made little difference to the oxygen cost of walking, but a height difference of 30 cm altered the cost by 14 percent. Workman and Armstrong also investigated the oxygen cost of grade walking. It was expected that the added oxygen cost of climbing the grade would be related to body weight times the vertical lift, the latter being equal to percent grade times belt speed. However, in practice the excess $\dot{V}O_2$ for grade walking was equal to 4.88 times percent grade times speed in km/h and was independent of body weight.

When the oxygen costs of the commonly used Bruce treadmill test[10] (Table 2-II) are calculated from the Workman nomogram, the values are quite close to those published by Bruce, except for stage 4. This discrepancy may arise because most subjects are running in stage 4 and running may be more efficient than walking at this speed and grade. Predictions also favor the taller subject. Margaria's data[11] for graded treadmill walking show energy costs of 13, 21, and 35 ml/kg-min, low for the first two stages of the Bruce test but appropriate for the third stage in comparison with those shown in Table 2-II.

In Table 2-III, the energy cost of the Bruce treadmill test has been predicted for a 160 cm/70 kg adult, using the Workman nomogram. The cost is divided into resting, horizontal, and grade-walking components. A resting $\dot{V}O_2$ of 3.5 ml/kg-min was assumed, and the relative costs of the horizontal and grade-walking components were then compared. The relative percentages of the net cost were quite similar at stages 2, 3, and 4, with the grade accounting for slightly more of the total $\dot{V}O_2$ than level walking at stages 3 and 4.

TABLE 2-I

OXYGEN COST (ML/KG-MIN) OF LEVEL WALKING AT 4.8 km/h. ESTIMATED FROM THE WORKMAN-ARMSTRONG NOMOGRAM

| | *Oxygen cost* | |
Body Weight *(kg)*	*(height* *160cm)*	*(height* *190cm)*
50	14.0	12.4
100	14.5	12.5

TABLE 2-II

A COMPARISON BETWEEN THE PUBLISHED OXYGEN COST OF THE BRUCE
TEST AND NOMOGRAM ESTIMATIONS OF $\dot{V}o_2$ (ml/kg-min)

	Published oxygen cost	Workman Nomogram Adult 70 kg		Silverman Nomogram Child	
	(Bruce)	*Height 160 cm*	*Height 190 cm*		
Stage				*25 kg*	*45 kg*
1	17.4	17.4	15.4	20.6	19.0
2	24.8	26.0	23.0	28.6	27.0
3	34.3	37.1	33.3	41.6	40.0
4	43.8	52.6	48.0	58.6	57.0

TABLE 2-III

HORIZONTAL AND VERTICAL COST COMPONENTS OF GRADED WALKING.
THE ENERGY COST OF THE BRUCE TEST HAS BEEN PREDICTED FOR A 160
cm/70 kg ADULT, USING THE WORKMAN NOMOGRAM

	Bruce Test		Oxygen Cost		Exercise Cost % due to components	
Stage	*Speed (km/h)*	*Grade %*	*Total*	*Net**	*Grade*	*Level*
			(ml/kg-min)	*(ml/kg-min)*		
1	2.72	10	17.4	13.9	39	61
2	4.00	12	26.0	22.5	50	50
3	5.44	14	37.1	33.6	55	45
4	6.72	16	52.6	49.1	53	47

*Assuming a resting oxygen consumption of 3.5 ml/kg-min

Treadmill tests in children

The oxygen costs of walking and running in children have not been studied extensively. Silverman and Anderson[12] constructed a nomogram from data on three girls and one boy, ranging in age from 6 to 11 years and weighing 22 to 53 kg. Robinson[13] studied nineteen boys at only one work load. The substantial population of Cassels and Morse[14] yielded values 5 ml/kg-min below those of Silverman and Anderson and of Robinson. The estimated cost of the Bruce protocol, using the Silverman nomogram, is shown in Table 2-II. At stage 3, calculated values are about 18 percent higher than estimated by Bruce.[10] Are these differences real or is this an example of the problems of obtaining comparable $\dot{V}o_2$ measurements from laboratory to laboratory? The oxygen cost of the Bruce test in the author's laboratory (Table 2-IV) is much lower than that calculated from the Silverman nomogram, being very close to the values published by Bruce, and confirmed in the laboratory for the Bruce protocol.

Differences between walking and running

Using the Silverman-Anderson nomograms, there are marked differences of estimated oxygen consumption between walking and running (Table 2-V). Compared to walking, running requires 50 percent more energy expenditure at stage 1, the same energy expenditure for stage 3, and 17 percent less for stage 4.

TABLE 2-IV
BRUCE TREADMILL TEST IN CHILDREN*
OXYGEN COST OF 3RD MINUTE (ml./kg. min)

Stage	Sex	Age 7 (3)†	Age 9-10 (11)†	Age 11-12 (10)†	Age 13-14 (8)†
I	M	20.2±2.0	18.7±2.0	18.2±1.3	18.5±1.7
	F	—	18.5±2.3	17.9±3.2	17.9±1.3
II	M	26.4±2.5	25.9±3.1	24.6±2.5	28.3±3.2
	F	—	25.1±2.8	24.1±2.3	23.5±2.6
III	M	40.2±0.4	36.1±5.4	36.8±3.2	39.2±5.2
	F	—	36.8±5.3	33.5±3.2	36.2±2.5

*From, Cumming and Glenn—unpublished data
†Number of subjects

TABLE 2-V
COMPARISON OF WALKING AND RUNNING
ESTIMATED OXYGEN COST OF THE BRUCE TEST (ml/kg-min)
IN A CHILD WEIGHING 30 kg
(FROM THE SILVERMAN-ANDERSON NOMOGRAM)

Bruce stage	$\dot{V}O_2$ Walking	$\dot{V}O_2$ Running	Running/Walking Ratio
1	20.8	30.5	1.47
2	28.0	35.0	1.25
3	40.5	41.0	1.01
4	57.5	48.0	0.83

At speeds over 7.5 km/h, running is known to be more efficient than walking (Bøje[15]). For level walking of 7.5 km/h, runners have the same efficiency—but for speeds over 8 km/h walking becomes very inefficient, using over twice as much energy as running. The changeover point is very likely to differ between subjects and may be dependent on height and stride length. Kagaya[16] reported a crossover at 7.5 to 8.3 km/h in sixteen– to twenty-one-year-old Japanese students. This problem has considerable bearing on the prediction of $\dot{V}o_2$ max from treadmill tests.

Performance tests

When measuring working capacity and physical performance, it is necessary to consider extraneous factors such as the learning of technique, prior experience with similar types of exercise, motivation, understanding, maturity factors in children, and functional decay in older adults.

In children, the range of values observed declines from age six to twelve, possibly because certain learning and experience factors are progressively eliminated. Ball throw and speed situps have a coefficient of variation of over 40 percent at age 6, but this declines to less than 25 percent by the age of 12 years.[17] Of any measurement, height has the lowest and most constant coefficient of variation in this age group—5 percent. Weight, on the other hand, has a coefficient of variation of 14 percent at age 6, and this increases to 22 percent by age 12.

Methods of size standardization

The relationship of body dimensions to physical performance and muscular work has interested researchers for many years, including Hill in 1950,[18] Asmussen,[19, 20] Von Döbeln,[21, 22] and Åstrand and Rodahl.[23] The oxygen cost of doing submaximal work has been discussed above, and a brief discussion of $\dot{V}o_2$ (max) in relation to body size is in order. Von Döbeln and Eriksson[24] used the arguments of Newton to show

that the force exerted by a muscle should be propor
cross sectional area; that time and length scales we
tional; that given uniform density mass should be p
to length cubed; and that flow per unit time, i.e. $\dot{V}O_2$ max
should be related to length squared. After five months of
training, the correlations between $\dot{V}O_2$ max and height, total
hemoglobin, and total body potassium in nine boys more closely
approached the theoretical exponents. It was thus argued that
training had eliminated the effects of differing initial levels of
physical condition, revealing more clearly the dependency of
$\dot{V}O_2$ max on the dimensions of the oxygen transport system.
From the theoretical reasoning, it was suggested that $\dot{V}O_2$ max
was best expressed per m^2 of body height to adjust for size
differences.[24] However, few investigators present their data in
this way, and $\dot{V}O_2$ max in ml/min per kg of body weight remains
the common basis of reporting results. The latter has the
advantage of simplicity and is of some practical value, since the
cost of locomotion for walking and running is most nearly
related to body weight. It is of interest that jockeys have $\dot{V}O_2$
(max) values of 50 to 65 ml/kg-min,[25] some approaching the
values found in endurance trained athletes. Perhaps the jockeys
are athletic, but the fact that they weigh only 50 kg probably has
some bearing on these high values.

Recent evidence indicates that in ectomorphs and
mesomorphs $\dot{V}O_2$ (max) is highly correlated with body weight,
while in endomorphs such a relationship is almost nonexis-
tent.[26] Depending on whether $\dot{V}O_2$ (max) is presented as ml/min
per kg BW, or ml/min per m^2 height, the aerobic power of girls
can be described as decreasing by 20 percent or increasing by
10 percent from age 10 to 14 years. There is plainly a need for
further understanding and standardization of the units used in
presenting $\dot{V}O_2$ (max); at present, the data can be manipulated
to serve the bias of the investigator.

Predictions of $\dot{V}O_2$ (max)

$\dot{V}O_2$ (max) depends a great deal not only on the body mass
but also on the amount of fat in this mass.[27] When assessing the

value of tests to predict $\dot{V}O_2$ (max) in persons with a large range of body weights and corresponding variation in the percentages of body fat, the correlation of $\dot{V}O_2$ (max) to fat free weight should not be overlooked.

Data for the twelve-minute run (Table 2-VI) provide an example of the dependency of $\dot{V}O_2$ (max) and performance on body size. The twelve-minute test used by Cooper is a very reasonable predictive test for $\dot{V}O_2$ (max) if conducted properly with well-motivated subjects. In seven groups of subjects, correlations between $\dot{V}O_2$ (max) and the twelve-minute run distance were highly significant, individual correlation coefficients ranging from .27 to .85.

However, almost equally high correlation coefficients were obtained by relating $\dot{V}O_2$ (max) to weight and percent body fat; thus in any of these seven groups, weight and skinfolds would have been almost as accurate a predictor of $\dot{V}O_2$ (max) as the run.

Size factors are dominant when evaluating methods of predicting $\dot{V}O_2$ (max) in children aged 8 to 16. $\dot{V}O_2$ (max) shows such a high correlation with height, weight, and lean body mass (Table 2-VII) that little is gained by adding a predictive test such as PWC 170.[28] However, if the age range is narrowed to 14 to 16 years so that the size range is also reduced, the correlation of $\dot{V}O_2$ (max) to size almost disappears, and the predictive power of PWC 170 becomes apparent. Size must be factored out when studying children over a large age range; when assessing the value of predictive tests it is probably more appropriate to concentrate on a narrow age group of only one to two years. In the study just discussed, more elaborate size indices such as height in m^2 or weight to the power of 0.67 were of no added advantage. Davies et al.[29] emphasized the importance of body composition in predicting the aerobic power of children, but they used ninety-two child "volunteers" 6 to 16 years of age. While the 0.85 correlation coefficient between LBM or leg volume and $\dot{V}O_2$ (max) seemed quite impressive, the correlation coefficient for the relationship between body weight and $\dot{V}O_2$ (max) was 0.84; these investigators would have been better advised to concentrate on a narrower age range.

TABLE 2-VI

PREDICTION OF V̇O₂ (MAX) FROM TWELVE-MINUTE RUN DISTANCE AND ANTHROPOMETRIC DATA

Group*	n	$\dot{V}O_2$ (max) (ml/kg-min) ± SD	Anthropometric alone		12-Minute Run		Both		Factors
			r	SE	r	SE	r	SE	
1.	7	33.4±4.2	.99	0.3	.25	4.4	—	—	Insufficient number
2.	58	48.1±6.6	.69	5.1	.63	5.2	.80	4.2	Run, age†, weight†
3.	15	31.7±3.7	.61	3.9	.47	3.9	.62	3.9	None
4.	27	35.0±7.1	.73	5.4	.74	4.9	.90	3.5	Run, weight†
5.	23	49.5±6.0	.77	4.9	.53	5.3	.80	4.3	Run, fat†, weight†
6.	10	60.6±6.1	.67	8.5	.75	4.2	.98	2.2	Run, weight†, fat†
7.	12	44.1±6.9	.47	13.3	.87	4.8	.90	4.0	Run

*1. YMCA Health Club members aged 61-72 (mean 65)—Only one trained regularly

2. Health Club members 22-60 years of age, all training regularly.

3. Volunteers from Home Economics Faculty, mean age 19 years, who participated in a "get-fit" home exercise study

4. (Girls) & 5. (Boys) Students; 7-10 obtained by selecting every third student from grades 5, 7 and 12; ages 10 to 17 years

6. (Boys) & 7. (Girls) Athletes selected from a track camp, ages 13-16 years.

†negative correlation

TABLE 2-VII

CORRELATION BETWEEN $\dot{V}_{O_2}$ (MAX) IN l/min AND SELECTED BODY DIMENSIONS (28)

	Boys 8-16 years (n = 58) Correlation Coefficient	Boys 14-16 years (n = 19) Correlation Coefficient
Height	.84	.29
Weight	.89	.04
LBM	.91	.08
^{40}K	.80	.40
PWC 170	.84	.78
PWC 170 + ^{40}K	.87	.84

Track and field studies

For a few years, we were able to study track and field athletes aged 13 to 17 years who were attending a summer camp. We sought to correlate laboratory measurements such as $\dot{V}_{O_2}$ (max), PWC_{170}, heart volume, calf x-ray measurements, pulmonary function, and bone age with track and field performance.[30] Over this age range, performance of many test items was significantly correlated with height and weight, the level of correlation often exceeding that for laboratory tests. For example, in the girls (Table 2-VIII) track and field performance was more closely correlated with overall body size than with radiographically measured calf muscle width.[31]

In another study at the track camp, performance of 13– to 17-year-old girls in the decathlon, 100 meter, 880 meter, and cross-country running, and in the hurdles and long jump all

TABLE 2-VIII

TRACK AND FIELD PERFORMANCE IN GIRLS AGED 13–17 YEARS—CORRELATION WITH ANTHROPOMETRIC DATA AND CALF MUSCLE WIDTH

Correlation Coefficients

	Age, Height, Weight	Calf Muscle Width
Shot put	.63	.49
Javelin thrown	.46	.27
High jump	.91	.76
100 yard run speed	.35	.38

showed a positive correlation with height and a negative correlation with weight. There were no grossly obese girls in this series—all were fit and had experience in the track events. This is further evidence that in some performance events, as well as in laboratory tests, the long and the lean are favored.

References

1. Tanner, J. M.: *The Physique of the Olympic Athlete.* George Allen and Unwin, London, 1964.
2. Cotes, J. E.: Relationships of oxygen consumption, ventilation and cardiac frequency to body weight during standardized submaximal exercise in normal subjects. *Ergonomics, 12*:415-427, 1969.
3. Åstrand, I., Åstrand, P. O., and Stunkard, A.: Oxygen intake of obese individuals during work on a bicycle ergometer. *Acta Physiol Scand, 50*:294-299, 1960.
4. Wyndham, C. H.: Influence of body size and composition on oxygen consumption during exercise and on maximal aerobic capacity of Bantu and Caucasian men. *Arch Phys Med Rehab, 52*:539-554, 1971.
5. Williams, C. G., Wyndham, C. H., and Morrison, J. F.: The influence of weight and of stature on the mechanical efficiency of men. *Int Z angew Physiol einschl Arbeitsphysiol, 23*:107-124, 1966.
6. Passmore, R. and Durnin, J. V. G. A.: Human Energy Expenditure. *Physiol Rev, 35*:801-810, 1955.
7. Workman, J. M. and Armstrong, B. W.: Oxygen cost of treadmill walking. *J Appl Physiol, 18*:798-803, 1963.
8. Workman, J. M. and Armstrong, B. W.: A nomogram for predicting treadmill-walking oxygen consumption. *J Appl Physiol, 19*:150-151, 1964.
9. Jankowski, L. W. et al.: Accuracy of methods for estimating O_2 cost of walking in coronary patients. *J Appl Physiol, 33*:672-673, 1972.
10. Bruce, R. A., Kusumi, F., and Hosmer, D.: Maximal oxygen intake and nomographic assessment of functional aerobic impairment in cardiovascular disease. *Am Heart J, 85*:546, 1973.
11. Margaria, R. et al.: Energy cost of running. *J Appl Physiol, 18*:367, 1963.
12. Silverman, M. and Anderson, S. D.: Metabolic cost of treadmill exercise in children. *J Appl Physiol, 33*:696-698, 1972.
13. Robinson, S.: Experimental studies of physical fitness in relation to age. *Arbeitsphysiologie, 10*:251, 1938.
14. Cassels, D. E. and Morse, M.: *Cardiopulmonary Data for Children and Young Adults.* Springfield, Thomas, 1962.

15. Bøje, O.: Energy production, pulmonary ventilation and length of steps in well trained runners working on a treadmill. *Acta Physiol Scand, 1*:362, 1944.

16. Kagaya, H.: Cardiorespiratory responses to optimal speed of walking and to metabolic intersection of speed of walking and running. *International Congress of Physical Activity Sciences 1976*. Quebec, CISAP 1976, pp. 108.

17. Borms, J., Hebbelinck, M., and Duquet, W.: On the variability of some physical fitness parameters in boys 6–13 years of age. In Seliger, V. (Ed.): *Physical Fitness*, Praha, Universita Karlova, 1973.

18. Hill, A. V.: The dimensions of animals and their muscular dynamics. *Proc Royal Inst Great Britain, 34*:450, 1950.

19. Asmussen, E. and Heeboll-Nielsen, K. R.: A dimensional analysis of physical performance and growth in boys. *J Appl Physiol, 7*:593-603, 1955.

20. Asmussen, E. and Heeboll-Nielsen, K. R.: Physical performance and growth in children. Influence of sex, age and intelligence. *J Appl Physiol, 8*:371-380, 1956.

21. Von Döbeln, W.: Maximal oxygen intake, body size and total hemoglobin in normal man. *Acta Physiol Scand, 38:*193, 1956.

22. Von Döbeln, W.: Human standard and maximal metabolic rate in relation to fat-free body mass. Acta Physiol Scand, 37 Suppl:126, 1956.

23. Åstrand, P. O. and Rodahl, K.: *Textbook of Work Physiology*. New York, McGraw-Hill, 1970.

24. Von Döbeln, W. and Eriksson, B.: Physical training, growth and maximal oxygen uptake of boys aged 11-13 years. In Bar-Or, O. (Ed.): *Proceedings of the Fourth International Symposium of Pediatric Work Physiology*. Natanya, Israël, Wingate Institute, 1973, p. 93.

25. Wilmore, J.: Small is beautiful but difficult. *Physician and Sports Medicine, 4*:88, 1976.

26. Walt, W. H. von der, et al.: The relationship of $\dot{V}O_2$ max to gross body mass and somatotype. *International Congress of Physical Activity Sciences 1976*. Quebec, CISAP, 1976, p. 150.

27. Buskirk, E. and Taylor, H. L.: Maximal oxygen intake and its relation to body composition, with special reference to chronic physical activity and obesity. *J Appl Physiol, 11*:72-78, 1957.

28. Cumming, G. R.: Maximum oxygen uptake and total body potassium in children. In Taylor, A. W. (Ed.): *Application of Science and Medicine to Sport*. Springfield, Thomas, 1975.

29. Davies, C. T. M., Barnes, C., and Godfrey, S.: Body composition and maximal exercise performance in children. *Human Biology, 44*: 195-214, 1972.

30. Cumming, G. R.: Correlation of athletic performance and aerobic power in 12 to 17 year old children with bone age, calf muscle, total body potassium and heart volume and two indices of anaerobic power. In

Bar-Or, O. (Ed.): *Proceedings of the Fourth International Symposium of Pediatric Work Physiology*, Natanya, Israël, Wingate Institute, 1973, p. 109.

31. Cumming, G. R. et al: Calf X-ray measurements correlated with age, body build and physical performance in boys and girls. *J Sports Med Phys Fitness, 13*:90-95, 1973.

Chapter 3

BODY DIMENSIONS AND PHYSIOLOGICAL INDICATORS OF PHYSICAL FITNESS DURING ADOLESCENCE

Š. Šprynarová and R. Reisenauer

Abstract

Indicators of functional capacity were followed longitudinally in several groups of subjects. Relationships between body dimensions and such indicators were tested by correlation coefficients, linear regressions ($y = a + bx$) and exponential regressions ($y = a \times x^b$). Lines and curves relating maximal aerobic power to body weight and height (repeated measurements between the ages of 11 and 15) were practically identical in successive years. However, in older boys aerobic power was greater than in younger boys having the same body weight. Exponents relating functional indicators to height and to weight were close to the theoretical values of 2 and 0.67 respectively. It is argued that the prediction of functional capacity from body dimensions should be elaborated separately for each age group of children and youth. The relationship of functional capacity to body dimensions during adolescence is more marked in well-trained boys than in groups with varying levels of fitness.

PHYSIOLOGICAL INDICATORS of physical fitness such as maximal aerobic power depend on body dimensions (Von Döbeln, 1957) and on the training of the subjects examined. In geometrically similar and qualitatively identical individuals, longitudinal dimensions (L) should be proportional; surface dimensions should then vary as L^2 and volumes as L^3. Functional indicators assessed in units of volume (e.g. maximal oxygen pulse, maximal respiratory capacity) in turn should be proportional to L^3 or to weight$^{1.0}$. Finally, accepting that time is proportional to length, functional indicators assessed as volumes per unit time (e.g. maximal oxygen uptake, maximal pulmonary ventilation) should be proportional to L^2 or weight$^{0.67}$ (Åstrand and Rodahl, 1970).

We were concerned to what extent this hypothesis applied to youth in different stages of adolescence and at different levels of training. We thus compared the relationships between indicators of functional capacity and body dimensions in several groups followed longitudinally. Functional capacity was measured during graded treadmill work (Šprynarová and Pařízková, 1963). Correlation coefficients, linear regressions ($y = a + bx$) and exponential regressions ($y = a \times x^b$) were fitted to the data for ninety boys who were tested repeatedly.

The shapes of estimated lines and curves for individual years (ages 11 to 15) were practically identical (Fig. 3-1). Within a given year it was thus possible to express maximal oxygen consumption as a function of weight or of height using a linear regression. Boys of different ages, however, were not qualitatively equal, older boys of a given body weight having a greater maximal aerobic power than younger boys. If prediction equations ignore this fact and use data obtained on children of different ages, they introduce an error which increases with the age range of the group.

In two groups of boys ($n = 90$ and $n = 39$) studied between the ages of 12 and 15 years, exponents relating functional indicators to height fell close to the theoretical value of 2, while weight exponents were near the theoretical value of 0.67 (Table 3-I).

On the other hand, functional indicators given in units of volume (such as maximal oxygen pulse) had very similar exponents, contrary to hypothesis.

Relationships were also investigated in trained youths who were followed longitudinally (eight basketball players, and eight boy and ten girl swimmers, Table 3-II). In these small and functionally homogeneous groups, exponents differed markedly from hypothesis.

The relationship between functional indicators and body dimensions should be most obvious in groups of subjects who are equally trained, since differences in training then cannot mask the relationship between body dimensions and functional

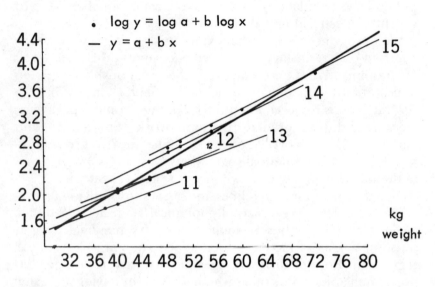

$$y = 249.42 + 57.89 \; x$$

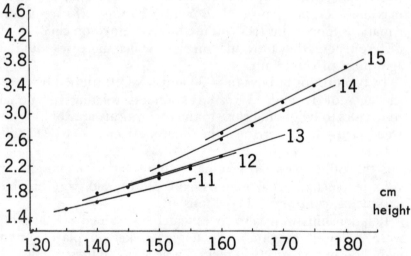

Figure 3-1. $\dot{V}_{O_2}$ (max) l/min is represented by the y-axis.

capacity. Comparison of correlation coefficients relating body weight and height to functional indicators in trained, functionally homogeneous groups and in boys with varying levels of physical fitness (Table 3-III) confirmed this assumption. The

TABLE 3-I

FUNCTIONAL VARIABLES. RELATIONSHIP TO BODY DIMENSIONS IN TWO GROUPS OF BOYS

(n = 90 and n = 39).

Exponent b in the equation $y = a \times x^b$

x	*weight*						*height*					
	expected value	observed value age (years)					expected value	observed value age (years)				
y		11	12	13	14	15		11	12	13	14	15
n = 90												
$\dot{V}O_2$ max	0.67	0.66	0.86	0.70	0.87	0.88	2.00	1.89	2.09	2.04	2.63	2.72
$\dot{V}$ max	0.67	0.61	0.79	0.56	0.72	0.64	2.00	1.79	2.38	1.95	2.34	1.97
O_2 pulse max	1.00	0.66	0.81	0.66	0.83	0.88	3.00	1.99	2.08	2.12	2.63	2.79
n = 39												
$\dot{V}O_2$ max	0.67	0.70	0.82	0.69	0.82	0.94	2.00	1.69	1.80	1.79	2.74	2.82
$\dot{V}$ max	0.67	0.53	0.54	0.49	0.67	0.67	2.00	1.59	1.98	1.90	2.67	2.29
O_2 pulse max	1.00	0.73	0.78	0.66	0.82	0.95	3.00	1.92	1.80	1.86	2.76	3.06

TABLE 3-II

FUNCTIONAL VARIABLES. RELATIONSHIP TO BODY DIMENSIONS IN GROUPS OF TRAINED YOUTH. EXPONENT B IN THE EQUATION

$$y = a \times x^b$$

x	*weight*					*height*				
	expected value	observed value age (years)				expected value	observed value age (years)			
y		12	13	14	15		12	13	14	15
basket-ball (n = 8)										
$\dot{V}O_2$ max	0.67	2.07	2.03	2.03	2.00	2.00	1.52	1.53	1.57	1.58
$\dot{V}$ max	0.67	1.13	1.15	1.16	1.16	2.00	0.83	0.86	0.90	0.92
O_2 pulse max	1.00	0.64	0.65	0.70	0.71	3.00	0.47	0.49	0.54	0.56
boy swimmers (n = 8)										
$\dot{V}O_2$ max	0.67	2.09	2.05	2.00	2.01	2.00	1.52	1.53	1.54	1.58
$\dot{V}$ max	0.67	1.17	1.18	1.16	1.16	2.00	0.85	0.88	0.89	0.81
O_2 pulse max	1.00	0.63	0.65	0.66	0.69	3.00	0.46	0.48	0.50	0.54
girl swimmers (n = 10)										
$\dot{V}O_2$ max	0.67	2.01	1.97	1.94	1.85	2.00	1.49	1.50	1.51	1.45
$\dot{V}$ max	0.67	1.11	1.12	1.11	1.13	2.00	0.82	0.85	0.86	0.89
O_2 pulse max	1.00	0.59	0.61	0.61	0.64	3.00	0.44	0.46	0.47	0.51

TABLE 3-III

CORRELATION OF FUNCTIONAL VARIABLES WITH BODY DIMENSIONS IN GROUPS OF YOUTH (SIGNIFICANT CORRELATION COEFFICIENTS MARKED BY ASTERISKS)

group		weight age (years)				height age (years)			
		12	13	14	15	12	13	14	15
differently trained and untrained boys (n=39)	$\dot{V}o_2$ max	0.659*	0.667*	0.747*	0.844*	0.422*	0.517*	0.724*	0.742*
	$\dot{V}$ max	0.400*	0.566*	0.647*	0.681*	0.436*	0.629*	0.745*	0.650*
	O_2 pulse max	0.599*	0.655*	0.708*	0.834*	0.398*	0.549*	0.705*	0.745*
basketball players (n=8)	$\dot{V}o_2$ max	0.840*	0.630	0.948*	0.908*	0.728*	0.608	0.959*	0.942*
	$\dot{V}$ max	0.888*	0.953*	0.877*	0.778*	0.888*	0.878*	0.897*	0.732*
	O_2 pulse max	0.893*	0.783*	0.957*	0.942*	0.893*	0.635	0.975*	0.975*
boy swimmers (n=8)	$\dot{V}o_2$ max	0.938*	0.863*	0.705	0.803*	0.740*	0.731*	0.611	0.823*
	$\dot{V}$ max	0.855*	0.776*	0.538	0.583	0.850*	0.714*	0.471	0.704*
	O_2 pulse max	0.920*	0.879*	0.690	0.756*	0.658	0.724*	0.623	0.755*
girl swimmers (n=10)	$\dot{V}o_2$ max	0.349	0.040	0.554	-0.198	0.335	0.548	0.487	-0.505
	$\dot{V}$ max	0.380	0.106	0.774*	0.320	0.133	0.310	0.271	0.034
	O_2 pulse max	0.436	0.265	0.347	-0.167	0.464	0.636*	0.535	0.059

closest relationships were found in trained boys; in the boys with varying fitness the relationship was less close; and in the trained girls significant correlation coefficients were encountered only rarely.

From the above results, we would conclude the following: (1) Within a one year age range, the relationship between functional indicators and body dimensions can be expressed satisfactorily by means of a linear regression. (2) Predictions of functional capacity based on the body dimensions of children and youth should be elaborated, treating data for each annual age group separately. (3) Hypotheses relating body dimensions to functional capacity apply only roughly during adolescence. (4) The relationship of functional capacity to body dimensions during adolescence is more marked in boys than in girls and is also more marked in functionally homogeneous groups of well-trained boys than in groups with varying levels of fitness.

References

Åstrand, P.-O. and Rodahl, K.: *Textbook of Physiology.* New York, McGraw-Hill, 1970.

Döbeln, W. von: Human standard and maximal metabolic rate in relation to fat free body mass. *Acta Physiol Scand, 37*:suppl. 126, 1956.

Šprynarová, Š. and Pařízková, J.: Changes in the aerobic capacity and body composition in obese boys after reduction. *J Appl Physiol, 20*:934-937, 1965.

Chapter 4

BODY WEIGHT AND ITS RELATIONSHIP TO PERFORMANCE ON THE BICYCLE ERGOMETER AND TREADMILL

D. Van Gerven, M. Ostyn, and B. Vanden Eynde

Abstract

This chapter investigates the relationship between body weight and performance on bicycle ergometer and treadmill tests. Data have been collected on two groups of male first-year physical education students, (group 1: thirty-three persons with a mean body weight of 60.1 kg; group 2: thirty-three persons with a mean body weight of 81.6 kg). The heavy subjects performed significantly better than the light subjects on the bicycle ergometer, whereas no intergroup difference of performance was found for the treadmill-run.

SEVERAL PREVIOUS authors [1, 4-6, 8-10] have discussed the influence of body weight on bicycle ergometer tests. We thus decided to verify whether effects of body weight differed between bicycle ergometer and treadmill tests. Our hypothesis was that heavy subjects would have an advantage on the standard bicycle ergometer procedure, but that in treadmill tests lighter persons would be favored.

Methods

From a group of male first-year undergraduates in physical education, we selected sixty-six students (mean age of 20 years) on the basis of extreme body weight; thirty-three subjects weighed at least one SD less than the average for the total group and thirty-three subjects weighed at least 1 SD more than the mean. The bicycle ergometer was a Siemens/Elema 380 machine with an electrical braking system that was compensated for variations of pedal frequency; nevertheless, the students were required to cycle at a rhythm between 53 and 63 pedal rotations per minute. The test was performed according to Hollmann,[2] with a starting load of 70 W and a final cardiac frequency of 170 beats/minute, as measured by auscultation. The treadmill test was executed according to the instructions of I.C.P.F.R. (super standard treadmill test), using a constant speed of 6 km/h and a starting slope of 4°, increased by 2° per minute of effort. The cardiac frequency was measured by telemeter (Hellige 19®).

TABLE 4-1: MEANS, STANDARD DEVIATION, AND COEFFICIENTS OF VARIATION FOR VARIABLES MEASURED IN BOTH WEIGHT GROUPS.

VARIABLES	LIGHTWEIGHTS				HEAVYWEIGHTS			
	N	$\bar{X}$	S.D.	V	N	$\bar{X}$	S.D.	V
BODY WEIGHT BEFORE BICYCLE TEST	33	60	2.8	5	33	82	3.3	4
PULSE RATE AT REST BEFORE BICYCLE	33	71	9.5	13	33	73	11.7	16
PULSE RATE LOAD LEVEL 70 W (3RD.MIN.)	33	107	10.8	10	33	100	10.3	10
PULSE RATE LOAD LEVEL 110 W (6TH.MIN.)	33	126	11.4	9	33	124	10.8	9
PULSE RATE LOAD LEVEL 150 W (9TH.MIN.)	33	145	13.3	9	33	129	11.4	9
PULSE RATE LOAD LEVEL 190 W (12TH.MIN.)	22	160	9.8	6	33	146	13.0	9
PULSE RATE LOAD LEVEL 230 W (15TH.MIN.)	4	164	5.3	3	25	157	10.2	6
PULSE RATE LOAD LEVEL 270 W (18TH.MIN.)	-	-	-	-	9	162	7.8	5
PULSE RATE LOAD LEVEL 310 W (21TH.MIN.)	-	-	-	-	1	-	-	-
EXECUTION TIME ON BICYCLE (SEC.)	33	756	108.1	14	33	939	144.6	15
BODY WEIGHT BEFORE TREADMILL RUN	33	60	2.7	4	33	82	3.4	4
PULSE RATE AT REST BEFORE TREADMILL	33	78	9.7	12	33	75	10.3	14
PULSE RATE 1ST MINUTE TREADMILL 4°	33	129	8.8	7	33	130	8.8	7
PULSE RATE 2ND MINUTE TREADMILL 6°	33	140	9.1	6	33	137	9.2	7
PULSE RATE 3RD MINUTE TREADMILL 8°	33	149	9.1	6	33	144	12.0	8
PULSE RATE 4TH MINUTE TREADMILL 10°	33	157	9.4	6	32	153	11.0	7
PULSE RATE 5TH MINUTE TREADMILL 12°	31	164	10.0	5	31	161	9.5	6
PULSE RATE 6TH MINUTE TREADMILL 14°	23	168	6.7	4	24	166	7.3	4
PULSE RATE 8TH MINUTE TREADMILL 16°	14	171	5.4	3	16	171	6.8	4
PULSE RATE 9TH MINUTE TREADMILL 18°	5	172	5.7	3	4	172	1.3	1
PULSE RATE 10TH MINUTE TREADMILL 20°	1	-	-	-	-	-	-	-
RUNNING TIME ON TREADMILL (SEC.)	33	374	73.5	19	33	374	71.9	19

TABLE 4-II: F- AND T-RATIO;
DIFFERENCE BETWEEN LIGHT WEIGHTS AND HEAVY WEIGHTS

VARIABLES	$\bar{X}$		F	T
	LEIGHT W.	HEAVY W.		
BODY WEIGHT BEFORE BICYCLE TEST	60	82	1.341	28.384**
PULSE RATE AT REST BEFORE BICYCLE	71	73	1.515	0.839
PULSE RATE LOAD LEVEL 70 W (3RD.MIN.)	107	100	1.130	2.702**
PULSE RATE LOAD LEVEL 110 W (6TH.MIN.)	126	124	1.101	4.560**
PULSE RATE LOAD LEVEL 150 W (9TH.MIN.)	145	129	1.366	5.244**
PULSE RATE LOAD LEVEL 190 W (12TH.MIN.)	160	146	1.802	4.406**
PULSE RATE LOAD LEVEL 230 W (15TH.MIN.)	164	157	4.826	1.476*
WORKING CAPACITY 130	3.745 KGM	6.201 KGM	2.019*	5.079**
WORKING CAPACITY 170	10.269 KGM	16.050 KGM	2.456**	7.215**
EXECUTION TIME ON BICYCLE (SEC.)	756	939	1.789	7.231**
BODY WEIGHT BEFORE TREADMILL RUN	60	82	1.613	27.828**
PULSE RATE AT REST BEFORE TREADMILL	78	75	1.129	1.253
PULSE RATE 1ST MINUTE TREADMILL 4°	129	130	1.010	0.490
PULSE RATE 2ND MINUTE TREADMILL 6°	140	137	1.040	1.640
PULSE RATE 3RD MINUTE TREADMILL 8°	149	144	1.722	1.760
PULSE RATE 4TH MINUTE TREADMILL 10°	157	153	1.364	1.765
PULSE RATE 5TH MINUTE TREADMILL 12°	164	161	1.119	1.263
PULSE RATE 6TH MINUTE TREADMILL 14°	168	166	1.206	1.042
PULSE RATE 8TH MINUTE TREADMILL 16°	171	171	1.589	0.225
PULSE RATE 9TH MINUTE TREADMILL 18°	172	172	21.895*	0.095
RUNNING TIME ON TREADMILL (SEC.)	374	374	1.043	0.0

(* SIGNIFICANTLY DIFFERENT AT THE 0.05 LEVEL)
(** SIGNIFICANTLY DIFFERENT AT THE 0.01 LEVEL)

Results

There was a progressive elimination of subjects at higher work loads in both bicycle and treadmill tests (Table 4-I and 4-II). On the treadmill, the elimination affected light– and heavyweight groups in a parallel way. However, on the bicycle ergometer, the elimination of lightweight subjects started after the ninth minute (at a work load of 190 W) and was complete by the fifteenth minute (at a work load of 270 W). In the group of heavyweights, elimination only began in the thirteenth minute (at a load of 230 W) and the number of participants gradually decreased until twenty one minutes (at a load of 310 W).

The heavyweights thus had a better performance curve than the lightweights on the standard bicycle ergometer procedure (Fig. 4-1). However, there were no weight-related differences in treadmill performance (Fig. 4-2).

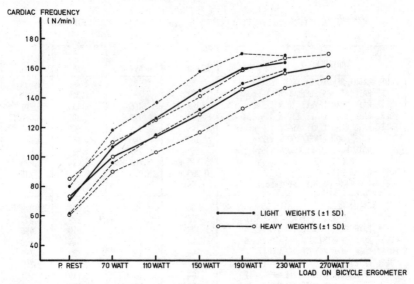

Figure 4-1. Cardiac frequency during bicycle ergometer test for both weight groups.

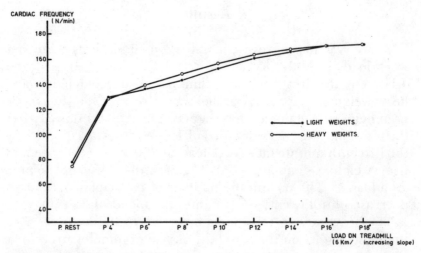

Figure 4-2. Cardiac frequency during treadmill run test for both weight groups.

Conclusion

Our test group was not representative of an average population and results thus cannot be generalized; nevertheless, we think, as does I. Ryhming,[7] that a light person puts more effort into bicycle ergometer procedures with a fixed external work load. Katch et al.[4] have suggested that a stepwise increase of the bicycle loading requires increasing static effort. Tolerance of static effort is certainly recognized as related to body weight.

References

1. McArdle, W. D. and J. R. Magel: Physical work capacity and maximum oxygen uptake in treadmill and bicycle exercise. *Med Sci Sports,* 2:118-123, 1970.
2. Hollman, W.: *Höchst– und Dauerleistungsfähigkeit des Sportlers.* Munich, J. Ambrosius Barth, 1963.
3. International Committee for Standardization of Physical Fitness Tests: *International manual for performance test and physique, body composition measurements.* Tokyo, 1973, pp. 21-36.
4. Katch, F. I., Girandola, R. N., and Katch, V. L.: The relationship of body weight on maximum oxygen uptake and heavy-work endurance capacity on the bicycle ergometer. *Med Sci Sports,* 3:101-106, 1971.
5. Mocellin, R.: Untersuchungen über die Abhängigkeit der Herzfrequenz bei relativ gleichen Leistungen von Alter bei 5-18 jährigen Herwachsenden, *III Internationales Seminar für Ergometrie.* Berlin, Institut für Leistungsmedizin, 1972, pp 60-64.
6. Ostyn, M., Van Gerven, D., and De Bruyn-Prevost, P.: Influence of body weight on results, obtained by sportsmen in submaximal work tests. *III Internationales Seminar für Ergometrie,* Berlin, Institut für Leistungsmedizin, 1972, pp. 201-204.
7. Ryhming, I.: A modified HARVARD step test for the evaluation of physical fitness. *Arbeitsphysiol, 15*:235-250, 1954.
8. Schönholzer, G., Bieler, G., and Howald, H.: Ergometrische Methoden zur Messüng der Aeroben und Anaeroben Kapazität. *III Internationales Seminar für Ergometrie.* Berlin, Institut für Leistungsmedizin 1972, pp. 84-97.
9. Shephard, R. J.: Standard tests of aerobic power. In Shephard, R. J. (Ed.): *Frontiers of Fitness.* Springfield, Thomas, 1971, pp. 233-264.
10. Usami, M.: Erfahrungen mit einer ergometrischen standardleistung von 1 Watt/kg Körpergewicht in Japan, *III Internationales Seminar für Ergometrie,* Berlin, Institut für Leistungsmedizin, 1972, pp. 102-105.

Chapter 5

KINANTHROPOMETRY TERMINOLOGY AND LANDMARKS*

W. D. Ross, S. R. Brown, M. Hebbelinck, and R. A. Faulkner

IN PREPARATION FOR the Montreal Olympic Games Anthropological Project (MOGAP), a study group[†] on kinanthropometric techniques met at the University of British Columbia in July 1973. The purpose of the group was to decide on terminology and landmarks for MOGAP and subsequent international cooperative kinanthropometric studies. The format was essentially a critical review of working papers assembled by the senior author in collaboration with S. R. Brown, N. C. Wilson, and M. V. Savage. Substantial changes were made to arrive at a consensus.

While traditional anthropometric techniques and various international agreements and standardization committee reports were well known to the participants, the final decisions represented an interplay of precedent and utility. For example, the definition of the ACROMIALE was based on the Geneva Convention (1912). The reason for selecting the "superior-external border" rather than the "most lateral aspect" (Martin) or "inferior-external border" (IBP) was a recognition that the most critical location was for acromiale height and upper

---

*This chapter is based on agreements reached by a Leon and Thea Koerner Foundation Study Group held at the University of British Columbia, July 1973.

†The group, which was convened by Dr. S. R. Brown (University of British Columbia), included MOGAP directors Dr. J. E. L. Carter (San Diego State University), Dr. M. Hebbelinck (Vrije Universiteit, Brussels), and Dr. W. D. Ross (Simon Fraser University), and consultants Dr. A. R. Behnke Jr. (San Francisco) and M. V. Savage (Simon Fraser University).

extremity and arm length, rather than biacromial breadth (where the anthropometrist manipulates the anthropometer to find the widest diameter, which would be somewhat inferior to our designated landmark for lengths). While techniques and terminology, in general, reflect classical anthropometry, the study group's primary orientation was not physical anthropology, but KINANTHROPOMETRY, the measurement of human *size, shape, proportion, composition, maturation* and *gross function* as related to research on *normal* and *atypical growth, exercise, physical performance* and *nutrition.* The participants were also concerned with the practical problem of how to analyse kinanthropometric data in order to get the greatest possible return of information. Thus, the techniques and proforma were selected to provide for somatograms, somatotypes, and proportionality profiles which go beyond routine parametric analyses.

TERMINOLOGY AND LANDMARKS

Because the body can assume an infinite variety of postures and attitudes, all descriptions of positions, directions, and relations are referred to a standard *anatomical position.* This is arbitrarily taken to be standing erect with the head and eyes directed forward, the upper extremities hanging by the sides with the palms forward, the thumbs away from the sides, the fingers directed downward and the feet together with the toes directed forward.

Planes and Axes

Three primary planes describe position:
(1) An ANTEROPOSTERIOR or SAGITTAL PLANE runs parallel to the vertical plane which divides the body into right and left halves. The sagittal plane which thus bisects the body is the MIDSAGITTAL PLANE.
(2) A FRONTAL or CORONAL PLANE runs at right angles to a sagittal plane, dividing the body into front and rear portions.

(3) A Transverse Plane runs at right angles to the other two
planes, dividing the body into upper and lower parts. Axes
of the body are formed by the intersection of planes as
follows:
  (x) A Lateral Axis is any line formed by the intersect of a
  frontal and a sagittal plane.
  (y) A Longitudinal Axis is any line formed by the
  intersect of a frontal and a sagittal plane.
  (z) An Anteroposterior or Sagittal Axis is any line
  formed by the intersect of a sagittal and a transverse
  plane.

Landmarks

‡Vertex (v). The most superior point on the skull, in the
midsagittal plane, when the head is held in the Frankfurt plane.

‡Gnathion (gn). Fr.: point mentonnier. Chin. The most
inferior border of the mandible in the midsagittal plane.

*Suprasternale (sst). Fr.: fourchette sternale. Suprasternal
notch. The superior border of the sternal notch (or incisura
jugularis) in the midsagittal plane.

*Mesoternale (mst). Point located on the corpus sterni at the
intersect of the midsagittal plane and the horizontal plane at
the midlevel of the IV chondrosternal articulation. One starts
counting at the manubriosternal joint, which corresponds to
the level of the second costal cartilage.

*Epigastrale (eg). Point located on anterior surface at the
intersect of the midsagittal plane and the horizontal plane
through the most inferior point on the tenth ribs.

‡Thelion (th). Breast nipple.

‡Omphalion (om). Midpoint of naval or umbilicus.

‡Symphysion (sy). Fr.: bord supérieur de la symphyse
pubienne. The superior border of the symphysis pubis at the
midsagittal plane. This is located by having the subject place his
index fingers about four centimeters apart and proceed
downward from the navel, palpating the abdominal wall gently
until the bony surface of the pubis is located. The anthropometrist can then palpate the "subject-located" landmark
with his left thumb, avoiding the foreside of the subject's

symphysis and genital parts which are inferior to the landmark. Generally, the landmark is at the upper level of the pubic hair zone and can be located through light clothing with no difficulty.

*Acromiale (a). Acromial point. The point at the superior and external border of the acromial process when the subject is standing erect with relaxed arms. This definition is in accord with the 1912 Geneva Convention (Stewart, 1952) but is not identical with "the most lateral" description of Martin and Saller (1957) or the "inferior-external border" found in the I.B.P. Handbook (Weiner and Lourie, 1969). The location of the point may be facilitated by having the subject bend laterally at the trunk, thus relaxing the deltoid muscle.

†Radiale (r). The point at the upper and lateral border of the head of the radius. It can be located by palpating downward in the lateral dimple at the elbow; the rotating head can be determined easily when the subject slightly pronates and supinates his forearm under the stationary condyle of the humerus.

†Stylion (sty). Fr.: apophyse styloide. The most distal point of the styloid process of the radius. It is located in the so-called "anatomical snuff box" (Fr.: tabatière anatomique), the triangular area formed when the thumb is extended laterally and the area defined by the raised tendons of abductor pollicus longus and extensor pollicus brevis with the extensor pollicus longus. For measurements on the ulna, the stylion ulnare can be used.

‡Dactylion (da). Fr.: extrémité intérieure du doigt medius. Tip of the middle finger. The most distal point of the middle finger or digit when the arm is hanging and the fingers are stretched downwards. The corresponding tips of the other fingers are designated as dactylion I, II, IV, and V.

‡Metacarpale Radiale (mr). The outermost point of the distal head of metacarpal II of the stretched hand, i.e. the most lateral point in reference to the anatomical position or the radial side of the hand.

‡Metacarpale Ulnare (mu). The outermost point on the distal head of the metacarpal V of the outstretched hand, i.e. the most medial point in reference to the anatomical position or the ulnar side of the hand.

‡ILIOCRISTALE (ic). Fr.: crête iliaque. The most lateral point of the crista iliaca. This landmark is usually encompassed when obtaining bi-iliocristal breadth with an anthropometer, although it is not usually identified unless a projected measurement for iliocristal length is required.

†ILIOSPINALE (is). Fr.: épine iliaque antéro-supérieure. The anterior superior iliac spine. The pronounced tip and not the most frontally curved site of the crista iliaca is the designated landmark.

†TROCHANTERION (tro). The most superior point on the greater trochanter of the femur. It cannot be located easily on fleshy subjects, especially women. However, an acceptable approximation may be achieved by having the subject slightly abduct his leg and move it forward and backwards while the anthropometrist palpates the femur progressively upwards with his finger to determine the landmark on the uppermost point of the greater trochanter.

†TIBIALE (ti). Tibiale internum. Fr.: ligne articulaire du genou. Superior extremity of the tibia. The most proximal point of the margo glenoidalis on the medial border of the head of the tibia. This landmark is hard to locate on subjects with thick subcutaneous fat layers around the knee joint, particularly women. To find the tibiale, the upper border of the tibia is located by palpating the quadriceps tendon at the distal end of the patella. This may be facilitated by having the subject slightly flex his leg. The index finger is moved inward pressing the skin to locate the tibial point of the articulation at the frontal border of the ligamentum collaterale tibiale. The level at this point should be marked as the reference.

†TIBIALE EXTERNUM (te). This point corresponds to the tibiale above but is located on the lateral border of the head of the tibia. It is above the capitulum fibulare. The location of the landmark may be facilitated by having the subject flex his knee. The point is located at the center of the triad formed by the epicondylar femur, the epicondylar tibia, and the head of the fibula. Both tibial landmarks are situated in practically the same transverse plane.

†SPHYRION (sph). Malleolare mediale or malleolare internum. The most distal tip of the malleolare medialis (tibialis). This

landmark may be located most easily from beneath and dorsally. It is the distal tip and not the outermost point of the malleolus.

†SPHYRION FIBULARE (sph f). Malleolare laterale or malleolare externum. The most distal tip of the malleolare laterale (fibularis). The sphyrion fibulare is more distal than the sphyrion tibiale.

‡PTERNION (pte). The most posterior point on the heel of the foot when the subject is standing.

‡AKROPODION (ap). The most anterior point on the toe of the foot when the subject is standing. This may be the I or II phalange. The subject's toenail may have to be clipped to make a measurement.

‡METATARSALE TIBIALE (mt t). The outermost point on the head of metatarsale I of the foot when the subject is standing.

‡METATARSALE FIBULARE (mt f). The outermost point of the head of metatarsale V when the subject is standing.

*CERVICALE (c). The most posterior point on the spinous process of the seventh cervical vertebra. To locate this landmark, the subject nods his head forward; the spinous process of the seventh cervical vertebra moves away from the spinous process of the usually more prominent first thoracic vertebra; once the cervicale is located, the subject assumes an erect standing position and its location is marked.

‡GLUTEALE (ga). Midgluteal arch. This point is at the sacrococcygeal fusion in the midsagittal plane. It is located by placing the thumb at the top of the gluteal furrow and palpating in a downward direction with the thumb. The fingers should be spread upwards over the lumbar region of the subject and the landmark can be located with minimal adjustment of clothing.

---

*dermatographic mark at midsagittal plane.
†dermatographic mark on right side only.
‡landmark located at the time of measurement.

References

Hrdlicka, A.: *Practical Anthropometry,* 4th ed. Philadelphia, Wistar Institutes of Anatomy and Biology, 1952.

Martin, R. and Saller, K.: *Lehrbuch der Anthropologie.* Band 2. Stuttgart, Gustav Fischer, 1959.

Weiner, J. S. and Lourie, J. A. (Ed.): *Human Biology.* Oxford, Blackwell Scientific Publications, 1969.

Chapter 6

RACIAL DIFFERENCES IN FUNCTIONAL CAPACITY

V. Klissouras

THIS DISCUSSION WILL focus on the following question: To what extent are variations in functional capacity based on genetic differences between individuals or populations? The performance criterion of functional capacity examined will be the maximal aerobic power and the thesis will be developed on the basis of data derived from regional and twin studies.

Regional Studies

We recently had opportunity to study (Chan Onn Leng et al., 1974; Thinakaran et al., 1974) in their natural environment Malayan aborigines, the Temiars, a primitive community of Nomadic hunters inhabiting the jungle along the Ninggiri tributary of the Kelantan River. Some city dwellers (Malays, Chinese, and Indians) exposed to the same variety of environment were also tested. These three populations are genetically different in the sense that they are culturally isolated and maintain distinct corporate gene pools through a high rate of endogamy.

The maximal oxygen uptake was measured directly, using the Douglas bag method. Gas volumes were determined with a calibrated gasometer and gas concentrations with a Haldane gas analyzer. Blood samples were taken for pH and lactate determinations. Heart rate was recorded throughout the test. Exercise was carried out using a step test with two risers, each

0.4 m high. The average ambient temperature was 26°C. Subjects were made to perform three work loads of 18, 23, and 28 ascents per minute on the single step, and subsequently two work loads, at 22 and 26 ascents per minute on the double step. Work loads were performed for five minutes with ten minute rest intervals; however, the duration of the last stage depended upon the work tolerance of the individual. In order to control the stepping rate, a metronome was used for the city dwellers and the more familiar bamboo beat for the Temiars. The bamboo beat is used in all-night bomo dances and seems to induce mental concentration; several dancers were observed to go into a trance during maximal testing.

The jungle dwellers consisted of twenty-five boys (12 to 18 years) and ten men (20 to 40 years); the city dwellers consisted of twenty-six boys (12 to 18 years), nine of Malay, nine of Indian, and eight of Chinese origin, all selected from the same school. The mean values for maximal oxygen uptake, blood lactate, and pH, and heart rate did not differ significantly among the three ethnic groups (Table 6-I), neither were there significant intergroup differences in these measurements at submaximal work loads.

It was anticipated that the Temiars might have a high maximal aerobic power as compared to city dwellers. However, although they lead a physically active life, it is at a leisurely pace. For the period of time they were observed, they spent the morning clearing the jungle and planting tapioca, bananas, and

TABLE 6-I

METABOLIC RESPONSES TO MAXIMAL EFFORT IN DIFFERENT ETHNIC GROUPS IN MALAYSIA (CHAN ONN LENG et al., 1974; THINAKARAN et al., 1974).

Ethnic Group	Oxygen Uptake $ml\text{-}kg^{-1} min^{-1}$	Blood lactate $mg\%$	Heart rate beats/min	Blood pH
Malays	49.5 ± 10.6	78.2 ± 29.6	193 ± 10	7.24 ± 0.04
Indians	47.2 ± 5.1	68.6 ± 29.6	198 ± 5	7.27 ± 0.05
Chinese	43.6 ± 4.6	85.0 ± 29.7	196 ± 3	7.23 ± 0.06
Temiars				
boys	45.9 ± 6.7	75.0 ± 18.0	194 ± 4	
men	53.2 ± 2.0	94.0 ± 32.4	187 ± 10	

hill padi. There was a short break for a lunch consisting of two pieces of baked tapioca root; then they set about hunting with their blow pipes and poisoned darts. Telemetric monitoring seldom revealed heart rates exceeding 130 beats per minute (Fig. 6-1). However, people going into a trance during the all-night bomo dances reached close to maximal heart rates.

The comparability of functional capacity observed among the different ethnic groups tested is in agreement with several other regional studies. For example, Robinson and his associates (1941) found practically the same maximal aerobic power in American Caucasian and Negro sharecroppers who were living under the same environmental conditions and with similar levels of habitual activity. Wyndham (1966) was impressed with the remarkable similarity of physiological responses between physically active Caucasians, Bantu, and Bushmen in Southern Africa. He noted no differences in $\dot{V}o_2$ max and only small differences in reactions to standard heat and cold stresses, in spite of differences between the three

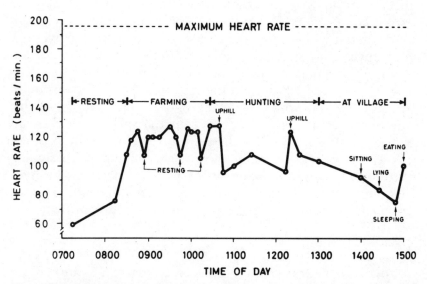

Figure 6-1. Telemetric monitoring of heart rate of jungle dweller during daily activity. Reproduced with permission of editor. From Onn-leng Chan et al.: The cardiorespiratory fitness and energy expenditure of the Temiars. *Med J Malaysia, 28*:267-272, 1974.

ethnic groups with respect to morphology, nutrition, patterns of activity, and the use made of shelter for protection against climatic extremes. Davies and co-workers (1972) observed no differences of maximal aerobic power between young adult Kurdish and Yemenite Jews, both groups being active agricultural workers, living under identical environmental conditions, and with a similar nutritional state. Neither did they observe any differences between these groups, sedentary Caucasians, and Yoruba villagers.* A mean maximal aerobic power of the same order has been reported for several other ethnic groups including arctic Indians (Andersen et al., 1960), Eskimo hunters (Andersen et al., 1963; Rode and Shephard, 1971; Lammert, 1972), the Ainu and other Japanese inhabitants of Hokkaido (Ikai et al., 1971), the Tarahumara Indians of Mexico (Balke and Snow, 1965), Nomadic Lapps (Andersen, 1962), the Pascuans of Easter Island (Ekblom and Gjessing, 1968), and Dorobo, Turkana and other African natives (Prampero et al., 1969).

It would appear from these various studies that there are no differences in $\dot{V}O_2$ max among ethnic groups that can be attributed to genetic factors. It must be admitted, however, that the variation within any ethnic group far exceeds the average differences among groups and to compare them in terms of mean values is misleading. Note, for example, that the $\dot{V}O_2$ max expressed in ml-kg^{-1}-min^{-1} ranged from 40 to 62 in the Arctic Indians, from 43 to 84 in the Eskimos, from 29 to 52 in the Ainu, and from 38 to 78 in the Temiars. In fact one Temiar had a $\dot{V}O_2$ max of 78, while the respective value for his brother was 47. Both men were in their early twenties with similar nutritional states and patterns of physical activity, strongly suggesting that genetic factors played an important role in producing the wide difference of $\dot{V}O_2$ max between them.

Twin Studies

$\dot{V}O_2$ max, like any other polygenic variable, is under the control of many genes and we can expect it also to be affected

---

*Other authors have disputed the interpretation that Davies et al. made of this data, suggesting that there were small differences between these populations.—Ed.

by the previous history of the individual and by a host of other nongenetic factors. It is necessary to resort to statistical analysis in order to separate the effects of these various factors. Consider an experiment of nature that allows the separation of nongenetic from genetic elements. This is the occurrence of two types of twins: twins that are genetically identical and twins that are genetically different. Differences between identical twins indicate how much two individuals differ because of environmental influences alone. The intrapair difference in $\dot{V}o_2$ max between nonidentical twins shows a greater spread than between identical twins (Fig. 6-2), indicating that the addition of genetic diversity to the purely environmental influences increases the overall difference between members of a pair.

A comparison of the intrapair variance between identical and nonidentical twins provides a measure of the relative contribution of genetic and nongenetic factors to the total interindividual variation observed in a given attribute. This measure is known as the heritability estimate (H_{est}). We have derived such H_{ests} for a number of physiological attributes. The H_{est} of $\dot{V}o_2$ (max) for one sample of twins was about 93 percent. Unfortunately, a H_{est} applies only to the population studied

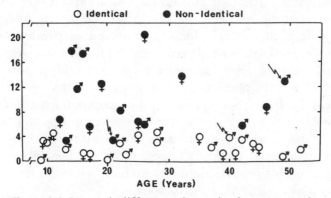

Figure 6-2. Intrapair differences in maximal oxygen uptake in identical and non-identical twins of different age. Reproduced with permission of the editor. From V. Klissouras et al.: Adaptation to maximal effort. *J Appl Physiol*, 33:288-293, 1972.

and to its particular environment. It cannot be extrapolated and used to explain differences observed between ethnic groups. Such an extrapolation would assume first, that the intragroup and intergroup environmental influences are comparable, and second, that each ethnic group is distinguished by a different genotype with respect to the variable under study. In fact, there is no basis for either of these assumptions, and, hence, an intrapopulation H_{est} cannot indicate the relative contribution of genetic and nongenetic factors to interpopulation variability.

"Ethnic group differences are compounds of individual differences; they are more often relative than absolute; ethnic groups differ in the frequencies of some genes more often than in that a certain gene is wholly absent in one group and present in every individual of another" (Dobzhansky, 1968). Thus, any given genetic combination may be found in almost any ethnic group, but the frequency with which it is found may vary from one ethnic group to another. Any genetic differences between ethnic groups must be small, since "an individual is the product of about 44,000 pairs of genes. Of these, 90 percent are held constant by everybody; of the remaining 5,000 or so, at least half must be allowed for sexual differences and only about 2,500 genes—i.e. 3.5 percent of the whole—remain to account for individual variations and ethnic variations" (Cole, 1965).

Since natural selection is the principal agent of genetic change, it is this force which is expected to produce ethnic variations in adaptability. Possible examples of selective adaptation are (a) the morphological differentiation produced by climatic loads applied over many generations and (b) the functional differentiation observed in populations which have been indigenous to high altitudes for several thousand years.

The average body size increases from warmer towards cooler biotopes (Roberts, 1953). It appears that the loss of heat from an organism is proportional to its surface, while the production of heat is proportional to its mass.

Under this assumption greater and bigger individuals have an advantage in cooler biotopes, for they first can produce more heat than smaller and lighter ones, and secondly, due to their relatively smaller surface, they can resist the effects of cooling much better than bigger ones. It seems evident, that such differences in heat regulation are of significant value with respect to climatic adaptation in man. Therefore it also seems to be evident, that the observed morphological variability in man may be seen as a result of selective adaptation (Walter, 1971).

With regard to hypoxic loads, Morpurgo and co-workers (1970) studied Indian natives of the Peruvian highlands and Europeans resident at high altitudes and at sea level. They confirmed the reported shift to the right of the oxygen dissociation curve at high altitude and they further observed this shift at both pH 7.4 and pH 6.7. In the latter case, however, they noted that the mean P_{50} and P_{80} values (partial pressures of oxygen required for 50 percent and 80 percent saturation of hemoglobin) of the Europeans at high altitudes were lower than those of the Peruvian Indians (Table 6-II). Thus, at P_{50} and P_{80} the Peruvians had a higher Bohr effect than the Europeans. The change in the oxygen affinity of hemoglobin at high altitude may result from an increase of 2,3-diphosphoglycerate. Whatever the mechanism, a higher Bohr effect should facilitate life at low oxygen pressures, because it enables the tissues to withdraw large amounts of oxygen from blood for relatively small decreases of Po_2. According to the authors, the identity of the Bohr effect among Europeans living at high altitudes for years and those living at sea level means that the phenomenon observed in highland natives is more than a simple physiological adaptation and should be interpreted as an evolutionary adaptive phenomenon.

Although more data are needed for a better understanding of man's adaptive variations, it is doubtful whether selective pressures currently prevailing in any biotope are sufficient to cause genetic adaptation of the structures and functions which support maximal physical effort.

References

Andersen, K. L.: Ethnic group differences in fitness for sustained muscular exercise. *Can Med Assoc J*, *96*:832-835, 1967.

Andersen, K. L.: Work capacity of selected populations. In Baker, P. T. and

TABLE 6-II

COMPARISON OF PARTIAL OXYGEN PRESSURES REQUIRED FOR 50 PERCENT (P_{50}) AND 80 PERCENT (P_{80}) SATURATION OF HEMOGLOBIN IN HEMOLYSATES DILUTED IN O.1 M PHOSPHATE BUFFER, AT pH 7.4 AND pH 6.7, FROM EUROPEANS AND PERUVIAN INDIANS (WITH STANDARD DEVIATIONS OF THE MEAN). THE BOHR EFFECT IS CALCULATED AS THE DIFFERENCE BETWEEN THE VALUES OBTAINED AT pH 6.7 AND 7.4 (MORPURGO et al., 1970).

Population	No. of individuals	P_{50}			P_{80}		
		pH 7.4	pH 6.7	Bohr effect	pH 7.4	pH 6.7	Bohr effect
Europeans at sea level	18	10.5 ± 1.30	26.4 ± 1.48	6.9	27.0 ± 1.91	37.9 ± 2.80	10.9
Europeans at high altitudes (above 3,500 m)	8	24.8 ± 2.23	31.3 ± 3.21	6.5	35.1 ± 2.86	46.3 ± 4.14	11.2
Peruvian Indians at high altitudes (above 3,500 m)	28	25.0 ± 2.80	33.7 ± 2.94	8.7	35.5 ± 4.83	52.7 ± 5.98	17.2

Weiner, J. S. (Ed.): *The Biology of Human Adaptability.* Oxford, Clarendon Press, 1966, pp. 67-90.

Andersen, K. L. et al.: Physical fitness of Arctic Indians. *J Appl Physiol,* 15:645-648, 1960.

Andersen, K. L. and Hart, J. S.: Aerobic working capacity of Eskimos. *J Appl Physiol, 18*:764-768, 1963.

Balke, B. and Snow, C.: Anthropological and physiological observations on Tarahumara endurance runners. *Am J Phys Anthropol, 23*:293-302, 1965.

Chan, O. et al.: The cardiorespiratory fitness and energy expenditure of the Temiars. *Med J Malaysia, 28*:267-272, 1974.

Cole, S.: *Races of Man.* Trustees of the British Museum, London 1965.

Davies, C. T. M. et al: Ethnic differences in physical working capacity. *J Appl Physiol, 33*:726-732, 1972.

Dobzhansky, R.: Biological aspects of race in men. In Mend, M. et al. (Eds.): *Science and the Concept of Race.* New York, Columbia University Press, 1968.

Ekblom, B. and Gjessing J.: Maximal oxygen uptake of the Easter Island population. *J Appl Physiol, 25*:124-129, 1968.

Ikai, M. et al.: Aerobic Capacity of Ainu and other Japanese of Hokkaido. *Med Sci Sport, 3*:6-11, 1971.

Klissouras, V., Pirnay, P., and Petit, J. M.: Adaptation to maximal effort: Genetics and Age. *J Appl Physiol, 35*:288-293, 1972.

Lammert, O.: Maximal aerobic power and energy expenditure of Eskimo hunters in Greenland. *J Appl Physiol, 33*:184-188, 1972.

Morpurgo, G. et al.: Higher Bohr effect in Indian natives of Peruvian highlands as compared with Europeans. *Nature (Lond.), 227*:387-388, 1970.

Prampero, P. E. Di and Cerretelli, P.: Maximal muscular power (aerobic and anaerobic) in African natives. *Ergonomics, 12*:51-59, 1971.

Roberts, D. E.: Body weight, race and climate. *Am J Phys Anthropol, 11*:533-558, 1953.

Robinson, S. et al.: Adaptation to exercise of negro and white share croppers in comparison with Northern whites. *Human Biol, 13*:139-158, 1941.

Rode, A. and Shephard, R. J.: Cardio-respiratory fitness of an Arctic community. *J Appl Physiol, 31*:519-526, 1971.

Thinakaran, T. et al.: Ethnic differences in physiological responses to maximal effort in Malaysian adolescents. *Proc. XXth World Congress in Sports Medicine.* Melbourne, 1975.

Walter, H.: Remarks on the environmental adaptation of man. *Humangenetik, 13*:85-97, 1971.

Wyndham, C. H.: Southern African ethnic adaptation to temperature and exercise. In Baker, P. T. and Weiner, J. S. (Eds.): *The Biology of Human Adaptability.* Oxford, Clarendon Press, 1966, pp. 201-244.

Chapter 7

HEIGHT-WEIGHT COMPARISON OF CANADIAN SCHOOLCHILDREN

M. K. Rajic, H. Lavallée, R. J. Shephard, J. C. Jéquier, R. Labarre,

and C. Beaucage

Abstract

Height and weight data have been collected on 546 children aged 6 to 12 years and living in the Trois-Rivières region. Differences in these variables due to sex, area of residence (urban or rural industrial), and participation in five additional hours of vigorous activity per week are shown to be slight. However, the French Canadian children are significantly smaller than several recent samples from English Canada. Account must be taken of such regional differences when assessing the normality of child growth and development.

Introduction

THE PURPOSE OF this work was to compare the age course of two important growth variables, i.e. standing height and weight, in French Canadian children with similar data from other Canadian surveys, and with the widely used growth and development charts of Tanner & Whitehouse.*

Our information was collected in the course of a longitudinal study of children in the Trois-Rivières region.[7] The prime purpose of this study was to measure the effects of added physical activity on physical growth and psychological development. The additional physical activity was standardized

---

*Growth and Development Record, University of London, Institute of Child Health, Great Ormond St., London W.C.I.

60

and integrated into the academic program at the elementary school level.[7, 8] Each year, a considerable number of measurements of physical performance,[10] cardiorespiratory efficiency,[15] motor skills,[1] and anthropometry were made on the children within fifteen days of their birthday. The material presented here is a cross sectional analysis of results obtained during the first five years of the study.

Our population comprised 546 children of both sexes drawn from a "rural-industrial" village (Pont-Rouge) and an urban community (Trois-Rivières). One half of the sample (the "experimental" group) received a nominal sixty minutes of physical activity five times per week. The other half (the "control" group) received only the usual weekly period of physical education given at all elementary schools in Québec.

Measurements of height and weight were collected in accordance with International Biological Program recommendations.[21] Because readings were taken annually, the number of data points substantially exceeded the number of subjects.

Where previous authors have provided detailed statistics, the significance of differences in height between the present population and these earlier samples can be calculated according to standard statistical principles.

Since the weight is not usually normally distributed, it is not possible to use the two first tests. Nevertheless, weight has a normal distribution after logarithmic transformation.

In all comparisons, it is important to verify that the "age" of the child corresponds closely with his birthday, so that the variance of the measurement time does not add to the variance of the factor under study.

Statistical tests

To compare different populations, we used standard statistical tests, taking advantage as much as possible of the information available. Given M_1, S_1, and n_1 (the mean, the standard deviation, and the size of the first population) and m_2, S_2, and n_2 (the mean, standard deviation, and size of a second population) the tests are

(1) t-test for normally distributed variables with equal variances:

$$t = \frac{M_1 - M_2}{\left[\dfrac{S_1^2 (n_1-1) + S_2^2 (n_2-1)}{(n_1 + n_2 - 2)} \cdot \dfrac{(n_1 + n_2)}{n_1 n_2}\right]^{\frac{1}{2}}}$$

(2) t-test for normally distributed variables with unequal variance:

$$t = \frac{M_1 - M_2}{\left[\dfrac{S_1^2}{n_1} + \dfrac{S_2^2}{n_2}\right]^{\frac{1}{2}}}$$

(3) If only the mean of the second population is known, we can verify if this mean falls within the 95% confidence interval for the mean of the first population. This confidence interval is given by the following:

$$\left[M_1 - \left(t_{x/2}, n_1 - 1\right) \frac{S_1}{\sqrt{n_1}}\right] \quad \text{and} \quad \left[M_1 + \left(t_{x/2}, n_1 - 1\right) \frac{S_1}{\sqrt{n_1}}\right]$$

(4) Finally, if only the median of the second population is known, the confidence interval for the median of the first population can be found, and it is possible to verify if the median falls within this interval or not.

Results

After analysis of descriptive statistics, we checked the distribution of our variables for normality (Tables 7-I and 7-II). As expected, standing height did not depart significantly from a normal distribution. However, absolute values for gross body weight failed to follow a Gaussian distribution.[9] Application of the Kolmogorov-Smirnov test showed that a logarithmic transformation (base 10) of the weight readings was sufficient to yield a normal distribution curve (Table 7-III). All compari-

Table 7-I. Height (cm) of Subjects Examined in the Trois-Rivières Regional Study

Years	GIRLS						BOYS					
	N	Mean	S.D.	S.E.	G_1*	G_2*	N	Mean	S.D.	S.E.	G_1*	G_2*
6	62	112.8	5.58	0.708	-0.878	4.94	76	114.1	4.78	0.548	0.125	2.677
7	125	118.7	5.17	0.462	-0.268	2.854	155	119.9	4.83	0.387	0.133	3.056
8	163	124.7	5.50	0.430	-0.131	2.921	208	125.4	5.06	0.350	0.107	2.659
9	164	130.0	5.91	0.461	-0.122	3.145	185	130.9	5.15	0.378	-0.028	2.522
10	157	134.8	6.55	0.522	0.324	4.192	170	135.4	5.18	0.397	0.204	2.795
11	123	140.9	6.73	0.606	0.273	3.370	114	140.4	5.29	0.495	0.292	3.085
12	42	148.2	7.00	1.080	0.236	3.364	51	144.7	6.09	0.852	0.414	3.636

* Normality tested by Kolmogorov-Smirnov test.

Table 7-II. Weight (kg) of Subjects Examined in the Trois-Rivières Regional Study.

Years	GIRLS						BOYS					
	N	Mean	S.D.	S.E.	G_1*	G_2*	N	Mean	S.D.	S.E.	G_1*	G_2*
6	62	19.46	2.57	0.326	1.034	5.192	76	20.64	2.76	0.316	1.337	5.912
7	127	21.74	3.41	0.302	1.592	7.807	157	22.61	2.91	0.232	1.001	4.741
8	164	24.66	4.20	0.327	1.512	7.617	208	25.14	3.46	0.239	1.026	5.001
9	164	27.41	5.29	0.413	1.576	7.188	185	28.14	4.02	0.295	0.851	3.542
10	158	30.34	6.14	0.488	1.587	7.302	170	30.51	4.91	0.376	1.394	6.055
11	123	34.06	6.50	0.586	0.770	2.857	114	33.53	5.79	0.542	1.221	4.689
12	42	38.44	6.41	0.989	0.315	2.206	51	36.76	8.05	1.127	1.430	4.454

* Hypothesis of normality rejected by Kolmogorov-Smirnov testing.

Table 7-III. Logarithmic of Weight (kg) of Subjects Examined in the Trois-Rivières Regional Study.

Years	GIRLS						BOYS					
	N	Mean	S.D.	S.E.	G_1*	G_2*	N	Mean	S.D.	S.E.	G_1*	G_2*
6	62	1.29	0.55	0.069	0.492	3.969	76	1.31	0.55	0.063	0.735	4.886
7	127	1.33	0.63	0.055	0.812	4.891	157	1.35	0.54	0.043	0.725	3.812
8	164	1.39	0.69	0.053	0.684	4.542	206	1.40	0.57	0.039	0.481	3.879
9	164	1.43	0.76	0.059	0.743	4.442	145	1.44	0.60	0.049	0.486	2.979
10	157	1.47	0.81	0.064	0.784	4.076	170	1.48	0.65	0.049	0.784	4.149
11	123	1.52	0.80	0.072	0.429	2.434	114	1.52	0.70	0.065	0.729	3.528
12	42	1.58	0.72	0.111	0.460	2.116	51	1.56	0.86	0.120	1.030	3.429

* Normality tested by Kolmogorov-Smirnov test.

sons of weight to be discussed here were made after completion of such a logarithmic transformation.

Data for our several subgroups of subjects allowed consideration of three primary factors: sex, place of residence (rural or urban), and the added physical education program (control or experimental group). There were significant sex differences of standing height ($p<0.05$). At the age of 7, the boys were taller than the girls, while at the age of 12 the girls were taller than the boys (Fig. 7-1). The children living in the urban milieu were taller than those from the rural-industrial region, significantly so at the ages of 6, 7, and 8 ($p<0.05$). We have previously found a somewhat larger urban height advantage when comparing Trois-Rivières with a rural nonindustrial area.[16] Weight differences between the groups were small. However, boys were heavier than girls at the ages of 6 and 7 years, and at the age of 6, urban children were heavier than rural ones (Fig. 7-2). The experimental factor, five added periods of physical education weekly, did not modify either height or weight significantly. Only the sex factor has been retained when making comparisons with other investigations. Our mean values of standing height and weight were almost identical with those found by Demirjian[3, 4] during the late 1960s; his subjects were Francophone children living in Montreal. The height and weight values obtained in the Canadian study of Pett and Ogilvie[11] some twenty years ago were also similar to ours. Relative to our 95 percent confidence limits, the boys studied by Pett and Olgivie were smaller than ours at 8 years of age, whereas their body weights were greater at 8 and 10 years of age. Similarly, their girls were heavier than ours at 8 and 12 years of age.

The growth curve of our sample fell below that for the English Canadian boys of Edmonton studied by Howell in 1964/5[5] but above that for Eskimo boys[13] who were measured in 1969/70 (Fig. 7-3). Findings for the girls were similar (Fig. 7-4). The values of Demirjian and Pett and Ogilvie have been excluded from the figures, because they would be superimposed on data for the Trois-Rivières region. The weights of the Edmonton children were greater than those of our sample, both in boys (Fig. 7-5) and in girls (Fig. 7-6).

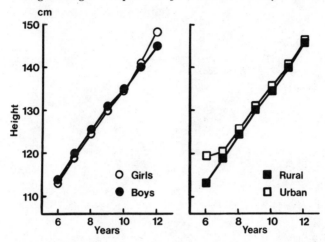

Figure 7-1. Heights of children examined in the Trois Rivières regional study.

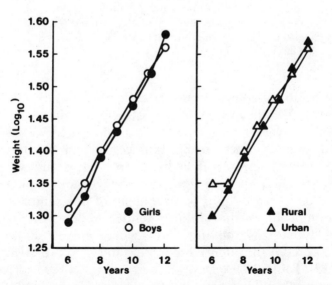

Figure 7-2. Weights of children examined in the Trois-Rivières regional study study—normalized data ($\log_{10}$ transformation).

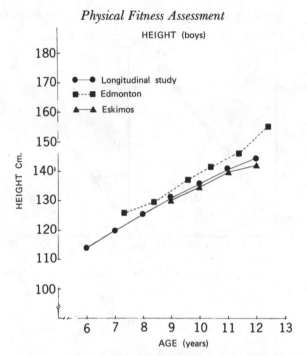

Figure 7-3. Comparison between height of boys enrolled in longitudinal study, "white" anglophone boys of Edmonton, and Canadian Eskimo boys. Data from M. L. Howell et al. (1966) and A. Rode and R. J. Shephard (1971).

The statistical comparisons for children living in Edmonton (Tables 7-IV and V) were made after interpolation of height and weight values to ages identical with the Trois-Rivières regional sample. Such formal tests confirmed the impression drawn from the graphs that the mean heights and weights of Edmonton children aged eight to twelve years exceeded the 95 percent confidence limits for the mean of our sample.

Although the Eskimo children tended to be shorter than the French Canadians, the only points where mean data lay below our 95 percent confidence limits were in girls aged 10 and boys aged 12 (Table 7-IV). Despite their smaller size, Eskimo girls were consistently heavier than Quebec children (Table 7-V).

The median height of English Canadian children studied by Stennett and Cram[19] was slightly greater than that of the

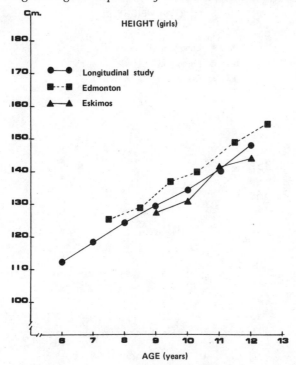

Figure 7-4. Comparison between height of girls enrolled in longitudinal study, "white" anglophone girls of Edmonton, and Canadian Eskimo girls. Data from M. L. Howell et al. (1966) and A. Rode and R. J. Shephard (1971).

Trois-Rivières regional sample, with significant differences for boys aged 10 and 12 years and girls aged 6 and 11 years. The children of Ontario were also slightly heavier than the French Canadians. After logarithmic transformation of the weights cited by Stennett and Cram,[19] we observed significant differences for boys between the ages of 7 and 12 years, and for girls at 7, 10, and 11 years of age. The weight of the English Canadian girls at 6, 9, and 12 years also exceeded the 95 percent confidence limits for our French Canadian population.

The C.A.H.P.E.R. survey of 1965[6] covered a random sample of Canadian youth; presumably, 70 to 75 percent were Anglophone, 25 to 30 percent Francophone, and a small

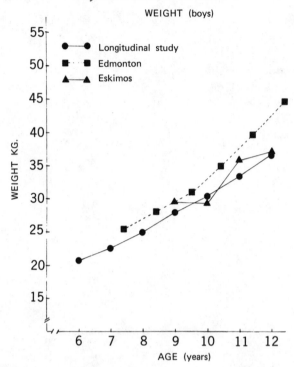

WEIGHT (boys)

Figure 7-5. Comparison of weights between boys
enrolled in longitudinal study, "white" anglophone
boys of Edmonton, and Canadian Eskimo boys. Data
from M. L. Howell et al. (1966) and A. Rode and R. J.
Shephard (1971).

proportion were of North American Indian parentage. Unfortunately, heights were not measured in the C.A.H.P.E.R. survey. Body weights were significantly higher than in our sample between 7 and 10 years of age.

Although there were substantial differences between the present sample and children from English Canada, our data were more comparable with findings from western Europe, differences of height and weight being less significant relative to the widely used scales of Tanner and Whitehouse (Fig. 7-7 and 7-8) or a recent study from Belgium. Girls of 10 and 11 and boys of 8, 10, and 11 were significantly taller in England than in French Canada; further, perhaps because his sample was less

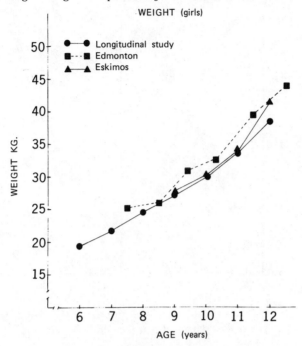

Figure 7-6. Comparison of weights between girls enrolled in longitudinal study, "white" anglophone girls of Edmonton, and Canadian Eskimo girls. Data from M. L. Howell et al. (1966) and A. Rode and R. J. Shephard (1971).

homogenous, the 90th percentile of Tanner's population deviated further from the mean, with significantly greater heights at all ages from 7 to 12. The English girls had a significant weight advantage at all ages from 6 to 12, but differences between the boys of London and the Trois-Rivières region were insignificant.

Discussion

Our three experimental variables of sex, milieu, and added physical education program all had small and inconsistent effects on the weight and height of children living in the

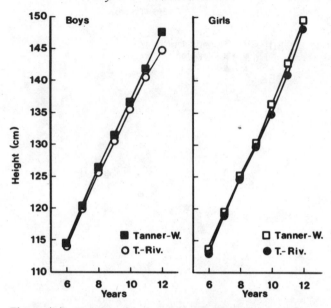

Figure 7-7. Height of boys and girls from Trois-Rivières region relative to norms of Tanner–Whitehouse.

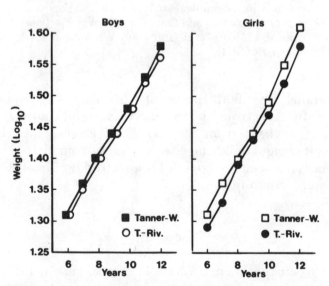

Figure 7-8. Weight of boys and girls from Trois-Rivières region relative to norms of Tanner–Whitehouse.

Table 7-IV. Previously Published Data for Height of Children (Girls).

Girls	Demirjian (3,4)	Pett & Ogilvie (11)	Howell et al. (5)	Rode & Shephard (13)	Stennet & Cram (19)	Tanner & White-house	Belgium Study (12)
6	112.68	112.3			114.30+	113.8	116.47*
7	118.54	118.1			119.38	119.6	122.05*
8	124.26	124.2	126.93+	127.5	124.46	125.2	127.27*
9	129.05	129.5	132.98+	131.0	130.81	130.5	132.36*
10	135.43	135.4	139.12+	141.8+	135.89	136.5+	137.69*
11	141.53	140.5	145.46+	144.3	146.05+	142.8+	145.11*
12	147.58	147.8	151.81+		148.59	149.6	151.50*

+ 95% Confidence interval
* t-test at 5%
** After interpolation

Table 7-IV. Previously Published Data for Height of Children (Boys).

Boys	Demirjian (3,4)	Pett & Ogilvie (11)	Howell et al. (5)	Rode & Shephard (13)	Stennet & Cram (19)	Tanner & White-house	Belgium Study (12)
6	113.87	113.3			114.30	114.4	116.96*
7	119.74	119.4+			120.65	120.5	123.76*
8	125.52	124.7	128.42		125.73	126.4+	128.92*
9	130.17	130.3	133.34	130.0	130.81	131.6	133.42*
10	135.60	135.9	139.05	134.8	137.16+	136.8+	138.69*
11	139.99	140.7	144.08	140.0	142.24	142.0+	143.68*
12	145.39	145.8	151.28	142.1+	147.32+	147.8+	148.41*

+ 95% Confidence interval
* t-test at 5%
** After interpolation

Trois-Rivières region. However, the current generation of English Canadian children seem generally taller and heavier than the children of Québec, both with respect to those we have tested and relative to others seen by Demirjian in Montréal.

Many of the statistical comparisons described here were of necessity made relative to the 95 percent confidence limits of our estimated mean values. We have thus made a rather conservative estimate of the statistical significance of growth differences between the English, French, and Eskimo populations of Canada.

Table 7-V. Previously Published Data for Weight of Children (Log$_{10}$ kg — Girls).

Girls	Demirjian (3,4)	Pett & Ogilvie (11)	Howell et al. (5)	Howell & McNab (6)	Rode & Shephard (13)	Stennet & Cram (19)	Tanner & White-house	Belgium Study (12)
6	1.30	1.30+				1.30 -	1.31*	1.33+
7	1.33	1.35+		1.40+		1.35*	1.36*	1.37+
8	1.41+	1.41+	1.41+	1.42+		1.39	1.40*	1.42+
9	1.43	1.45+	1.46+	1.48+	1.44	1.44	1.44*	1.46+
10	1.49+	1.50+	1.51+	1.53+	1.48	1.49*	1.49*	1.52+
11	1.54	1.54+	1.56+	1.56+	1.53	1.55*	1.55*	1.57+
12	1.59	1.62+	1.62+	1.61+	1.62+	1.60	1.61*	1.63+

+ 95% Confidence interval for mean,
* 95% Confidence interval for mean.
** After interpolation.

Table 7-V. Previously Published Data for Weight of Children (Log$_{10}$ kg — Boys).

Boys	Demirjian (3,4)	Pett & Ogilvie (11)	Howell et al. (5)	Howell & McNab (6)	Rode & Shephard (13)	Stennet & Cram (19)	Tanner & White-house	Belgium Study (12)
6	1.30	1.32				1.31	1.31	1.33+
7	1.35	1.36		1.41+		1.36*	1.36	1.38+
8	1.39	1.41+	1.43+	1.44+		1.41*	1.40	1.42+
9	1.44	1.46+	1.47+	1.48+	1.48+	1.46*	1.44	1.46+
10	1.48	1.50+	1.52+	1.53+	1.47	1.50*	1.48	1.51+
11	1.52	1.54+	1.58+	1.58+	1.56+	1.54*	1.53	1.55+
12	1.59+	1.58	1.63+	1.62+	1.57	1.59*	1.58	1.59+

+ 95% Confidence interval for mean.
* 95% Confidence interval for mean.
** After interpolation

Various authors have attributed 35 to 65 percent of variations in size to inheritance. We are reluctant to attribute this large a part of the apparent ethnic differences to genetic factors, since (1) in cultures like the Candian Eskimo such differences are rapidly being obliterated by secular growth trends[13, 14, 17] and (2) in many series, differences due to socioeconomic factors outweigh those described here. Current thinking is that a change of diet—either an improvement in its general balance (Suzuki, personal comm. to R.J.S.) or an increase in the content of refined carbohydrate[14, 17]—has played a major role in augmenting the size of individuals living in underprivileged communities. However, further study will be necessary before we can identify the precise environmental factors responsible for either existing differences of growth or secular alterations in such patterns.

The main lesson to draw from the present observations is that irrespective of causation, there are significant regional differences of growth in Canada, and account should be taken of these variations when evaluating the normality of development in a given child.

References

1. Beaucage, C.: Relations entre les sous-tests non-verbaux de WISC et les gnosies digitales. *VII International Symposium of Paediatric Work Physiology.* 6-10 October, 1975. Univ. du Québec à Trois-Rivières, Trois-Rivières. Québec, Editions Le Pélican, In Press, 1977.
2. Conover, W. J.: *Practical Nonparametric Statistics.* New York, John Wiley and Sons, 1971.
3. Demirjian, A., Dubuc, M. B., and Jenicek, M.: Etude comparative de la croissance de l'enfant canadien d'origine française à Montréal. *Can J Public Health, 62*:111-119, 1971.
4. Demirjian, A., Jenicek, J., and Dubuc, M.B.: Les normes staturoponderales de l'enfant urbain canadien-français d'âge scolaire. *Can J Public Health, 63*:14-30, 1972.
5. Howell, L. M., Loiselle, D. S., and Lucas, W. G.: *Strength of Edmonton School Children.* Unpublished report, Fitness Research Unit, University of Alberta, Edmonton, 1966.
6. Howell, M. L. and Macnab, R. B. J.: Capacité de travail des écoliers canadiens. Ottawa, Ont. CAHPER, 1968.
7. Jéquier, J. C. et al.: Influence de l'activité physique intégrée au programme scolaire sur la croissance et le développement de l'enfant: protocole et problèmes méthodologique. *La vie mèdicale au Canada Français: 4*,513-516, 1975.
8. Jéquier, J. C. et al.: History and protocol of the longitudinal study of Trois-Rivières. *VII International Symposium of Paediatric Work Physiology.* 6-10 October, 1975. Univ. du Québec à Trois-Rivières, Trois-Rivières. Québec, Editions Le Pélican, In Press, 1977.
9. Jéquier, J. C. et al.: The assumption of normality in longitudinal studies. *VII International Symposium of Paediatric Work Physiology.* 6-10 October, 1975. Univ. du Québec à Trois-Rivières, Trois-Rivières. Québec, Editions Le Pélican, In Press, 1977.

10. Lavallée, H. et al.: Influence of a primary school physical activity program on some tests of performance. *VII International Symposium of Paediatric Work Physiology.* 6-10 October, 1975. Univ. du Québec à Trois-Riviéres, Trois-Rivières. Québec, Editions Le Pélican, In Press, 1977.
11. Pett, L. B. and Ogilvie, G. F.: The Canadian weight-height survey. *Human Biology, 28*:177, 1956.
12. Rajic, M. et al.: *Quelques difficultés des comparaisons staturo-pondérales.* Québec, Editions Le Pélican. In Press, 1977.
13. Rode, A. and Shephard, R. J.: The cardiorespiratory fitness of an arctic community. *J Appl Physiol, 31*:519-526, 1971.
14. Draper, H. H., A review of recent nutritional research in the arctic. pp 120-129. In Shephard, R. J. and Itoh, S. (Eds.) *Circumpolar Health.* Toronto, University of Toronto Press, 1976.
15. Shephard, R. J. et al.: Influence of added activity classes upon the working capacity of Quebec schoolchildren. *VII International Symposium of Paediatric Work Physiology.* 6-10 October, 1975. Univ. du Québec à Trois-Rivières, Trois-Rivières. Québec, Editions Le Pélican, In Press, 1977.
16. Shephard, R. J. et al: La capacité physique des enfants canadiens: Une comparaison entre les enfants canadiens-français, canadiens-anglais et esquimaux. II Anthropométrie et volumes pulmonaires. *Union Médicale du Canada, 104*:259-269, 1975.
17. Shephard, R. J.: Work physiology and activity patterns of circumpolar Eskimos and Ainu—a synthesis of IBP data. *Human Biol, 46*:263-294, 1974.
18. Shephard, R. J.: Human Physiological Work Capacity: *I.B.P. Synthesis,* vol. 4. Cambridge, University Press, 1978.
19. Stennett, R. G. and Cram, D. M.: Cross sectional height and weight norms for a representative sample of urban, school-aged, Ontario children. *Can J Public Health, 60*:465-470, 1969.
20. Twiesselmann, F.: *Développement biométrique de l'enfant à l'adulte.* Brussels, Presses Universitaires de Bruxelles, 1969.
21. Weiner, J. S. and Lourie, J. A.: *Handbook of Methodology for Field Testing.* Oxford, U. K., Blackwell Scientific Publications, 1969.

Chapter 8

LEARNING AND HABITUATION AS FACTORS AFFECTING FITNESS TESTING

C. T. M. DAVIES

Abstract

The physiological responses to repeated one-leg and two-leg exercise have been studied on a stationary ergometer. Repeated two-leg exercise produced a marked fall in cardiac frequency at given oxygen intake during the first three occasions of measurement in five sedentary subjects unaccustomed to laboratory procedures. The maximal aerobic power output and the O_2 cost of work did not change during this period. In a further four subjects, repeated one-leg work effected a decrease of f_h. This was specific to the limb being exercised, but facilitated habituation of the other limb and the effects of one-leg work could be transferred to normal two-leg exercise. Habituation may thus have a peripheral as well as a central cardiovascular component and may reflect the redistribution of blood flow to and within the working muscles. This could represent an inherent autonomic (nervous) adjustment of a hitherto "sedentary" cardiovascular system to the requirements of exercise, being an early manifestation of the training process. Thus, in practical terms, the subjecting of a sedentary person to exercise inevitably changes his physiological state and confounds the prediction of maximal performance from submaximal effort.

Introduction

EXERCISE TESTS ARE increasingly used for the evaluation of physical fitness in normal subjects and for diagnostic and investigative purposes in patients. They are also applied to training and rehabilitation programs and the clinical assessment of certain drugs. The most commonly used exercise tests are those based on measurements of cardiac frequency and oxygen intake. Usually a single test is given and invariably the subject or patient is used as his own control. The investigator assumes that the changes observed are due solely to the applied procedure, for example an injection of a drug or a training regimen, and ignores the possible influence of learning and habituation of the standard exercise test.

This chapter, which is based largely on previously published work (Davies, Tuxworth, and Young, 1970; and Davies and Sargeant, 1975), examines the nature of the habituation stimulus and the role of learning in exercise testing.

Material and Methods

The investigation was undertaken in two parts. In the first part, five healthy subjects were each studied on sixteen consecutive days. On the first visit to the laboratory, the subjects were instructed how to use the mouthpiece and pedal the bicycle, but they were not allowed to practice. During the preliminary period, ECG electrodes were fitted and at zero time the subject was asked to mount the bicycle and pedal for thirty minutes. The work load ($\dot{W}$) was increased every six minutes, the aim being to span the subject's exercise capacity range. On the second visit to the laboratory, a measurement of maximal aerobic power ($\dot{V}o_2$ max) was made as described by Davies (1968). The criterion for maximal performance was that $\dot{V}o_2$ showed no further rise with increasing $\dot{W}$. On subsequent visits to the laboratory, this pattern of submaximal followed by maximal work was maintained.

In the second part of the investigation, seven healthy male subjects were required to perform one-leg exercise, using a modified (Monark) bicycle ergometer (see Davies and Sargeant, 1975). There were eight sequential visits to the laboratory; on the first four occasions, the left or the right leg was used and on the second four occasions the other leg. On a further three occasions immediately following the one-leg work, they were measured in the normal way using both legs to pedal the ergometer. The responses to maximal exercise were measured after the first, fourth, and eighth occasion for one-leg work and after the ninth and eleventh occasion for two-leg work. Throughout both parts of the study, submaximal oxygen intake ($\dot{V}_{O_2}$) and carbon dioxide ($\dot{V}_{CO_2}$) were measured by the open circuit technique, using a dry gas meter (Parkinson-Cowan) in conjunction with paramagnetic and infrared analysers to determine respiratory minute volumes, O_2 and CO_2 concentrations respectively. Maximal oxygen intake was measured using the Douglas bag technique. Individual results obtained during submaximal two-leg work were expressed as $\dot{V}_{O_2}$ at a work load of 900 kpm-min ($\dot{V}_{O_2}$ 900), respiratory minute volume at a $\dot{V}_{CO_2}$ of 1.5 l-min^{-1} ($\dot{V}_{E}$ 1.5) and cardiac frequency at a $\dot{V}_{O_2}$ of 1.5 l-min^{-1} (f_h 1.5). The same analytical procedure was used for one-leg work, except that a work load of 450 kpm-min^{-1} rather than 900 kpm-min^{-1} was used for the expression of $\dot{V}_{O_2}$. The physical characteristics of the subjects are given in Table 8-I.

TABLE 8-I

PHYSICAL CHARACTERISTICS OF THE SUBJECTS PARTICIPATING IN PARTS I AND II OF THE INVESTIGATION (MEAN ± S.D.).

PART	Age (yr)	Wt (kg)	Ht (cm)
I	19.8 ± 2.6	75.7 ± 8.7	179.1 ± 2.0
II	25.5 ± 5.0	66.1 ± 5.9	169.8 ± 4.6

Results

The responses to submaximal and maximal exercise during Part 1 of the investigation are summarized in Table 8-II. From Day 1 to 16, $\dot{V}_{O_2}$ 900 remained unchanged. This was equally true of $\dot{V}_{E}$ 1.5, except between the first and second occasions of submaximal work when there was a small (-5 l-min^{-1}), but significant (P<0.05) decrease of minute ventilation. The f_h 1.5 on the other hand, showed a marked decline from a mean value of 145 beats-min^{-1} on Day 1 to 124 beats-min^{-1} on Day 7; thereafter, there was a smaller decline to 118 beats-min^{-1} on

Physical Fitness Assessment

TABLE 8-II

EFFECTS OF REPEATED EXERCISE ON OXYGEN INTAKE AT A WORK LOAD OF 900 kpm-min^{-1} ($\dot{V}O_2$ 900), RESPIRATORY MINUTE VOLUME ($\dot{V}E$ 1.5), CARDIAC FREQUENCY (f_h 1.5) AT A $\dot{V}O_2$ OF 1.5 l-min^{-1}, MAXIMAL OXYGEN INTAKE ($\dot{V}O_2$ max) AND THE CORRESPONDING MAXIMUM RESPIRATORY MINUTE VOLUME, VENTILATION ($\dot{V}E$ max), AND CARDIAC FREQUENCY (f_h max). MEAN ± S.D.

DAY	$\dot{V}E$ 1.5 (1.min^{-1})	$\dot{V}O_2$ 900 (1.min^{-1})	f_h 1.5 (beats.min^{-1})	$\dot{V}E$ max (1.min^{-1})	$\dot{V}O_2$ max (1.min^{-1})	f_h max (beats/min)
1	40.46 ±4.98	1.99 ±0.11	145 ±6			
2				142.8 ±15.3	3.18 ±0.17	197 ±7
3	35.79† ±2.53	2.04 ±0.10	134* ±9			
4				143.1 ±6.7	3.17 ±0.27	200 ±2
5	35.72 ±3.90	2.06 ±0.12	131* ±5			
6				152.2 ±15.7	3.23 ±0.20	197 ±7
7	37.85 ±3.83	2.01 ±0.05	129* ±10			
8				146.9 ±17.9	3.33† ±0.26	196 ±7
9	34.73 ±4.53	2.09 ±0.11	124 ±7			
10				149.2 ±23.3	3.42† ±0.17	197 ±7
11	34.45 ±4.80	2.04 ±0.08	125 ±10			
12				148.3 ±24.5	3.31 ±0.15	196 ±3
13	34.97 ±5.87	2.00 ±0.08	117† ±8			
14				149.9 ±22.4	3.41 ±0.15	195 ±7
15	35.42 ±5.46	1.98 ±0.08	118 ±8			
16				152.8 ±26.0	3.45 ±0.19	193 ±6

*P < 0.01
†P <0.05

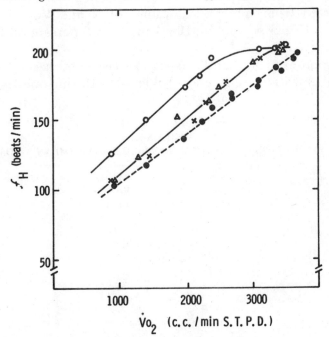

Figure 8-1. Relationship of heart rate to oxygen consumption in successive tests.

Day 15. The change from Day 1 to Day 5 was due entirely to a reduced intercept for the $f_h/\dot{V}o_2$ regression line; the slope remained unchanged. From Day 7 to Day 15, the situation was reversed, with a small decrease in the slope of the $f_h/\dot{V}o_2$ line while the intercept remained constant (Fig. 8-1).

Maximal oxygen intake ($\dot{V}o_2$ max) showed no significant changes during the first three occasions of maximal work (Days 2 to 6). Between the third and fourth and fifth measurements $\dot{V}o_2$ max increased by approximately 0.2 l-min^{-1} ($+5.5\%$), but it remained constant thereafter (Table 8-II).

The changes in f_h 1.5 from Day 1 to Day 5 had a marked effect on the predicted $\dot{V}o_2$ max. The asymptotic nature of the $\dot{V}o_2/f_h$ curve was pronounced on Days 1 and 2, but this feature gradually disappeared, being completely absent by the end of the investigation (Fig. 8-1). The accuracy of the $\dot{V}o_2$ max

Physical Fitness Assessment

predicted from submaximal values of f_h and $\dot{V}O_2$ increased from $- 15 \pm 9$ percent on Day 1 to $- 1 \pm 3$ percent on Day 15 (Table 8-III).

Responses to one– and two–leg exercise in the second part of the investigation are given in Table 8-IV. During one-leg work,

TABLE 8-III
PREDICTION OF MAXIMAL AEROBIC POWER. (MEAN ± S.D.)

DAY*	Observed $\dot{V}O_2$ max $(l\text{-}min^{-1})$	Predicted $\dot{V}O_2$ max $(l\text{-}min^{-1})$	Difference (%)
1		2.68 ±0.23	
2	3.18 ±0.17		−15.4 ±8.9
3		3.01 ±0.16	
4	3.17 ±0.20		−4.0 ±13.8
5		3.16 ±0.05	
6	3.23 ±0.20		−2.4 ±6.6
7		3.07 ±0.13	
8	3.33 ±0.26		−6.5 ±10.5
9		3.32 ±0.28	
10	3.42 ±0.17		−2.7 ±12.3
11		3.27 ±0.31	
12	3.31 ±0.15		−1.1 ±11.5
13		3.52 ±0.42	
14	3.41 ±0.15		+2.4 ±15.1
15		3.43 ±0.19	
16	3.45 ±0.19		−0.9 ±3.4

*For types of activity required on individual days, see text.

$\dot{V}O_2$ at 450 kpm-min^{-1} ($\dot{V}O_2$ 450) and $\dot{V}E$ 1.5 remain unchanged throughout the study. In contrast, f_h 1.5 remained constant during the first two occasions, showed a significant (P<0.05) fall on the third occasion, and remained constant thereafter. A small decrease of f_h 1.5 was observed in the second test on the opposite leg (Table 8-III). The magnitude of changes in f_h during one-leg habituation was related to the initial $\dot{V}O_2$ max, the greatest changes being seen in the more

TABLE 8-IV
EFFECTS OF REPEATED ONE-LEG EXERCISE.
SYMBOLS AS FOR TABLE 8-II. MEAN ± S.D. OF DATA.

| | | Submaximal work | | | Maximal work | $\dot{V}O_2$ | |
	Occasion	$\dot{V}E$ 1.5 (l-min^{-1})	$\dot{V}O_2$ 450 (l-min^{-1})	f_h 1.5 (beats-min^{-1})	$\dot{V}E$ max (l-min^{-1})	max net (l-min^{-1})	f_h max (beats-min^{-1})
1st leg.	1	50.38 ±6.84	1.43 ±0.12	125 ±18			
					124.1 ±19.6	2.41 ±0.19	179 ±12
	2	49.87 ±3.03	1.40 ±0.10	125 ±15			
	3	47.53 ±3.95	1.43 ±0.08	120* ±16			
	4	44.29 ±5.54	1.40 ±0.09	118 ±15			
					116.9 ±11.8	2.44 ±0.31	175 ±7
	5	49.23 ±2.20	1.44 ±0.11	125 ±16			
					105.5 ±13.2	2.23 ±0.23	175 ±6
2nd leg.	6	49.04 ±2.05	1.40 ±0.04	119* ±14			
	7	47.05 +3.79	1.38 +0.03	119 +12			
	8	46.27 ±4.27	1.42 ±0.06	120 ±12			
					111.0 ±11.2	2.22 ±0.29	174 ±5

*Significance (paired t test) P < 0.05

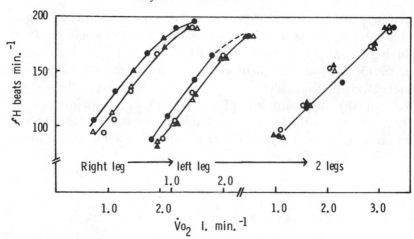

Figure 8-2. Changes of heart rate during one-legged habituation in relation to initial fitness.

sedentary subjects (Fig 8-2). During submaximal two-leg work (occasions 9 to 11 inclusive) all the physiological responses to exercise remained constant (Table 8-IV).

At maximal effort, the $\dot{V}o_2$ max of one-leg measured after the first, fourth, and eighth occasion and that of two-legs after the ninth and eleventh occasion showed no significant changes.

Discussion

The selection criteria for the two parts of the investigation differed significantly. In Part 1 of the study, the five subjects were normal healthy males, but none was in athletic training and four of the five took no regular exercise. Lack of physical fitness is reflected in their low $\dot{V}o_2$ max and high cardiac frequencies for a given work output (Table 8-II). A condition of entry into the study was that subjects had not attended a laboratory or pedalled a bicycle ergometer before. This was deliberate, because this is the type of subject one normally encounters in population studies of working capacity and in clinical laboratories where exercise tests are routinely applied.

In the second part of the investigation, the subjects were accustomed to laboratory procedures, although they had not used a bicycle ergometer previously. All were normally active, and two were in training.

The results of the first part of the study show clearly (Table 8-II) that although $\dot{V}o_2$ 900 and $\dot{V}o_2$ max remain unchanged over the initial three occasions of submaximal work, f_h 1.5 decreased from 145 to 124 beats-min^{-1} and $\dot{V}e$ 1.5 declined by 4 l-min^{-1}. The fall in f_h 1.5 cannot be attributed to a decrease in the external work performed due to a rise of mechanical efficiency nor to an increase in overall work capacity, since neither the $\dot{V}o_2$ at given work load nor the $\dot{V}o_2$ max changed over the seven-day period. Equally, it cannot be due to a decrease in fixed $\dot{V}o_2$ due to anxiety or emotional stress, since one would then have expected to see more pronounced changes of f_h at the lower work levels and for the effect to diminish with increasing severity of effort (Bevegard and Shepherd, 1967). The major changes in f_h 1.5 were due to a parallel displacement of the $f_h/\dot{V}o_2$ line. In part two of the investigation, a similar pattern of cardiac frequency changes was seen, although their magnitude was different. Repeated one-leg exercise had no effect on $\dot{V}o_2$ 450 or $\dot{V}e$ 1.5 and it produced a much smaller decrease of f_h 1.5 than seen with two-leg work (Table 8-IV). The change in f_h 1.5 was not seen until the third occasion of measurement and was not transferred directly to the second limb, although prior habituation of one limb appeared to facilitate that of the other; the same change of f_h 1.5 was detected during the second test on the second leg (Fig. 8-2). When two-leg work was performed having habituated each limb individually and sequentially, $\dot{V}o_2$ 900, $\dot{V}e$ 1.5, and f_h 1.5 were all unaffected by repetition of the test exercise.

It would seem from these results that habituation may be affected by both central (cardiovascular) and peripheral (muscle) factors. Unfortunately, the data do not allow a complete analysis of the physiological mechanisms underlying habituation. It could reflect in part a redistribution of blood to and within the working muscles, representing an inherent autonomic readjustment of the cardiovascular system to the requirements of exercise. Equally, it could be just an early manifestation of the accepted training phenomenon. In both cases the practical implications are clear; if the objective is simply to predict accurately $\dot{V}o_2$ max from submaximal measurements of f_h and $\dot{V}o_2$, at least two preliminary periods of test exercise should be given. On the other hand, if one is interested in the responses to exercise per se, subjecting a hitherto sedentary person to exercise inevitably changes his physiological state and this may well confound the variables one is trying to measure.

References

Bevegård, B. S. and Shepherd, J. T.: Regulation of circulation during exercise. *Physiol Rev, 47* (2):178-213, 1967.

Davies, C. T. M.: Determinants of maximum aerobic power in relation to age. *J Physiol, 197*:76-77, 1968.

Davies, C. T. M., Tuxworth, W., and Young, J. M.: Physiological effects of repeated exercise. *Clin Sci, 39*:247-258, 1970.

Davies, C. T. M. and Sargeant, A. J.: Effects of training on the physiological responses to 1– and 2-leg work. *J Appl Physiol, 38*:377-381, 1975.

Chapter 9

SEASONAL VARIATIONS OF C.A.H.P.E.R. PERFORMANCE TESTS

J. C. Jéquier, R. Labarre, R. J. Shephard, H. Lavallée, C. Beaucage, and M. Rajic

Abstract

The C.A.H.P.E.R. performance tests have been performed biennially by a large sample of boys and girls aged 6 to 12 years as part of the Trois-Rivières regional study of growth and development. Significant seasonal differences are demonstrated. Tests of muscle force and endurance (speed sit-ups, standing broad jump, and flexed arm hang) show the greatest gains over the winter (at a time when height and weight increases have been small). Tests involving agility (shuttle run, 50-yard run, and 300-yard run) also improve most over the winter (when the physical education programme is operating); however, if skill learning is responsible it becomes necessary to postulate that skills acquired are lost over a three-month summer vacation period.

THE TESTS OF physical efficiency introduced by the Canadian Association for Health, Physical Education and Recreation (C.A.H.P.E.R.) comprise a battery of six simple tests: the number of sit-ups per minute, the distance of a standing broad jump (feet), the maximal time for a flexed arm hang, a shuttle run (time to run 4 × 30 feet), and times for 50– and 300-yard runs. The techniques are standardized, and the results obtained on a random sample of Canadian school children between 7 and 17 years of age have been reported as percentiles.[1]

It is well recognized that physical performance is influenced by a great number of conditions. Beside practical variables of execution such as the weather, the environmental temperature, ground conditions, and the quality of data recording, results are affected by more individual factors such as the level of fitness, the motivation, and the body weight of the subject.

Scores for the C.A.H.P.E.R. tests are one important group of variables that have been measured regularly in a longitudinal study of the Trois-Rivières region initiated in 1970.[2] The prime purpose of the study is to measure the effect of added required physical education on the growth and development of children between the ages of 5 and 13 years. Since the physical education is integrated into the normal academic curriculum, it is given for about nine months of the year, between September and June. The C.A.H.P.E.R. tests are administered in June (at the end of the school year) and in October, one month after the beginning of the school year.

Parallel studies[3, 4] have shown significant seasonal variations of the increments in height, weight, and $\dot{V}O_2$ (max). A comparison of performance test scores in June and October was thus of some interest.

Method

The sample comprised 546 children, boys and girls participating in the Trois-Rivières region longitudinal study. A cohort has been followed since 1970. At that time, the group consisted of children aged 5 to 9 years. Two C.A.H.P.E.R. tests have been administered annually, in June and October; on both occasions, the 50-yard and 300-yard events were completed out of doors, in good weather. The other four test items were measured in the gymnasium. By 1976, we had collected twelve complete sets of repeated C.A.H.P.E.R. tests. Allowing for absences and defections, the final sample included approximately 3,500 complete sets of data on each of the six measurements.

A first breakdown of these results was made by age, grouping students by intervals of six months from 6 to 13 years of age. The second breakdown classified tests according to the time of testing (June or October) at each age level (Fig. 9-1). Based on these data, we tested the following hypothesis: There is an increase in two successive measurements of performance due to the intervening time interval, but the *difference* between two sequential measurements adjusted for this time interval (four months between June and October, and eight months between October and June) should be equal, unless there is a systematic seasonal effect. We thus compared the mean monthly changes in summer and winter, both globally over the whole age range and separately at each age level (Fig. 9-1).

For each of the six tests, two analyses of variance were performed. The first analysis considered only the effect of season, comparing the mean monthly differences in summer to those of winter, over the entire age range from 6 to 12 years. The second series of analyses included also the age effect (which is of course highly significant) and the age/season interaction (to test whether seasonal differences were equally important for each of the six-month age categories).

Results

Table 9-I examines seasonal differences, ignoring age effects. The first two columns show mean performance scores for June and October. Category I subjects performed the first measurement in June, whereas category II subjects performed first in October. The third column shows the change of performance from the first to the second measurement, expressed per month. Although the absolute changes per

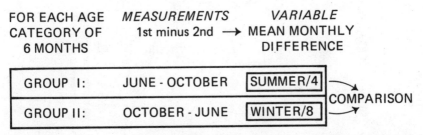

Figure 9-1. Design of study to assess seasonal differences in the growth and development of physical performance.

TABLE 9-I

SEASONAL DIFFERENCES IN PERFORMANCE. COMPARISON OF 2873 TESTS PERFORMED IN SUMMER AND WINTER ON BOYS AND GIRLS AGED 6–12 YEARS.

Performance measure	Category*	Performance Score		Average difference in Score per month	Average monthly change as % of first meas.	F†	p‡
		Spring	Fall				
1. Speed Sit-ups (number)	1	33.79	30.49	−.8822	−2.61	266.9	< 0.001
	2	33.72	29.82	.5036	+1.69		
2. Standing broad jump (feet)	1	4.416	4.194	−.0537	−1.22	391.7	< 0.001
	2	4.409	4.149	.0319	+0.77		
3. Shuttle run (sec)	1	13.39	13.80	.1010	+0.75	250.4	< 0.001
	2	13.36	13.88	−.0638	−0.46		
4. Flexed arm hang (sec)	1	28.51	24.88	−.9017	−3.16	100.2	< 0.001
	2	28.97	24.76	.5564	+2.25		
5. 50 yard run (sec)	1	9.45	9.78	.043	+0.46	75.6	< 0.001
	2	9.43	9.87	−.072	−0.73		
6. 300 yard run (sec)	1	77.00	77.67	.006	+0.01	5.47	.018
	2	77.20	78.35	−.285	−0.36		

*1 = First measurement in June, second in October (4 months)
 2 = First measurement in October, second in June (8 months)
†F: Fisher F ratio
‡p: Probability

month are small, because of the sample size the F ratios are large, all differences being highly significant.

Although all seasonal differences are significant (Fig. 9-2), there also exist clear inter-test differences. The largest effects are found for the flexed arm hang and the smallest for the 300-yard run. However, all tests show their increment in winter (Table 9-II).

What is the quantitative importance of these seasonal differences? As an example, the results for the standing broad jump are presented in Figure 9-3. Results for the other tests are similar. Mean scores are summarized annually to show the first and the second performance in a given year. The four

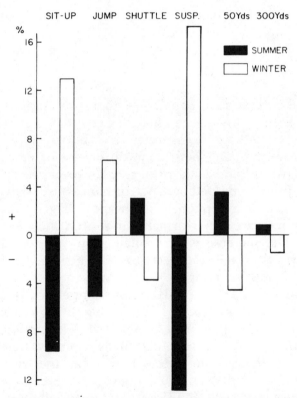

Figure 9-2. Seasonal variation of performance expressed as a percent of the first value for four summer months and eight winter months.

TABLE 9-II

A SUMMARY OF SEASONAL DIFFERENCES IN THE IMPROVEMENT OF
PHYSICAL PERFORMANCE.

IMPROVEMENT OF
PERFORMANCE DURING

WINTER
SPEED SIT-UPS
STANDING BROAD JUMP
FLEXED ARM HANG

SHUTTLE RUN
50-YARD RUN
300-YARD RUN

lines are almost parallel. The first performance is always poorer than the second, since each child has grown for about half a year between the two measurements. The age effect is also clearly identified, and there is no difference of performance between groups 1 and 2 at a given age. However, the difference between June and October performances is systematically present, the only exception being at age 6 (Fig. 9-4); typically there is an increase of performance in winter, and a decrease in summer. The increase is very small, being greatest in those under 8 years of age; the decrease is larger and has a more variable relationship to age.

Factorial analysis (Table 9-III) shows that effects due to age, season, and their interaction are all highly significant. The significance of the age effect is expected. The significance of the seasonal effect confirms that changes are systematic with season. The interaction effect shows that the decrease of performance over the summer is not equal at every age. All six performance tests yield significant F ratios for all three factors, with the exception that the 300-yard run shows no significant age/season interaction.

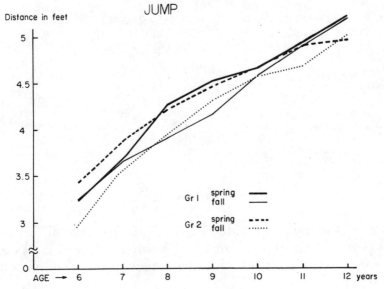

Figure 9-3. Standing broad jump scores.

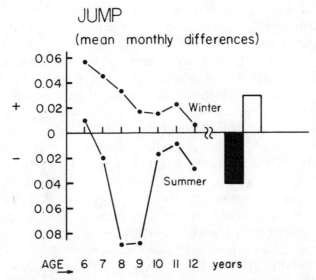

Figure 9-4. Difference between June and October performance.

TABLE 9-III

AN EXAMPLE OF THE FACTORIAL ANALYSIS USED. DATA FOR MEAN
MONTHLY DIFFERENCES IN STANDING BROAD JUMP SCORES, BROKEN
DOWN BY SEASON AND BY AGE.

Source of Variation	DF	Sums of Squares	F	Significance
Total	3474	63.67		
Age	13	1.99	9.72	<0.001
Season	1	5.69	362.29	<0.001
Age X Season	13	1.24	6.06	<0.001
Residual	3447	54.14		

Discussion

The absolute magnitude of most of the seasonal differences in performance is quite small. Nevertheless, the findings are consistent for each test, for most age classes, and for each season.

All tests show an increase of performance in the winter. At least two factors are probably operating—the specific training effect of the physical education program, given during the winter only, and the significant acceleration of height and weight gain during the summer. Cumming[5] has stressed previously that height and weight account for a large part of the variance in performance test scores.

Three of the performance tests (speed sit-ups, standing broad jump, and flexed arm hang) evaluate muscular strength and/or *endurance*. However, we cannot explain changes in scores on summer increases of height and weight. Standing heights were 0.52 cm shorter for a given age in the period April/June and 1.75 cm taller during the period July/ September. Equally, body weights were 0.44 kg lighter than predicted in the spring and 0.69 kg heavier in the summer. On the assumption that muscle force is proportional to the square of height[6], one would expect a 6 percent gain of muscular performance on the basis of this differential growth, whereas in fact scores deteriorated over the summer.

The weight gain may have partly offset the advantage of the larger muscles. This would be particularly true if the added weight is fat rather than muscle.

The remaining tests (50–, 300-yd run, shuttle run) all involve the element of *agility*. During the winter, the weight is relatively stable but the physical education program could be influencing the skill of the pupils. Aerobic power is also increasing,[4] with implications for the 300-yard run. If agility is indeed improved during the winter, it is interesting that this gain is lost over the succeeding summer, with a corresponding deterioration in scores for these three tests.

The definitive explanation of these seasonal differences requires further investigation. In particular, allowance should be made for the effects of parallel changes in weight and height, and normal and enhanced programs of physical education should be compared.

References

1. C.A.H.P.E.R.: *Le Manuel d'instructions du test d'efficience physique de la CAHPER à l'usage des garçons et filles de 7 à 17 ans.* Toronto, CAHPER, 1966.
2. Jéquier, J. C. et al.: The longitudinal examination of growth and development: history and protocol of the Trois-Rivières regional study. In Shephard, R. J. and Lavallèe, H. (Eds.): *Frontiers of Physical Activity and Child Health.* Quebec City, Editions Pelican, In Press 1977.
3. Rajic, M. et al.: Seasonal differences in height and weight. In preparation.
4. Shephard, R. J. et al.: Seasonal differences in working capacity. In Shephard, R. J. and Lavallèe, H. (Eds.): *Frontiers of Physical Activity and Child Health,* Quebec City, Pelican Press, In Press 1977.
5. Cumming, G. R.: Correlation of physical performance with laboratory measures of fitness. In Shephard, R. J. (Ed.): Frontiers of Fitness. Springfield, Thomas, 1971.
6. Shephard, R. J.: Human Physiologic Work Capacity : *I.B.P. Synthesis,* Vol. 4. London, Cambridge University Press, 1978

Chapter 10

ENVIRONMENTAL VARIABLES AFFECTING FITNESS TESTING

Abstract

The environmental factors that influence physical fitness testing are test specific. Increase in altitude above sea level decreases maximal oxygen intake and therefore influences endurance performance. At the same time, speed and throwing test results may be better at higher altitudes because of lower air resistance. Wind speed above certain values decreases or increases running times for short distances, depending on direction. Rain, snow, and ice conditions hamper fitness testing and normally no tests should be run under such conditions. Environmental heat influences heart rate, body temperature, and sweating responses and tests using heart rate as a variable for evaluating fitness or predicting aerobic power are markedly affected. Heat and cold, furthermore, have psychological influences and the necessary motivation may be lacking under such conditions. Because of the toxic effects of motor exhaust gases, running events should not be scheduled along busy roads and highways.

Introduction

MAN HAS SUCH REMARKABLE abilities to adapt himself to severe environmental conditions that it is almost inconceivable to talk about environment as handicapping fitness testing. Men are daily living and/or working at altitudes of 4000 m; others are delving as deep as 3000 m below the surface and furthermore, doing so at nearly saturated temperatures of 30 to 33°C; the tropical and desert areas of the world hold no fears to pastoral or industrial mankind; and the arctic and antarctic

94

regions were opened long ago. However, to work efficiently in such environments, man first has to acclimatize himself, because he is essentially a resident of cool to temperate regions situated close to sea level. Only a very small proportion of the world's inhabitants live at altitudes in excess of 1000 m.

As we are interested in the population at large and not necessarily in highly trained and adapted individuals, we have to consider the influences that environmental variables would have on ordinary subjects being subjected to physical fitness tests. The tests with which we will concern ourselves are those given in Larson's book, *Fitness, Health and Work Capacity*.[4] The considerations given prominence in this chapter do not necessarily apply to athletic performance.

Altitude

Although the percentage of oxygen in the earth's atmosphere does not vary from place to place, the partial pressure of oxygen decreases with increase in altitude above sea level. The drop in partial pressure handicaps the physically active man because the amount of air he now breathes yields insufficient oxygen. About 3 percent of the population are unable to adapt to the hypoxic conditions of altitude, while others may initially develop acute mountain sickness. Smokers and those who have a low $\dot{V}o_2$ max show the worst reactions and tasks normally rated as submaximal now shift into the maximum category.

At medium altitudes (1800 m, 630 mmHg), man has to breathe 30 percent more air (BTPS) than at sea level to deliver the same quantity of oxygen to the alveoli. In theory, he could increase respiratory rate, respiratory depth, or both. Observations indicate, however, that an athlete cannot make such changes without upsetting running rhythm, so that initially at least he elects to keep respiratory minute volumes unchanged.

Respiratory absorption of oxygen is reflected in the partial pressure of oxygen in arterial blood (Po_2). This value normally increases slightly with an increase of energy expenditure, only to fall again at maximum effort.[9] At medium altitudes, the Po_2 at rest is already 18 to 20 mmHg lower than at sea level, and it decreases further with increase in physical activity. Reported values for sea level, 1800 m, 3100 m, and 4300 m are 96, 80, 55, and 54 mmHg respectively. Altitudes higher than these fall outside the scope of present considerations.

A decrease in Po_2 results in hypoxic conditions (and thus a marked change of acid/base balance) setting in earlier during sustained exercise. There is an associated decrease of stroke volume, probably due to inadequate oxygenation of the myocardium. Increases in heart rate are insufficient to prevent a decrease of cardiac output. Fatigue and/or shortness of breath is therefore noticed earlier when physical exercise is done at altitude, but some of this must be attributed to the cold, which usually accompanies altitude. Two performance tests, the distance run and the shuttle run, would certainly show lower scores at altitude, and others may be affected.

As sprint events are normally run anaerobically, performance in these events is not influenced by hypoxia. However, because of the lower wind resistance at medium altitudes, scores for such events may be improved.[5]

Another physiological variable influenced by altitude is maximum heart rate; this decreases with an increase of altitude. This seems paradoxical because heart rates for submaximum activity are substantially increased when we go from sea level to 2000 m or higher.

All the above-mentioned facts point to a significant influence of altitude on aerobic power. This is true whether measuring the $\dot{V}o_2$ max directly or predicting it from heart rate responses to submaximal exercise. The linear relationship between barometric pressure and $\dot{V}o_2$ max is illustrated in Figure 10-1; this represents the average results obtained on twenty-five men.[8] Clearly, the subjects tested at altitude have a disadvantage. However, correction factors have been worked out for different atmospheric pressures; indeed, the results in Figure 10-1 could be used for this purpose.

Cold

Conditions sufficient to reduce core temperature are not conducive to physical fitness testing and will not be considered.

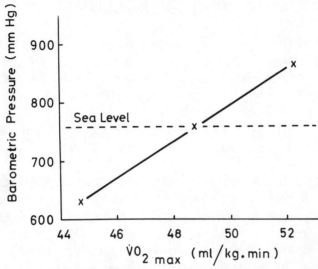

Figure 10-1. Increase in maximum oxygen intake with increase in barometric pressure.

Exposure to cold initially cools the body surface and leads to shivering. The major concern is cooling of the extremities. Cooling of the body surface does not impair manual dexterity, provided that the hands are kept warm.[2] Cold hands always lead to reduced performance in dexterity tasks, regardless of whether the rest of the body is warm or not. Cold upper and lower extremities are stiff due to an increase in the viscosity of the fluids and tissues of the tendons and joints. Needless to say, as long as core temperature is maintained at normal or above normal levels, cold hands and feet will not occur even in subzero temperatures.

Warm-up exercises should always be part and parcel of a fitness testing program. Unfortunately, there are usually long delays between test items when large groups have to be tested. Performance will suffer from chilling if the environment is uncomfortably cold. Trying to counter the cold by additional clothing makes the test subject clumsy and restricts his movements. Most tests of physical performance, physique, and body composition, along with the medical examination, should be done in environments of 20 to 24°C.

Heat and Humidity

Most of the physical fitness tests recommended by I.C.P.F.R. do not involve long continued exercise, so that the major concern of exercise in the heat (heat stroke) does not enter the picture. The majority of tests are not affected seriously by heat but some difficulty may be experienced in completing the whole series of performance tests in one session. As in all severe environments, the limiting factor may be lack of interest and motivation.

The maximum oxygen intake should not be predicted from heart rate responses if the wet-bulb temperature is in excess of 24°C. Relative humidity has only a negligible influence on human responses such as heart rate and body temperature, provided that the wet-bulb temperature is below 24°C.[1] However, there is a significant decrease in predicted $\dot{V}o_2$ max

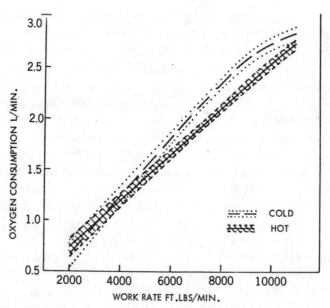

Figure 10-2. Oxygen consumption as related to increases in work rate under hot and cold conditions, with 95 percent confidence limits.

whenever this wet-bulb temperature is exceeded.[3] Dry bulb temperatures up to 30°C have no influence on the test results. People differ markedly in respect to their state of heat acclimatization and, therefore, the predicted $\dot{V}O_2$ max test should be restricted to environmental temperatures within the range 19 to 24°C. If tests have to be done in the heat, attention must be given to water intake, as a water-deficit leads to poor performance.

The influence of heat on the heart rate responses of highly acclimatized men during graded exercise[7] is shown in Figure 10-2. Taylor et al.[6] observed even more dramatic responses on unacclimatized subjects.

The directly measured $\dot{V}O_2$ max is, however, uninfluenced by heat exposure (Fig. 10-3). The body elects to provide blood and

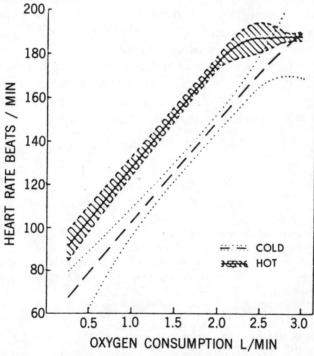

Figure 10-3. Heart rate as a function of oxygen intake during work in cool and in hot environments, with 95 percent confidence limits.

oxygen to working muscle even though a large proportion of the available cardiac output is required for body cooling. The consequent increase of body temperature is obvious and warns against the scheduling of endurance events in hot environments. Even the best of acclimatization procedures cannot protect the athlete fully against severe heat.

Atmospheric pollution

Whereas man can safely adapt or acclimatize to heat, cold, and a decreased partial pressure of oxygen, there is less possibility of adaptation to most forms of air pollution. The best tactic is to remove ourselves from the source or major concentration of such pollution.

Physical fitness testing requires that our subject increase his pulmonary ventilation. Pollutants such as those emanating from car exhaust systems are thus absorbed in larger quantities than in the sedentary subject, and the dose may be excessive. Physical fitness testing in which distance running has to be done along a busy highway or street is not to the advantage of the testee. The synergistic effect of altitude plus pollution may be enough to incapacitate a number of subjects.

References

1. Clarke, R. E., Orkin, L. R., and Rovenstein, E. A.: Body temperature studies in anaesthetized man. *JAMA, 154*:311-319, 1975.
2. Fox, R. H.: Local cooling in man. *Br Med J, 17*:14-18, 1961
3. Ketusinh, O. et al.: Influence of environmental temperature and humidity on oxygen uptake capacity. Proceedings, I.C.P.F.R. Meetings, Jyväskylä, Finland, 1973.
4. Larson L. (Ed): *Fitness, Health and Work Capacity.* New York, Macmillan Publishing Co. Inc, 1974, 593 pp.
5. Shephard, R. J.: The athlete at high altitude. Can Med Assoc J; 109:207-209, 1973.
6. Taylor, H. L. et al.: The standardisation and interpretation of submaximal and maximal tests of working capacity. *Pediatrics 32* (Supplement), 703-722, 1963.

7. Williams, C. G. et al.: Circulatory and metabolic reaction to work in heat. *J Appl Physiol, 17*:625, 1962.
8. Wyndham, C. H. et al.: Effects on maximal oxygen intake of acute changes in altitude in a deep mine. *J Appl Physiol, 29*:552-555, 1970.
9. Wyndham, C. H. et al.: Physiological effects of acute changes in altitude in a deep mine. *J Appl Physiol, 30*:232-237, 1971.

Chapter 11

AN ASSESSMENT OF EXERCISE AND HEAT ORTHOSTATISM

E. Shvartz, A. Meroz, A. Magazanik, Y. Sheonfeld, and
Y. Shapiro

Abstract

Nineteen young men were administered an orthostatic test (twenty minutes of standing, leaning against a wall) five times: before exercise, after exercise at 40 W and 80 W, after a $\dot{V}o_2$ max test, and after exercise in the heat. An additional group of eight subjects underwent the same procedure before and after eight days of heat acclimation. Among the nineteen subjects, the number of fainters before exercise, after exercise at 40 W and 80 W, after the $\dot{V}o_2$ max test, and after heat exposure were 1, 2, 4, 0, and 9 respectively. Heart rate and blood pressure responses corresponded to the number of fainting episodes, the worst responses being found after heat exposure and the best responses before exercise and after the $\dot{V}o_2$ max test. Orthostatic responses in the five conditions were interrelated. Subjects with a high $\dot{V}o_2$ max showed less fainting episodes and better orthostatic heart rates and blood pressure responses than subjects with an average $\dot{V}o_2$ max. Heat acclimation resulted in substantial improvements in all five orthostatic tests. Orthostatism is largely a function of physical fitness and heat tolerance. Exhaustive exercise is a useful antigravity method of preventing orthostatic collapse.

Introduction

M ANY STUDIES HAVE shown that man's orthostatism is imperfect. About 10 to 15 percent of normal young men faint during head up tilting or standing.[4, 5, 9, 10, 17] Eichna and Bean[3] and Eichna, Horvath, and Bean[4] noted that immediately antecedent exercise resulted in an adverse orthostatic response, probably because blood was pooled in the dilated blood vessels of the legs after exercise. Many studies have also shown that heat stress increases the tendency to orthostatic collapse, because peripheral vasodilatation places a substantial initial load on the cardiovascular system;[1, 3, 5, 6, 7, 9, 11, 12] likewise heat acclimatation results in an improvement of heat orthostatism.[1, 11] The relationship between physical fitness and orthostatism has not been clear. Early observations by Crampton[2] suggested that physically fit people had better responses during standing than unfit ones, but only minor improvements in tilt-table responses were seen after a moderate training program[8] and only small correlation coefficients were found between $\dot{V}O_2$ max and tilt tolerance.[10] No information has been available concerning the relationship between exercise and heat orthostatism and physical fitness. The purposes of the present study were to determine the relationship between orthostatism before exercise, after exercise of different intensities, and after exercise in heat, and to examine the influence of physical fitness and heat acclimatation on such reactions.

Methods

SUBJECTS: The main subjects were nineteen healthy young men, aged 18 to 20 years. Their mean weight, height, and body surface area were 67.2 kg, 1.74 cm, and 1.81 m² respectively. Their $\dot{V}O_2$ max ranged from 50 to 65 ml-kg^{-1}-min.$^{-1}$ An additional eight subjects, with almost identical physical characteristics but a lower $\dot{V}O_2$ max (42 to 56 ml-kg^{-1}-min^{-1}) were also tested.

PROCEDURES: On the first day of the experiment, tests were conducted in a temperate environment (23°C DB, 16°C WB). After reporting to the laboratory at about 8 AM, the subject rested for at least one hour, after which his reclining heart rate and blood pressure were determined. He was then asked to stand for twenty minutes with his feet 15 cm away from a wall, leaning motionless against it with the upper part of his back. Heart rate and blood pressure were recorded every five minutes. In cases of syncope, acute dizziness, or nausea, the subject was put immediately in a reclining position and his legs were raised. Following this orthostatic test, the subject rested for thirty minutes, after which he performed one hour of stepping onto a bench 30 cm high, at a rate of twelve steps-min^{-1}. The average work load was 40 W. Immediately after cessation of exercise, the subject was again given a twenty-minute orthostatic test. This was followed by thirty minutes of rest and fifteen minutes of exercise at a load of 80 W (twenty-four steps-min^{-1}). The same orthostatic test was administered after this work load. In the afternoon, after two hours of rest, the $\dot{V}o_2$ max was determined by graded treadmill exercise to exhaustion (constant speed of 10 km-hr^{-1}, with elevation of grade every two minutes, causing exhaustion within seven to eight minutes). Oxygen consumption was determined during the last minute of exercise. The orthostatic test was again administered after this test.

On the second day of the experiment, the subjects were tested in the heat (39.4°C DB, 30.3°C WB). Three hours of bench-stepping was performed at an average load of 40 W, after which the orthostatic test was administered as on the first day. During all exercise conditions, heart rate, rectal temperature, oxygen consumption, and sweat rate were determined. The subjects wore shorts only and drank water freely.

The second group of eight subjects undertook the above procedures both at 23°C and in the heat, before and after eight days of daily exposure to the same hot conditions.

MEASUREMENTS. The heart rate was measured using an ECG or by stethoscope. Blood pressures were determined by a mercury sphygmomanometer. Rectal temperatures were recorded with thermistors. Oxygen consumption was determined by the collection of expired air in Douglas bags, analyzing samples with the Beckman apparatus. The sweat rate was determined from the weight differences of nude subjects before and after exposure, making corrections for water intake and urine output.

Results

RESPONSES TO EXERCISE IN THE DIFFERENT CONDITIONS. In the first group of nineteen subjects, the mean heart rate and oxygen consumption after exercise at 40 and 80 W were 107 and 1.1, and 132 and 2.1 beats-min^{-1} and l-min^{-1} respectively. The mean heart rate during the $\dot{V}o_2$ max test was 190 beats-min^{-1}. After three hours of exercise in the heat, the mean heart rate and rectal temperature were 136 beats-min^{-1} and 38.5°C respectively. Acclimation of the second group of subjects resulted in the usual decreases in heart rate and rectal temperature (27 beats-min^{-1} and 0.7°C respectively) and an increase of 13 percent in sweat rate.

RELATIONSHIP BETWEEN ORTHOSTATISM IN THE DIFFERENT CONDITIONS AND THE EFFECT OF $\dot{V}o_2$ MAX AND HEAT ACCLIMATION. Table 11-I shows that exercise at 40 W resulted in slightly poorer orthostatism than that experienced before exercise. There were two fainting episodes after exercise as compared with one such episode before exercise; heart rates were also slightly higher and systolic blood pressures were lower. More adverse orthostatism was noticed after exercise at 80 W, where four subjects fainted. After the $\dot{V}o_2$ max test, the orthostatic heart rate was higher than after exercise at 80 W, but the blood pressure was maintained at preexercise levels and there were no fainting episodes. Poor orthostatism was noticed after heat exposure, where nine out of the nineteen subjects fainted. Table 11-I shows that subjects twelve and thirteen fainted in three conditions and subject sixteen fainted in two conditions, while the rest of the subjects fainted only once.

Differences between the responses of the fainters and the nonfainters are shown in Table 11-I. The fainters showed higher heart rates and lower systolic blood pressures in all conditions. The intergroup difference of $\dot{V}o_2$ max was not significant. However, when the responses of all subjects were considered, the five subjects with the highest $\dot{V}o_2$ max values had three times less fainting episodes than the five subjects with the lowest $\dot{V}o_2$ max. The acclimation group, whose orthostatic responses before acclimation (a total of ten fainting episodes) were poorer than those of the first group, showed impressive improvements after acclimation, the total decreasing to two faints, both during heat exposure.

Table 11-III shows that the orthostatic heart rate responses in the different conditions were interrelated and negatively

TABLE 11-I

ORTHOSTATIC RESPONSES AND FAINTING EPISODES IN DIFFERENT CONDITIONS (N = 19)*

Condition	Heart rate, (beats-min^{-1})	Systemic blood pressure (mm Hg)	Fainting episodes	Subject No.†
Before exercise	±85 11.3	±123/90 6.2 5.2	1	12
After exercise 40 Watts	±90 16.1	±115/90 10.5 9.1	2	12, 13
80 Watts	±96 18.7	±111/89 9.3 8.1	4	5, 13, 16, 18
V̇o$_2$ max test	±116 20.2	±123/94 10.5 6.2	0	
Heat exposure	±122 22.5	±113/86 14.7 7.5	9	6, 8, 10, 11, 12 13, 14, 15, ·16

*Data are means ± SD of average responses during the 20-min of standing with the number of fainting episodes.

†Subject No. refers to individual subjects from 1 to 19.

TABLE 11-II

ORTHOSTATIC RESPONSES OF "FAINTERS" AND "NON-FAINTERS" IN DIFFERENT CONDITIONS*

	"Fainters" (N=11)		"Non-fainters" (N=8)	
	Heart rate, (beats-min^{-1})	Systemic Blood Pressure (mm Hg)	Heart rate, (beats-min^{-1})	Systemic Blood Pressure (mm Hg)
Before exercise	±88 10.3	±121/90 7.5 5.5	±82 7.6	±129/93 6.2 5.5
After exercise 40 Watts	±96 12.2	±114/89 10.9 7.8	±85 13.4	±115/94 9.6 7.8
80 Watts	±100 17.8	±109/88 10.7 6.8	±95 16.3	±118/92 8.7 9.7
V̇o$_2$ max test	±117 21.1	±122/94 9.6 6.6	±112 21.9	±132/95 9.5 9.2
Heat exposure	±123 23.3	±107/87 15.2 7.5	±113 22.2	±119/85 16.6 6.7
V̇o$_2$ max, ml-kg^{-1}-min^{-1}	±54 7.5		±57 10.4	

*Data are means ± SD of average responses during the 20-min orthostatic tests

TABLE 11-III

CORRELATION COEFFICIENTS BETWEEN ORTHOSTATIC HEART RATES IN THE DIFFERENT CONDITIONS, AND $\dot{V}O_2$ MAX

	Before exercise	After exercise			
		40 Watts	80 Watts	$\dot{V}O_2$ max test	Heat exposure
After exercise					
40 Watts	0.62*				
80 Watts	0.42	0.85*			
$\dot{V}O_2$ max test	0.22	0.44	0.64*		
Heat exposure	0.20	0.62*	0.69*	0.26	
$\dot{V}O_2$ max, ml-kg^{-1}-min^{-1}	−0.31	−0.43	−0.38	−0.32	−0.35

*Significant at $P < 0.05$

TABLE 11-IV

CORRELATION COEFFICIENTS BETWEEN ORTHOSTATIC SYSTOLIC BLOOD PRESSURES IN THE DIFFERENT CONDITIONS, AND $\dot{V}O_2$ MAX

	Before exercise	After exercise			
		40 Watts	80 Watts	$\dot{V}O_2$ max test	Heat exposure
After exercise					
40 Watts	0.65*				
80 Watts	0.72*	0.66*			
$\dot{V}O_2$ max test	0.33	0.32	0.57*		
Heat exposure	0.30	0.47*	0.31	0.51*	
$\dot{V}O_2$ max, ml-kg^{-1}-min^{-1}	−0.07	−0.15	−0.01	−0.13	−0.01

*Significant at $P < 0.05$

correlated with $\dot{V}O_2$ max. Similar but lower correlation coefficients were noticed for systolic blood pressure (Table 11-IV).

Discussion

When man changes from a reclining to a standing position, the compensatory increase in peripheral resistance and heart rate maintain a sufficient cardiac output to offset the hydrostatic effect of gravity, preventing collapse in most, but not all, normal people. If orthostatism is preceded by moderate exercise (40 W), the cessation of effort probably results in more blood pooling in the dilated vessels of the leg muscles than that experienced before exercise because of the cessation of the venous pump. More strenuous exercise (80 W) results in poorer responses with more fainting episodes (Table 11-I), in agreement with the results of previous studies.[3, 4] The absence of orthostatic responses after the $\dot{V}O_2$ max test was surprising. Possibly, exhaustive exercise confers orthostatic protection. During exhaustive exercise, there is a tremendous increase of cardiac output, with a maximal heart rate of 190 beats-min^{-1} and a pulse pressure of 90 mmHg (as determined immediately after exercise), the latter reflecting a very large stroke volume. The relatively large pulse pressure was maintained during recovery (Table 11-I) and heart rate was also high so that cardiac output may have remained sufficient to prevent orthostatic collapse. In fact, the data of Table 11-I suggests that the cardiac output during orthostasis after the $\dot{V}O_2$ max test was higher than that during preexercise orthostatism. Exhaustive exercise may therefore be a very good method to prevent orthostatic collapse.

Tables 11-II, III, and IV show that orthostatism is a general, rather than a specific, phenomenon. Those not fainting also show more favourable heart rate and blood pressure responses than the fainters (Table 11-II). Orthostatic heart rates and systolic blood pressure are also related in the different conditions. Although these relationships range from poor to moderate only, if orthostatic heart rate and systolic blood pressure and the incidents of fainting are considered simultaneously, we obtain the general picture of a relationship between orthostatism before exercise, after submaximal exercise, and after exercise in the heat. Orthostatism after exhausting exercise is less closely related to the other orthostatic conditions, because the large increase in heart rate and pulse pressure which occurs during this type of exercise decreases the differences between individuals during subsequent orthostatism.

Among the nineteen subjects with a high $\dot{V}O_2$ max (50 to 65 ml-kg^{-1}-min^{-1}) there were few differences of orthostatism, but the group showed substantial differences from subjects with lower $\dot{V}O_2$ max (42 to 56 ml-kg^{-1}-min^{-1}). The results show that physical fitness has a beneficial effect on orthostatism, but it takes a very strenuous training program or subjects with very high $\dot{V}O_2$ max to reveal this effect. Orthostatism is a passive position, and this may explain why it takes very strenuous training to cause beneficial changes. Nevertheless, the results of this study support the early observation of Crampton[2] that physical fitness is positively related to orthostatic tolerance.

In contrast, orthostatism was improved by only eight days of heat acclimation, and indeed when the heat acclimated subjects were compared with the high $\dot{V}O_2$ max group, the responses of the former were slightly better. This is probably related to the increase of plasma volume and stroke volume with the decrease of thermal strain that occur during heat acclimation. Only strenuous training can yield such increases of stroke volume and blood volume. When all subjects were rated from 1 to 27 on the basis of their performance on the five orthostatic tests, and this was correlated with composite scores based on $\dot{V}O_2$ max and heat tolerance, a high correlation coefficient ($r = 0.92$) was obtained. The results of this study, therefore, show that orthostatism is largely a function of heat tolerance and aerobic power. It should be noted, however, that $\dot{V}O_2$ max and heat tolerance are related capacities. In short, physically fit and heat acclimated people show good orthostatism, while physically unfit and unacclimated individuals tend to faint during prolonged standing before and after exercise.

References

1. Bean, W. B. and Eichna, L. W.: Performance in relation to environmental temperature. *Fed Proc* 6:144-158, 1943.
2. Crampton, W. C.: The gravity resistive ability of the circulation: Its measurement and significance (blood ptosis). *Am J Med Sci*, 160:721-737, 1920.
3. Eichna, L. W. and Bean, W. B.: Orthostatic hypotension in normal young men following physical exertion, environmental thermal loads, or both. *J Clin Invest*, 23:942, 1944.

4. Eichna, L. W., Horvath, S. M., and Bean, W. B.: Post-exertion orthostatic hypotension. *Am J Med Sci, 213*:641-654, 1947.
5. Greenleaf, J. E., Bosco, J. S., and Matter, M., Jr.: Orthostatic tolerance in dehydrated, heat-acclimated men following exercise in the heat. *Aerospace Med, 45*:491-497, 1974.
6. Lind, A. R., Leithead, C. S., and McNicol, G. W.: Cardiovascular changes during syncope induced by tilting men in the heat. *J Appl Physiol, 25*:268-276, 1968.
7. Scott, J. C., Bazett, H. C., and MacKie, G. C.: Climatic effects on cardiac output and the circulation in man. *Am J Physiol, 129*:102-122, 1940.
8. Shvartz, E.: Effect of two different training programs on cardiovascular adjustments to gravity. *Res Quart, 40*:575-581, 1969.
9. Shvartz, E. and Meyerstein, N.: Effect of heat and natural acclimatization to heat on tilt tolerance of men and women. *J Appl Physiol, 28*:428-432, 1970.
10. Shvartz, E. and Meyerstein, N.: Relation of tilt tolerance to aerobic capacity and physical characteristics. *Aerospace Med, 43*:278-280, 1972.
11. Shvartz, E., Strydom, N. B., and Kotze, H.: Orthostatism and heat acclimation. *J Appl Physiol, 39*:590-595, 1975.
12. Taylor, H. L., Henschel, A. F., and Keys, A.: Cardiovascular adjustments of man in rest and work during exposure to dry heat. *Am J Physiol, 139*:583-591, 1943.

Section Two

FITNESS TESTING AND THE PREDICTION OF ATHLETIC PERFORMANCE

Chapter 12

THE PREDICTION OF ATHLETIC PERFORMANCE BY LABORATORY AND FIELD TESTS—AN OVERVIEW*

Roy J. Shephard

Abstract

The determinants of athletic performance are analyzed briefly with respect to psychological factors (motivation, release of central inhibition, and arousal), constitution (muscle bulk, body mass, form, and center of gravity), neuromuscular performance (speed and acceleration), skill, flexibility (static and dynamic), strength (explosive, dynamic, and static force), and the ability to sustain work (anaerobic capacity, aerobic power, food stores, tolerance of thermal stress, and maintenance of fluid and mineral reserves).

Application of these concepts to the prediction of swimming performance is illustrated for sprint and for medium-distance competitors; the combination of scores from an appropriate battery of physiological tests yielded a performance index that had a high coefficient of correlation with the coach's rating (0.89 for the sprinters, 0.98 for the middle-distance performers). Parallel analyses yielded coefficients of 0.87 for white-water paddlers, 0.92 for dinghy sailors in calm weather, and 0.95 for dinghy sailors in rough weather.

The value of translating laboratory performance tests into corresponding field procedures is stressed in terms of objectivity, assessment of group and individual training responses, motivation, and the regulation of rehabilitation. The physiological demands of soccer are described, and details are given of a battery of field tests developed for the Canadian Soccer Association.

A plea is made for internationally standardized methods of data collection, in order to provide a reliable scientific foundation for assessments of athletic performance.

*It is a pleasure to acknowledge the contribution of several colleagues and graduate students to the process of data collection in the water sports, including Robin Campbell, Gaetan Godin, Geoffrey Wright, Ken Sidney, and Veli Niinimaa.

113

Introduction

TESTING THE FITNESS of the average sedentary adult is fairly simple. One is concerned with the ability to perform physical work for a few minutes to an hour, with obesity, and with the risk of myocardial infarction (Shephard, 1969, 1972). For many purposes, it is sufficient to predict the aerobic power from the pulse rate during a standard step or bicycle ergometer test, to make caliper measurements of skinfold thicknesses, and to note abnormal rhythms and ST segmental voltages in the stress electrocardiogram.

However, for the athlete, fitness is sport and event specific, and we need a corresponding variety of tests to predict the superb performer. This article will discuss general determinants of athletic success, drawing illustrations from water sports: swimming, white-water paddling, and dinghy sailing. It will also discuss translations of the laboratory tests into field procedures, illustrating this process by tests developed for the Canadian Soccer Association.

DETERMINANTS OF ATHLETIC SUCCESS

Psychological factors

Often, the ultimate limitation of performance is psychological rather than physiological.

Motivation and Central Inhibition

Motivation is needed to sustain training, to excel in competition, to sacrifice safety to speed, to tolerate discomfort, and to subordinate personal glory to group objectives. An excess of central inhibition may keep a sportsman from realizing his physiological potential.

Arousal

Moderate arousal ensures a brisk cardiac and respiratory anticipation of effort, a brief reaction time, and adequate muscle tone to develop maximum force. Premature arousal can cause hyperventilation, sleeplessness, and general exhaustion before a major competition. Excessive arousal during competition gives jerky, poorly coordinated movements, particularly disastrous in such skilled sports as pistol-shooting and golf-putting.

The measurement and manipulation of such variables are the responsibility of the team psychologist. Formal tests are in their infancy, and often objective data on such items as motivation, cooperation, and over-arousal are best collected as the peer ratings of the coach and teammates.

Constitutional factors

Neither the physiologist nor the coach can alter genes. Nevertheless, an appropriate body build is vital to success in many sports.

Muscle Bulk

Muscle bulk is needed in contact sports; it gives the inertia to dislodge an opponent and also protects the bones and joints of the assailant. In sports such as swimming and rowing, body weight is largely supported, and an increase of body mass increases the available power. Cross-channel swimmers can even profit from the buoyancy and thermal insulation of thick subcutaneous fat. However, in many sports such as running, the body weight is raised and lowered at each pace. Muscle force and aerobic power should then be considered per unit of body weight.

The Body Form

Body form can also affect competitive skill; thus, the pace length of the runner varies with leg length, while the maximum frequency of economical, ballistic-type limb movements varies as the reciprocal of the square root of leg length. A taller person gains in distance events (where economy is the rule), but in the less economical forced movements of the sprint a shorter person has the advantage. A high *center of gravity* is a handicap for precisely coordinated activities such as skating and gymnastics. However, in basketball, a tall body and long arms help guide the ball to its objective, and height is also an advantage in dinghy sailing.

Gross measurements of body build require little more than a scales, tape meaures, and fat calipers, although precision of readings can be improved by using formal anthropometric kits.

Cellular Constitution

Needle biopsy has drawn attention to microscopic differences of constitution between successful and indifferent performers. For example, the distance runner has more slow twitch muscle fibers than the successful sprinter. This aspect of selection falls outside the scope of the present chapter.

Neuromuscular performance

Neuromuscular determinants of performance include speed, skill, flexibility, and strength.

Speed

Speed depends on the time to initiate a movement, acceleration, and subsequent deceleration.

REACTION TIME: The reaction time depends on the length of nerve pathways from the receptor, such as the ears or eyes detecting the starter's signal, to the reacting muscles. It is also influenced by delays in the central processing of information. International gymnasts, for example, make enough reversals of body movements to severely tax the information processing capacity of the brain. Measurements of reaction time and information processing are highly specific, not only to given movements but also to a given environment. It is thus best to make measurements by analysis of films taken under competitive conditions.

ACCELERATION: Acceleration depends on the relationship between body mass and driving force. The ideal sprinter, for example, has powerful legs with little weight elsewhere on the body. The explosive force of the muscles can be determined by jumping on a force platform, or by timing the ascent of a brief flight of stairs. On the track, the course of acceleration can be followed by analysis of films or by interruption of a series of suitably spaced mechanical or photosensitive timing devices.

DECELERATION: Deceleration occurs in the final three seconds or so of a sprint, as the body continues to battle wind resistance (proportional to the third power of speed), tissue viscosity, and the friction between the shoes and playing surface. The crucial physiological factor is a depletion of tissue phosphagen stores. Initial reserves could be assessed by muscle biopsy, but it is much simpler to measure deceleration directly by analysis of films or use of sequential timing devices.

Skill

Some components of skill are probably inherited, while others reflect cumulative athletic experience, stored as movement and response patterns in the cerebral cortex and cerebellum. Our studies show the dinghy sailor has a good perception of body posture[4, 10] and the same is true of the diver, the gymnast, and the soccer player.

Balance can be examined on the stabilometer, a sophisticated form of teeter-totter. More simply the athlete can stand on one leg with his eyes closed (as in the stork-stand test). Other aspects of skill are better quantified by peer-ratings of filmed or actual performances.

Flexibility

Flexibility includes static and dynamic elements. In some sports, such as gymnastics, both aspects of flexibility are extremely important. Static flexibility is determined very simply as the maximum possible rotation about each of the major axes of a joint. Dynamic flexibility is determined by fitting an electrically recording goniometer to the axis of rotation and noting the applied force and the potential range of movement at different speeds of rotation. Some research workers are also applying forced oscillations to limbs and noting the resultant movement, both under relaxed conditions and with varying intensities of muscle contraction.

Strength

Strength comprises explosive, dynamic, and static components.

EXPLOSIVE FORCE: Explosive force is vital to the jumper, the thrower, and the sprinter. Some aspects are constitutional: leverage and the proportion of fast and slow fibers. However, the effective force also depends on the number of actomyosin filaments per fiber (increased by training) and the number of fibers activated (increased by learning).

DYNAMIC FORCE: Dynamic strength depends on maintaining the energy initially stored in high energy phosphate bonds. These can release energy equivalent to an oxygen consumption of 250 ml/kg-min. However, total stores give a capacity of only 30 to 35 ml/kg, depleted in about eight seconds of maximum effort.[3]

The immediate replenishment of phosphagen is based on the breakdown of glycogen to pyruvate, which in the absence of oxygen accumulates as lactate. The equivalent oxygen consumption is about 70 ml/kg-min, sustained for forty seconds to give a capacity of about 45 ml/kg.[3] The power athlete usually has large muscles and a large blood volume. For this reason, he may build up a larger total oxygen debt than his endurance counterpart. However, the concentration of blood lactate at exhaustion (about 120 mg/100 ml) is relatively similar in most groups of athletes.

If effort is sustained, these energy resources are progressively supplemented by a steady transport of oxygen. Over a minute or so, this increases to 60 ml/kg-min in the average athlete, but to 80 to 85 ml/kg-min in the superb endurance competitor.

Both steady oxygen transport and oxygen debt are best measured by collection of expired gas during exhaustive treadmill running. Predictions of maximum oxygen intake from submaximum tests may differ from the true maximum oxygen intake by 10 to 15 percent even if care is taken to standardize office temperature, initial rest, learning, and anxiety.

In many team games, repeated sprints lead to a progressive depletion of the glycogen needed to sustain anaerobic work.

Replenishment takes one to two days, and for this reason some have suggested giving glucose solutions at half-time. While glycogen concentrations can be determined directly by muscle biopsy, a rough idea of glycogen exhaustion can be obtained from the "drop-off" in scores for repeated sprints and other forms of anaerobic work.

STATIC FORCE. Static strength is important in feats such as weight-lifting. Unless a muscle belly is greatly "diluted" by fat and connective tissue, potential force is related to cross section.

Dinghy sailing requires prolonged static contractions of the abdominal and thigh muscles. Blood flow to the active muscles is impeded at 15 percent of maximum voluntary force, and flow is completely blocked at more than 70 percent of maximum effort. The contraction must then be sustained by anaerobic metabolism. As with dynamic effort, glycogen depletion could be examined by needle biopsy, but it is simpler to time the endurance of the active muscles before and after a period of simulated sailing.

SUSTAINED WORK. With very sustained effort, performance is also influenced by the rate of mobilization of body fat, by the maintenance of body fluids, and by thermal homeostasis. Problems of thermo-regulation can arise in the distance cyclist, the marathon runner, and the North American footballer; a footballer is particularly at risk if his protective equipment is impermeable to sweat.

LABORATORY PREDICTIONS OF PERFORMANCE

Swimming

Specificity is important in swimming. Many physiologists have described swimmers without reference to distance. We obtained data on eighteen members of the University of Toronto men's swimming team.[5] Eight were participants in anaerobic-type contests of 20 to 110 second duration. Four were contestants in middle-distance events lasting around two minutes, and six were long distance men, competing over distances of 400 to 1500 meters.

We asked the coach to rate the overall performance of each individual on a 1 to 18 scale. We also asked him to make a numerical rating of swimming skill.

Constitutional factors were assessed by standard anthropometric techniques. Buoyancy was assessed from vital capacity, residual lung volumes, and body fat as determined by underwater weighing. Aerobic power was measured by uphill treadmill running.

It would have been nice to have the swimming treadmill developed by the group in Stockholm or to use techniques such as tethered swimming. However, we were looking for performance prediction procedures suitable for more general application. Fortunately, there is a fairly close correlation between uphill treadmill running and swimming flume data, particularly in well-trained subjects. Anaerobic capacity was determined from blood lactate and excess oxygen consumption following exhausting exercise. Muscle strength readings were obtained by standard tensiometers and dynamometers.

In order to develop a performance profile, we calculated coefficients of correlation between the coach's rating of performance and physiological results. Data were ranked in nonparametric form. The sprinters were awarded 1 to 8 points for each test (Table 12-I). A weighting factor of 2 was used for r values in the range 0.7 to 0.9, and 1 for r values of less than 0.7.

Skill merited a weighting of 2, and all other factors a weighting of 1. The cumulative score ranged from 14 in the

Table 12-I. Relationship between the coach's assessment of overall performance and physiological data: sprint swimmers. (5)

OVER-ALL PERFORMANCE	SKILL (r=0.86)	KNEE EXT. STRENGTH (r=0.49)	UPPER ARM CIRC. (r=0.45)	FEV$_1$/FVC % (r=-0.45)	RESTING f$_h$ (r=-0.75)	BLOOD LACTATE POST-EX (r=0.49)	CUMULATIVE SCORE
2	2	4	1	1	3	3	14
4	4	1	6	4	2	1	18
5	6	7	5	7	1	5	31
12	10	6	4	3	6	4	33
13	8	3	3	5	5	7	31
14	14	2	2	2	8	8	36
15	12	5	7	8	4	2	38
17	16	8	8	6	7	6	51

best swimmer to 51 for the poorest competitor. The correlation between the overall physiological score and the coach's rating of performance was 0.89. The main anomaly was a subject rated number 3 by the physiologists but number 5 by the coach. Apparently the physiologists gave too much significance to his knee extension strength and upper arm circumference.

The profile of the distance performer (Table 12-II) is more closely correlated with the coach's rating, with a correlation

Table 12-II. Relationship between the coach's assessment of overall performance and physiological data: distance swimmers. (5)

OVER-ALL PERFORMANCE	SKILL (r=0.86)	T.L.C. (r=0.97)	F.V.C. (r=0.86)	V$_{O_2}$ (r=0.84)	CHEST TRANS. DIAMETER (r=0.70)	CUMULATIVE SCORE
1	2	6	4	2	1	15
3	4	3	2	4	2	15
8	6	9	10	6	6	37
10	8	12	6	8	3	37
16	10	15	8	10	5	48
18	12	18	12	12	4	58

coefficient of 0.98. This seems a general experience. It is easier for the physiologist to pick out distance performers than sprinters, who rely heavily on specialized skills. Again, two pairs of fairly well-matched competitors were ranked equally in physiological terms. This problem might have been avoided if we had given a higher weighting to the coach's assessment of swimming skills.

We did not have opportunity to rate the swimmers under intense competition but suspect psychological factors were a problem for some of our team. In terms of aerobic powers, our distance men achieved near international standings (Table 12-III). They did quite well against other Canadian Universities, but fared rather poorly against United States teams that we suspect had better psychological training or made better use of their physiological endowment.

None of our competitors swam extremely long distances, and the majority were quite thin. Nevertheless, the buoyancy of a large vital capacity was important to performance, particularly in the distance men. Perhaps because the swimmer is weight-supported, muscle bulk was also important to success in distance as well as sprint competitors. Tolerance of lactates and oxygen debt contributed to sprint performance, but this was mainly a consequence of bulky and powerful muscles. When

Table 12-III. Comparison between aerobic power of University of Toronto distance swimmers and average data taken from world literature. (5)

	AEROBIC POWER	
	l./min STPD	ml./kg.min.
International class	4.53	60.5
Collegiate class	4.31	57.4
Recreational class	3.53	50.6
U of T men	4.53	60.0
(distance|men)	4.89	65.4

oxygen debt data were expressed per kilo of body weight, the correlation with performance became statistically insignificant. The ratio of wrist breadth to bicondylar diameter was high in all swimmers. We suspect it is more difficult to keep large-boned legs in a horizontal position in order to achieve efficient hydro-planing.

The White-water Paddler

We have applied the same type of analysis to white-water paddling.[8] There are two principal classes of white-water slalom. In the kayak class, a single competitor sits on his boat with the knees flexed about 30° and paddles with a double-ended blade. In the canoeing class, one or two competitors kneel in their boat, paddling with a single-ended blade. Physiological demands are similar for the two classes of events. The boats are paddled as rapidly as possible over a course of 400 to 800 meters. About two dozen gates are set in rough water. The score is computed from the elapsed time and ten to fifteen second penalties are awarded for hitting or missing gates. Four to five minutes of endurance type work are combined with frantic bursts of anaerobic paddling at the gates.

Table 12-IV. Whitewater paddlers, listed in order of coach's rating. Scores for physiological tests rated in nonparametric forum, with summation to give cumulative physiological score. (8)

Contestant	Force	Height	Vital capacity	Aerobic power	Oxygen debt	Lean body mass	Experience	Cumulative score
Po	4	8	6	10	10	8	10	56
Mu	9	9	9	6	8	7	8	56
Ke	10	10	10	9	5	10	9	63
Tw	7	8	8	7	7	6	8	51
He	8	8	7	9	6	9	1	48
Ho	2	5	3	4	9	4	5	32
Jo	5	5	4	4	2	3	8	31
McK	1	1	1	1	1	1	5	11
McC	3	2	5	2	3	5	2	22
Ha	6	3	3	6	4	2	5	29

The relationship between the coach's rating of overall performance and the physiological data is shown in Table 12-IV. Results are for ten male competitors from the Credit River club in southern Ontario. Each variable has been given equal weighting, so scores could run from 7 to 70. Muscle force was based on grip strength, knee extension, elbow flexion, trunk flexion, and trunk extension; correlations with the coach's rating were highest for knee extension ($r = 0.58$) and for the sum of all six forces ($r = 0.45$). The legs played an important isometric role in holding the competitor within his craft. However, absolute force was less important in the arm and back muscles, since they were used mainly in the rhythmic work of paddling. Height was useful in steering, giving a correlation of 0.57 with the coach's rating. Lung volumes were not particularly outstanding, but nevertheless they were related to overall ability, with a correlation of 0.64 for absolute vital capacity and 0.69 for the age- and height-adjusted values. Possibly, this reflects development of the chest muscles by paddling. The aerobic power was again measured on the treadmill. Arguments could be advanced for an arm work test. Nevertheless, the centrally limited treadmill test had a correlation of 0.67 with overall ability. As in other weight-supported sports, the correlation became insignificant when expressed per kilogram of body weight. The total oxygen debt was positively correlated both with blood lactate ($r = 0.73$) and with the coach's performance rating ($r = 0.68$); again, the correlation became insignificant if expressed per kg of body weight. The percentage body fat was computed from skinfold readings. The seven younger competitors had an average of 11.6 percent body fat, but two of the three older competitors were fatter, with 16 to 20 percent body fat. Because body weight was supported, this did not impair their competitive position. The younger competitors had a body mass 3.8 kg below the "ideal" predicted by the Society of Actuaries tables. On the other hand, the three older men carried an excess weight of 5.8 kg, much of which was muscle. The correlation between lean body mass and overall ability was 0.72. Our last objective criterion was years of experience of competitive paddling, chosen as one simple index of skill.

Adding the scores for individual variables, cumulative values ranged from 11 to 63. The correlation between the cumulative score and the coach's assessment was r=0.87. One interesting exception was Ke (Table 12-V). He was rated third by the coach, yet had the best cumulative score. In the 1971 Canadian national white-water contests, he did better than Mu and Po. However, in the Munich Olympics he finished a poor third to

Table 12-V. Competitive performance of whitewater paddlers of Table 12-IV in a Canadian National contest (1971) and the Munich Olympic Contest. (8)

Class and course	Contestant	Score (sec)[a]
K-I	Ke	325.4
	Po	362.6
	McC	465.0
	He	490.4
K-I Jr	Mu	428.0
K-I W	Pa	723.5
	Ho	850.0
C-I	Tw	683.4
C-I Jr	Ho	856.8
	Ha	895.0
	McK	901.7
C-II	Jo	628.8 (two contestants)

1972 Olympic contest

	Time (sec)	Penalty (sec)	Score (sec)[a]	
Winner	258.6	10	268.6	1/37
Mu	304.8	130	434.1	34/37
Po	309.9	160	469.9	
	319.3	140	459.3	35/37
Ke	290.5	350	650.5	
	305.5	290	595.5	37/37

[a] Including penalty points.

the other two. This suggests his main weakness was a poor tolerance of international competition, a point apparent to the coach but not brought out by the physiological testing.

Dinghy Sailing

In calm weather, there were few significant correlations between the captain's ranking of sailing performance and objective variables.[4, 10] We found a correlation of 0.87 with total years of sailing experience, and 0.93 with years of competitive sailing experience. Peer ratings of resistance to mental fatigue correlated 0.64 with performance, and resting blood glucose (possibly also an indicator of resistance to mental fatigue) showed a correlation of 0.80. Table 12-VI illustrates the composite performance index. Despite the difficulty in establishing objective variables for calm-wind sailing, there was a correlation of 0.92 between the captain's ranking and the performance index.

TABLE 12-VI

SUBJECTS LISTED ACCORDING TO CAPTAIN'S RANKING, TO SHOW DEVELOPMENT OF AN OBJECTIVE SCORE FOR SAILING PERFORMANCE IN A LIGHT WIND. PHYSIOLOGICAL AND OTHER VARIABLES RANKED IN NONPARAMETRIC FORM, WITH WEIGHTING OF 3 IF $r > 0.9$, 2 IF $r = 0.7$–0.9, AND 1 IF $r = 0.5$–0.7[10]

Subject	Captain's ranking for light wind	Competitive experience $(r = 0.93,$ weighting $= 3)$	Team rating of resistance to mental fatigue $(r = 0.64,$ weighting $= 1)$	Resting blood glucose $(r = 0.80,$ weighting $= 2)$	Overall weighted score
E	10	27	5	20	52
C	9	30	10	15	55
Bb	8	24	9	18	51
R	7	12	6	10	28
Ki	6	19.5	7	8	34.5
Br	5	12	8	8	28
K	4	4.5	3.5	15	26
M	3	19.5	1.5	12	33
Kh	2	4.5	3.5	4	12
T	1	12	1.5	2	15.5

In a high wind, performance was much more dependent on physiological variables. The captain's ranking had a correlation of 0.81 with quadriceps strength, 0.75 with absolute aerobic power, 0.59 with anaerobic capacity as measured by uphill treadmill running time, and 0.60 with scores on a stabilometer test. Putting these items into a performance index, we found a correlation of 0.95 with the captain's rating and 0.93 with the ratings provided by other team members (Table 12-VII).

TRANSLATION OF LABORATORY PROCEDURES INTO FIELD TESTS

The above examples illustrate the potential for taking laboratory tests and applying them to the ranking of contestants in many sports. Let us now examine the practical value of field tests and see how we can translate the laboratory procedures into simple field tools of value to the coach and trainer, taking as our example the sport of Association Football ("Soccer").

Value of Field Tests

The good coach, sports physician, team manager, or trainer can often select his team almost intuitively. Equally, he can regulate training, apparently with great precision. With such skills already at hand, why do we need field tests that mimic laboratory procedures? Field tests have the advantage of objectivity and can contribute to both program assessment and the monitoring of individual progress.

Objectivity

Individual, intuitive expertise is pooled and set on a uniform, reliable, and semiscientific basis. There is also a relative immunity from problems of personality and other sources of bias. Sometimes the coach knows more than the physiologist. We have noted already the discrepancy between the coach's rating and physiological scores for white-water paddlers. We

TABLE 12-VII

SUBJECTS LISTED ACCORDING TO CAPTAIN'S RANKING TO SHOW DEVELOPMENT OF AN OBJECTIVE SCORE FOR SAILING PERFORMANCE IN A HIGH WIND. PHYSIOLOGICAL VARIABLES AND PEER RATING RANKED IN NON-PARAMETRIC FORM, WITH WEIGHTING OF 2 IF COEFFICIENT OF CORRELATION WITH PERFORMANCE HAS $r = 0.7$-0.9, AND 1 IF $r = 0.5$-0.7.[10]

Subject	Captain's ranking for high wind	Quadriceps strength ($r = 0.81$, weight = 2)	Aerobic power l/min ($r = 0.75$, weight = 2)	Team rating of resistance to mental fatigue ($r = 0.80$, weight = 2)	Anaerobic endurance ($r = 0.51$, weight = 1)	Balance ($r = 0.60$, weight = 1)	Overall weighted score
Bb	10	18	12	18	4	10	62
R	9	6	18	16	7	8	55
Br	8	20	20	14	9	4	67
C	7	16	16	20	8	6	66
Kj	6	12	14	12	10	5	53
K	5	14	10	7	6	7	44
Kh	4	2	8	7	5	9	31
M	3	10	6	3	3	1	23
T	2	8	4	3	2	3	20
E	1	4	2	10	1	2	19

correlation with peer rating 0.91
correlation with captain's rating 0.92

wondered initially whether the coach was not biased against one paddler who was of German origin. However, the coach's verdict was vindicated by the Munich Olympic Games. Presumably, the coach perceived this man had a difficulty in handling top-level competitions that was not revealed by physiological tests. Nevertheless, the best of coaches can develop a bias, and simple objective tests provide a useful counterweight to this.

Program assessment

Objective tests provide a yardstick, not only when recruiting new players but also when testing the gains made through training. Weakness in both the program and individual responses can be identified and corrected. Thus, looking again at data for the white-water paddlers (Table 12-IV), we might conclude that Po could profit from stronger muscles, Mu from a development of aerobic power, and Ke from a development of anaerobic mechanisms.

In Canada, much of our rowing, paddling, and sailing preparation must be on dry land. Land-based training is essential to maintain the condition of our water sportsmen during the winter months.[4, 9] The program used by our Toronto rowing club is based on circuit training, with a strong cardiovascular emphasis.[9] How well does this prepare the rowers? We compared scores on physiological tests at the end of winter training and after a strenuous summer on the water. If the winter preparation had been ideal, we would have found no change of score from winter to summer months (Table 12-VIII). The men seemed well-prepared in terms of aerobic power, with no gain over the rowing season. Body fat decreased over the summer, but even their preseason readings were in no way indicative of obesity. Lung volumes showed no change. Hand grip and knee extension force increased over the rowing season, suggesting we need to augment our training of the corresponding muscle groups in the winter gymnasium. However, other muscle groups including knee flexion and arm pull became weaker over the summer; possibly our circuit directed too much attention to these muscles.

TABLE 12-VIII

DATA ON 6 OARSMEN, SHOWING CHANGES IN RESULTS OF PHYSIOLOGICAL TESTS BETWEEN THE END OF THE WINTER TRAINING PROGRAM AND THE END OF THE COMPETITIVE ROWING SEASON.[9]

	End of winter	End of summer	Δ
Skinfold (average of 8 sites, mm)	7.2 ± 1.8	5.5 + 1.0	− 1.7 ± 1.2
Muscle strength			
R. grip (kg)	52.6 ± 6.6	55.7 ± 8.4	+ 3.1 ± 5.8
L. grip (kg)	51.8 ± 9.5	53.3 ± 9.4	+ 1.5 ± 2.9
R. knee extension (kg)	75.5 ± 21.9	83.0 ± 18.5	+ 7.5 ± 21.2
R. knee flexion (kg)	77.6 ± 18.5	71.2 ± 13.4	− 6.4 ±10.2
R. arm pull (kg)	131.9 ± 9.6	121.5 ± 5.0	−10.4 ± 11.3
Forced expiratory volume, 1 sec, litres BTPS	5.10 ± 0.68	5.06 ± 0.63	− 0.04 ± 0.05
Forced vital capacity (l BTPS)	6.12 ± 0.71	6.15 ± 0.74	+ 0.03 ± 0.05
Aerobic power (l/min STPD)	4.93 ± 0.26	4.86 ± 0.16	− 0.07 ± 0.11

Monitoring Progress

Test scores encourage the player and motivate him to greater efforts, particularly if they show that his performance is improving with training. Objective measurements also allow monitoring of recovery following injury; in association with clinical review, they are helpful in judging what additional exercises are needed during rehabilitation and when it is appropriate for a team-member to return to play.

The Specific Demands of Soccer

The physiologist has a harder time devising tests for soccer than for some endurance-type sports. Soccer combines a need for readily measured components of organic fitness with demands for teamwork, group skills, and mastery of technique—items that not even a psychologist really knows how to measure. A typical game calls for 1500 to 4000 yards of jogging and from 250 to 2000 yards of all-out running. Individual all-out runs cover a median distance of 30 yards.

The average player also makes a succession of quick turns, dodging and twisting maneuvers, weaving, jumping, leaping, and rapid accelerations. He must receive and control the ball with precision, making accurate passes while anticipating a challenge from his opponents. Finally, the relative importance of skills such as running, weaving, and jumping vary with playing position. The physiological attributes contributing to top-level performance include strength, endurance, speed, agility, and flexibility:

Strength

Muscles such as the quadriceps, gastrocnemius, and hamstrings must develop the explosive forces used in jumping, kicking, and turning. Isometric strength is also needed for balance and ball control.

Endurance

Endurance must be both muscular and cardiovascular. Endurance of the calf and thigh muscles has a vital impact on fatigue during the final fifteen minutes of play. Cardiorespiratory endurance is particularly necessary under adverse ground or environmental conditions. If the weather is hot and humid, ninety minutes of vigorous activity places a severe stress on the cardiovascular system.

Speed

Many aspects of speed are needed by the successful soccer player. These include a fast reaction time, decision time, and movement time.

Agility

Speed must be combined with agility. Sensitive position receptors are needed in the inner ears, in the muscles, and in the joints of the limbs with a coordination of eye and leg movements, and an ability to balance on the flexed leg, often while this is under some torsion.

Flexibility

Joints, particularly in the legs, must have good flexibility, both under "static" conditions (that is, when moving very slowly) and under "dynamic" conditions (that is, when moving rapidly).

A Soccer Test Battery

It is a horrendous task to propose a test battery covering all of the above requirements. However, a relatively complete and simple practical battery has recently been developed by the Canadian Soccer Association (Table 12-IX).

Body build

Height, weight, and skinfold thicknesses are easily re-corded.[11] The popular image of body build for the wing-forward and the goalkeeper are well known: The goal-keeper is about 7 cm taller and 10 kg heavier than the wing-forward.[7] However, there is a need to accumulate more objective data for individual playing positions as a first single step in the selection of players.

Flexibility

Many playing positions call for an extreme range of movements. Unfortunately, flexibility is joint specific, and an adequate test battery would need to assess the potential range and speed of movement at each of the major joints. Constraints of time make it necessary to form impressions from one or two tests, making supplementary examination of injured joints.

Table 12-IX. Proposed test battery for laboratory and field assessment
of soccer players. (6)

FIELD	LAB
Body Build	
Height'	Height
Weight	Weight
	Skinfold
Flexibility	
Sit and reach	Goniometer
Hop , step & jump	
Balance	
Stork stand	Stabilometer
Strength	
Bent - knee sit up	Hip flexion
	Ankle plantar & dorsi - flexion
Standing broad jump	Anaerobic power
Vertical reach	Vertical force
Speed	
50 yard dash	50 yard dash
Crdio - respiratory endurance	
600 yard run	Anaerobic capacity
12 min distance	Aerobic power
Muscular endurance	
600 yard "drop off"	Anaerobic capacity "drop off"

Laboratory tests of flexibility are based on the goniometer.
One simple measure of static flexibility is the "sit and reach"
test. This measures the flexibility of the back. It provides a
measure of changes in the same person but unfortunately gives

some advantage to short players. Dynamic flexibility contributes to scores on a 50-yard run, and the "five hop, step, and jump" test. Scores for these last two procedures also reflect the explosive power of the leg muscles.

Balance

Laboratory tests of balance use a stabilometer. The field test is the "stork stand." This simulates the situation where a soccer player balances on one leg with his eyes occupied elsewhere.

Strength

Isometric strength is important in maintaining a player's balance on a slippery field. It also contributes to ball control. For the goal-keeper, the strength of almost all body muscles is important. In other playing positions, the muscles in the lower part of the trunk, the hip flexors, and the plantar and dorsiflexors of the ankle are used most frequently.

As with flexibility, the ideal procedure would be to measure the strength of many muscles. However, lack of norms and constraints of time force us to use only a few measurements. In the laboratory, cable tensiometry is used for such movements as hip flexion. A simple field measure of muscle strength and endurance is the number of bent-knee sit-ups performed in sixty seconds.

Explosive strength is needed for jumping, kicking, reaching, and turning. The quadriceps, gastrocnemius, and hamstring muscles are particularly important to the soccer player. Some laboratories have special platforms that can measure the force developed during a vertical jump. Possible field tests are the standing broad jump and the vertical "jump and reach." A heavy person is at a disadvantage in the latter test, but the penalty seems fair, as he experiences the same disadvantage when playing soccer. A more serious criticism is that a poor score may reflect short legs rather than a lack of explosive power.

Speed

While the laboratory worker explores details of reaction and movement times, the 50-yard dash provides a convenient overall assessment of speed and muscular coordination.

Endurance

CARDIORESPIRATORY ENDURANCE: Cardiorespiratory endurance reflects the ability to transport oxygen from the atmosphere to the working tissues. It provides stamina for repeated brisk jogging and is more important for the forwards than for the backs and goal-keeper.

The laboratory test is uphill running on a treadmill. One simple field alternative is to predict maximum oxygen intake from the heart rate and the work performed on a step test, using the nomogram of Åstrand and Ryhming.[1] An even simpler field test is to measure the distance run in fifteen or twelve minutes.[2] In well-motivated young men, such distances have a correlation of about 0.90 with maximum oxygen intake. In women and in children, problems of pacing and motivation are such that better results can often be obtained from the time needed to run 600 yards. The latter depends also upon the ability of the muscles to continue working in the absence of oxygen. For this reason, the 600-yard run is a useful test to apply to adult players.

MUSCULAR ENDURANCE: Muscular endurance depends partly on the extent of initial glycogen reserves within the active fibers. It also depends upon the demands made by a restriction of blood flow through the active muscles during the game. As stores are depleted, the capacity to carry out anaerobic work drops. In hockey games, blood lactate levels are often 30 to 50 percent down in the third period and similar changes are likely over a vigorous soccer game. Persuasive laboratory biochemists may convince a few hardy volunteers to submit to needle biopsy for direct estimations of muscle glycogen, but for many purposes useful information can be obtained by determining the tolerance of anaerobic work before and after the game. In the laboratory, the subject can be timed as he runs up a steeply inclined treadmill to exhaustion, while in the field one may compare 600-yard times before and after a vigorous training game.

Data Synthesis

Field tests have traditionally been expressed as percentiles. The average score for a normal population then lies at the 50th percentile. This has two disadvantages when dealing with the athlete. First, if several tests are carried out, we cannot add the percentiles together. The 99th percentile is much rarer and may have much greater significance for athletic success than the 95th percentile. One possible solution is to use a modified probit scale (Table 12-X). Individual test results are assigned a value of 1 to 11, according to the percentile attained. A second difficulty is that normal tables stop at the 90th or the 95th percentile, whereas the successful athlete may surpass the

Table 12-X. Transformation of percentile data to probit scale. (6)

Percentile of population	Qualitative rating	Standard performance score
99.9 or more	Top player	11
99.4 - 99.8	Good player	10
97 - 99.3	Very high	9
90 - 96		8
80 - 89	High	7
65 - 79		6
35 - 64	Average	5
20 - 34	Low	4
10 - 19		3
4 - 9	Very low	2
3 or less		1

99.9th percentile. Some type of extension of the tables is thus required. Since athletes are at the extreme end of a normal distribution curve, it is preferable to extend such a curve rather than attempt to establish a special distribution curve for a small and arbitrarily selected population of athletes. Subsequent data handling depends on accumulated knowledge of the sport; we need to know both the strength of correlations between individual field tests and peer-ratings of performance, and also overlap between the information provided by the various field tests. We have discussed above simple methods of combining data for the water sports. In soccer, the various playing positions are a further complication. To date, information is incomplete, and arbitrary weighting factors have been assigned. These must be revised as knowledge increases. A tentative schema for maximum oxygen intake is illustrated in Table 12-XI. As one might expect, the highest $\dot{V}O_2$ (max) values are found in the wings and the lowest in the goal-keepers. Some of the highest figures yet reported are those of de Rose (average $\dot{V}O_2$ (max) of 61 ml/kg-min). We have assigned a weighting factor of 3 to wing-forwards, with a potential range of scores from 3 for a very poor performance (3rd percentile or less) to 33 for an exceptional performance (99.9th percentile or

Table 12-XI. Probit scores for laboratory measurements of maximum oxygen intake. (6)

Males under 30	Males 30-39	Females under 39	Performance Index			
			Forward		Back	Goal
			Wing	Ins./ Semi		
72.0 or more	67.0 or more	62.0 or more	33	28	22	11
68.0 - 71.9	63.0 - 66.9	58.0 - 61.9	30	25	20	10
63.0 - 67.9	58.0 - 62.9	53.0 - 57.9	27	22	18	9
58.2 - 62.9	53.2 - 57.9	48.2 - 52.9	24	20	16	8
54.7 - 58.1	49.7 - 53.1	44.7 - 48.1	21	17	14	7
51.1 - 54.6	46.1 - 49.6	41.1 - 44.6	18	15	12	6
44.9 - 51.0	39.9 - 46.0	34.9 - 41.0	15	12	10	5
41.3 - 44.8	36.3 - 39.3	31.3 - 34.8	12	10	8	4
37.8 - 41.2	32.8 - 36.2	27.8 - 31.2	9	7	6	3
33.0 - 37.7	28.0 - 32.7	23.0 - 27.7	6	5	4	2
32.9 or less	27.9 or less	22.9 or less	3	2	2	1

better). However, the goal-keeper is given a weighting of only 1 (possible range of scores, 1 to 11). Simple addition of the scores for the various tests (Table 12-X) yields a potential scoring range of 106 to 583 for wing-forwards, 97 to 534 for inside– or semi-forwards, 74 to 407 for backs, and 106 to 583 for goal-keepers. [I have here used the traditional European classification, rather than the current Canadian classification of strikers, defence, and mid-field.]

Interpretation of results

A Typical Example

The way the scoring might work out for a wing-forward is illustrated in Table 12-XII. The individual in question achieved good ratings on flexibility (sit-and-reach), had a reasonable balance (stork-stand), an excellent endurance (twelve-minute run), and an excellent anaerobic capacity (600-yard run). However, his glycogen stores (600-yard drop-off) were less satisfactory, suggesting the need for an increase of dietary carbohydrate prior to contests. The main deficiencies were in muscular strength (bent-knee sit-ups), explosive force (standing broad jump, vertical jump and reach), and speed (50 yard run); the individual concerned could thus profit from specific muscle-building exercises (graded repetitions with weights) and wind-sprints that would develop his anaerobic power.

Limitations of Field Tests

Data from field tests must be interpreted with caution. The measurements are often made under less than ideal conditions. The testing room may be too hot or too cold. The track or the field may be dusty, slippery, rough, or have a strong headwind. The player may be fatigued from a recent match or practice. He may be restricted in his performance by a recent meal or lack of food. He may have business or domestic worries. He

Table 12-XII. Relationship between observed scores for a wing-forward and maximum possible scores for various traditional playing position.

	Observed	Maximum Possible Score			
		Wing	Inside semi	Back	Goal
SIT AND REACH	60	66	88	44	110
STORK STAND	63	77	77	77	77
BENT - KNEE SITUPS	42	77	77	77	77
BROAD JUMP	30	55	44	33	110
VERTICAL REACH	35	55	44	33	110
50 YARD RUN	56	88	66	44	44
600 YARD RUN	60	66	55	44	22
12 MIN RUN	33	33	28	22	11
600 YARD DROP - OFF	48	66	55	33	22
	435	587	534	407	583

may be anxious about the test result and its implications for his future with the team. He may be recovering from a recent injury or infection. Many of these problems can be overcome by careful standardization of test conditions. However, a poor result must be carefully verified before it is communicated to the player or translated into a training recommendation.

Certain tests are performed clumsily at a first attempt. Practice helps to teach the specific skills involved and overcomes the effects of anxiety.

It is also important to observe the motivation of the athlete. One player may be determined to impress his coach by a high test score. A second may fear that testing will prejudice performance in a subsequent game and perform at less than his best.

Lastly, general health must be noted. Even minor ailments may disturb test scores. No tests should be conducted if a player has an acute illness, and in any case of doubt, the team physician should be consulted.

A good result is encouraging but should not be an excuse to relax training. It may reflect the constitutional advantage of a specific body build, early maturation of an adolescent player, or familiarity with gymnasia and performance-type tests. Accordingly, the result achieved may be less than the individual's potential.

Mixed test results are not necessarily a contraindication to selection. Only an exceptional candidate could score highly on every test. Nevertheless, the test battery is helpful to the coach and trainer in indicating areas of organic fitness that need specific attention.

Lastly, when comparing results over the course of training, it is important to note that gains of organic fitness do not develop in a linear manner. It is much easier to progress from average to good than to take the next step from good to very good. A substantial jump in the composite performance index may be anticipated over the first few weeks of training, but gains will become progressively smaller as a player approaches peak condition. This point deserves emphasis so that players are not disheartened as the returns from their training regimen become smaller.

Potential for International cooperation

Much of what I have proposed is intuitive, and as yet lacks the firm base of detailed statistics. However, this shortcoming could be resolved quite rapidly if sports physicians throughout the world would agree on a minimum test battery for each type of sport and apply it for several years to all contestants within their care. A pooling of data would soon give us the norms we require. Perhaps one happy outcome of this Congress may be the initiation of such a project. If so, a real practical dividend could emerge from our gathering here in Trois-Rivières.

References

1. Åstrand, I.: Aerobic work capacity in men and women with special reference to age. *Acta Physiol Scand Supp, 169*:1-92 1960.
2. Cooper, K. H.: *Aerobics.* New York, Evans, 1968.
3. Margaria, R.: An outline for setting significant tests of muscular performance. In Yoshimura, H. and Weiner, J. S. (Eds.): *Human Adaptability and its Methodology.* Tokyo, Japan Society for the promotion of Sciences, 1966.
4. Niinimaa, V. M. J. et al.: *Physiological Profile of Competitive Dinghy Sailing.* Canadian Association of Sports Sciences, Edmonton, Alberta, 1974.

5. Shephard, R. J., Godin, C., and Campbell, R.: Characteristics of sprint, medium, and long distance swimmers. *Eur J Appl Physiol, 32*:99-116, 1974.

6. Shephard, R. J.: *Canadian Soccer Manual—Physical Performance Tests.* Ottawa, Canadian Soccer Association, 1975.

7. Shephard, R. J.: *Human Physiological Work Capacity I.B.P. Synthesis,* volume IV. Cambridge, Cambridge University Press, 1978.

8. Sidney, K. H. and Shephard, R. J.: Physiological characteristics of the white-water paddler. *Internat Z Angew Physiol, 31*:1-17, 1973.

9. Wright, G. R., Bompa, T., and Shephard, R. J.: Physiological evaluation of a winter training programme for oarsmen. *J Sports Med Fitness, 16*:22-37, 1976.

10. Niinimaa, V. et al.: Characteristics of the successful dinghy sailor. *J Sports Med Fitness, 17*:83-96, 1977.

11. Weiner, J. S. and Lourie J. A.: *Human Biology. A guide to field methods.* Oxford, Blackwell, 1969.

Suggested Additional Reading

Andersen, K. L. et al.: *Fundamentals of Exercise Testing.* Geneva, W.H.O., 1971.

Shephard, R. J.: *Frontiers of Fitness.* Springfield, Thomas, 1971.

Shephard, R. J.: *Alive, Man. The physiology of physical activity.* Springfield, Thomas, 1972.

Shephard, R. J.: *Endurance Fitness* (2nd ed.). Toronto, University of Toronto Press, 1977.

Shephard, R. J.: *The Fit Athlete.* Oxford, Oxford University Press, 1977.

Chapter 13

RELATIONSHIPS AMONG ANAEROBIC CAPACITY, SPRINT AND MIDDLE DISTANCE RUNNING OF SCHOOLCHILDREN*

O. Bar-Or and O. Inbar

Abstract

A thirty-second anaerobic cycling test was validated against running times (40, 300, 600 m, each in duplicate). The subjects were thirty-five boys (age 12.0 ± 1.7 years) who represented a random sample of 1000 nonathletic schoolchildren. Correlation coefficients between thirty-second power output (anaerobic capacity) and running times were 0.79, 0.79, and 0.15, respectively. The corresponding values for five-second power output (maximal anaerobic power) were 0.80, 0.81, and 0.16. Results for arm pedalling were very similar, the correlation between total arm power and total leg power being 0.97 and the corresponding value for five second power being 0.95. These findings, coupled with previous information, indicate that the thirty-second test is a fairly valid predictor of sprinting ability in nonathletic children. Its specificity for performance related to anaerobic capacity is high.

THE ROLE OF THE O_2 transport system as a factor determining physical performance has been widely studied. Less information is available on the contribution of anaerobic pathways to successful performance, although it is generally accepted that effort of high intensity and short duration is greatly dependent on such pathways.

One reason for the relative scarcity of information on anaerobic capacity and maximal anaerobic power is the nature

---

*Supported by the Sports Authority, Ministry of Education and Culture, Israel.

of existing laboratory tests. Some available tests, such as max O_2 debt, blood lactate, or pH, require well-trained staff and sophisticated laboratory equipment. Others, such as morphological and biochemical analysis of muscle-fiber characteristics, cannot be widely applied.

In the last fifteen years, much effort has been devoted toward the development of laboratory tests of anaerobic performance which are simple and short, yet accurate, reliable and valid. Samples are the step-climbing test of Margaria et al.[11] and the bicycle ergometer test of Ayalon et at.,[1] both of which estimate maximal anaerobic power. Other tests estimating the overall anaerobic capacity include the De Bruyn-Prevost supramaximal bicycle test[7] which lasts thirty to sixty seconds, a similar procedure described by Chaloupecky[5] which times eighty-five pedal revolutions against a resistance of 4 kp (Von Döbeln type ergometer), the one-minute pedalling test of Szögy and Cheribetiu,[12] and the thirty-second bicycle test described by Cumming.[6]

Borg[3] was the first to introduce a bicycle ergometer test of anaerobic capacity in which mechanical power output alone was measured. However, his test required a special ergometer[4] in which resistance was continuously increased at a predetermined rate.

The present study formed part of an evaluation of a thirty-second supramaximal pedalling test.[1, 2, 8-10] Unlike protocols described elsewhere, the resistance used in this test is adjusted relative to body weight. This report describes the validity of the test relative to running performance in sprints and middle distances; the subjects were twelve-year-old boys.

SUBJECTS: Thirty-five boys (12.0 ± 1.7 years) were selected out of some 1000 schoolchildren attending two urban schools in central Israel. A random-stratified sampling assured proportional representation of age groups and of ethnic origin of the grandparents.

Methods

Running Times were measured in duplicate over three distances: 40 m (low start), 300 m, and 600 m. Ten days

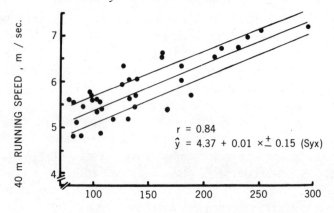

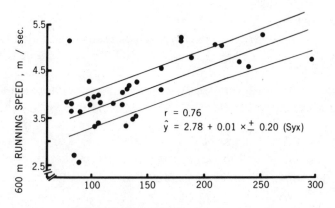

Figure 13-1. Relationship between 40 m running speed and maximal anaerobic power. Lines above and below the regression line represent ± two standard errors of the estimate.

Figure 13-2. Relationship between 600 m running speed and maximal anaerobic power. Lines above and below the regression line represent ± two standard errors of the estimate.

separated two consecutive measurements, and the better result of each pair was used for analysis.

The Anaerobic Test (AN 30″) was performed on a Fleisch bicycle ergometer. This ergometer is so constructed that one pedal revolution corresponds to a 10 meter movement of the flywheel circumference. A resistance of 30 gm/kg was adopted for the arm test and 40 gm/kg for the legs.

On the command to "start," the subject pedalled as fast as he could against a low resistance. This was quickly increased, reaching the desired level within three to four seconds. The electrically triggered counter and stopwatch were then activated and measurements began. The number of revolutions was recorded at five-second intervals for a total of thirty seconds. Total power output and output for each five second interval were computed.

Each subject performed an arm and a leg test, with thirty to forty-five minutes of rest between tests. The order of testing was counterbalanced.

Results

The running times of these subjects (Table 13-I) were comparable to values obtained from a larger survey of Israeli schoolchildren.

The five-second power output was linearly related to 40 m running speed. Linear relationships were also seen when the highest five-second power output was plotted against 300 m and 600 m running speeds, and when total thirty-second power output (overall anaerobic capacity[10]) was plotted against speeds

TABLE 13-I
RUNNING TIMES (SEC) AND RESULTS OBTAINED IN THE ANAEROBIC TEST (AN 30″)

	Running Times			AN. CAPACITY kpm/30″		MAX. ANAEROBIC POWER, kpm/5″		TOTAL REVOLUTIONS	
	40m (sec)	300m (sec)	600m (sec)	ARMS	LEGS	ARMS	LEGS	ARMS	LEGS
X̄	6.9	60.6	151.0	476.0	779.7	92.4	143.0	41.3	48.7
S.D.	0.8	13.1	27.0	171.4	312.8	37.6	55.3	7.4	8.0

TABLE 13-II
CORRELATION COEFFICIENTS BETWEEN RUNNING SPEEDS AND
RESULTS OF ANAEROBIC TESTS (n = 35)

| | Running Distance | | |
	40m	300m	600m
MAXIMAL ANAEROBIC POWER	0.84	0.85	0.76
ANAEROBIC CAPACITY	0.70	0.83	0.76

for each of the three runs (Table 13-II). As expected, success in the 40 m run is better reflected by anaerobic power than by anaerobic capacity, while the two anaerobic criteria are equally related to the 300 m and 600 m runs.

Discussion

Previous studies[1, 2, 8-10] have described some characteristics of the AN 30″ test. The test/retest reliability is 0.95 to 0.97. Success of performance is independent of motivation and possibly of heat and humidity (unpublished data). Scores respond favorably to warming up[9] and predict swimming performance fairly well in swimmers with a similar proficiency.[8] In young nonathletic adults, the highest five-second output has a correlation of 0.79 with the Margaria two-step test,[1] while the total thirty-second output has a correlation coefficient of 0.86 with the maximal O_2 debt of young trained females and males.[10] It may thus be assumed that the highest five-second output reflects maximal anaerobic power, and the total thirty-second output represents anaerobic capacity.

The present study shows a very consistent relationship (r = 0.99) between the five-second and the thirty-second output, suggesting that in nonathletic ten to fourteen-year-old children the two tests measure essentially the same physiological characteristics. It remains possible that in highly trained athletes, the five-second output could vary independently of the thirty second output.

References

1. Ayalon, A., Inbar, O., and Bar-Or, O.: Relationship among measurements of explosive strength and anaerobic power. In Nelson, R. C. and Morehouse, C. A. (Eds.): International Series on Sport Sciences, Vol. 1, *Biomechanics IV—Proceedings of the Fourth International Seminar on Biomechanics*. Baltimore, University Press, 1974.
2. Ben-Ari, E., Inbar, O., and Bar-Or, O.: *The Anaerobic Capacity of Men and Women 30-40 years old*. Presented at the International Congress of Physical Activity Sciences, Quebec City, July 1976.
3. Borg, G.: A work test for short-time work on the bicycle ergometer. In *Physical Performance and Perceived Exertion*. Gleerup, Lund, 1962, pp. 23-30.
4. Borg, G., Edström, C. G., and Marklund, G.: *A Bicycle Ergometer for Physiological and Psychological Studies*. Report No. 27 Inst of Appl Psychol, University of Stockholm, 1971.
5. Chaloupecky, R.: *An Evaluation of the Validity of Selected Tests for Predicting Maximal Oxygen Uptake*. Unpublished Doctoral Thesis. Stillwater, Oklahoma State University, 1972.
6. Cumming, G. R.: Correlation of Athletic Performance and Aerobic Power in 12 to 17 years old Children with Bone Age, Calf Muscle, Total Body Potassium, Heart Volume, and two Indices of Anaerobic Power. In Bar-Or, O. (Ed.). *Proceedings of the Fourth International Symposium on Pediatric Work Physiology*. Israel, Wingate Institute, 1972, pp. 109-134.
7. De Bruyn-Prevost, P.: *A Short Anaerobic Physical Fitness Test on the Bicycle Ergometer*. Unpublished paper. Louvain, Université Catholique de Louvain, Institut D'éducation Physique.
8. Inbar, O. and Bar-Or, O.: Relationships of anaerobic and aerobic arm and leg capacities to swimming performance of 8-12 years old children. *Proceedings of VIIth International Symposium: Pediatric Work Physiology, Trois-Rivières*. Québec, Pelican Press, in Press, 1977.
9. Inbar, O. and Bar-Or, O.: The effects of intermittent warm-up on 7-9 years old boys. *Eur J Appl Physiol, 34*:81-89, 1975.
10. Inbar, O., Dotan, R., and Bar-Or, O.: *Aerobic and Anaerobic Components of a 30 second Supramaximal Cycling Task*. Presented at the Annual Meeting of ACSM, Anaheim, May 1976.
11. Margaria, R., Aghemo, P., and Rovelli, E.: Measurement of Muscular power (Anaerobic) in Man. *J Appl Physiol, 21*:1662-1664, 1966.
12. Szögy, A. and Cheribetiu, G.; A 1 minute bicycle ergometer test for determination of anaerobic capacity. *Eur J Appl Physiol, 33*:171-176, 1974.

Chapter 14

OXYGEN DEBT AND INTEGRATED EMG DURING SPRINT RUNNING

T. Fukunaga, M. Kobayashi, A. Matsuo, and H. Fujimatsu

Abstract

The effect of running speed on oxygen debt and integrated EMG activity was observed in eight male subjects during 100 m sprint running. Oxygen debt per minute increased as about the 3.3rd power of the running speed. A curvilinear relationship was seen between running speed and the integrated EMG activity for three muscles (m. rectus femoris, m. biceps femoris, and m. tibialis anterior). Thus a highly significant correlation was found between the integrated EMG obtained from these three muscles and oxygen debt. It was concluded that the marked increase of oxygen debt during running at higher speeds was due to a corresponding increase of participating thigh and leg muscles.

IT HAS BEEN SUPPOSED that the electrical activity of a muscle during voluntary contraction is related in a simple way to the energy expended. Henriksson et al.[5] and Bigland et al.[3] showed a linear relationship between oxygen uptake and integrated EMG during bicycle exercise. The aim of this study was to observe the effect of speed on oxygen debt and integrated EMG activity during sprint running.

Methods

Seven healthy male athletes were selected as subjects. The average age was 25.7 yr (SD = 3.74), height 170 cm (6.03), and weight 78 kg (6.34). Each subjects was required to run a given distance (100 m) at a series of different speeds, corresponding to about 50, 60, 90, and 100 percent of maximal running speed.

The running speed was measured by means of photocells placed along a running track. At the beginning of each series of experiments, the subject's expired air was collected for five minutes, after an hour of rest in a recumbent position; this served as the resting value. The oxygen debt was measured in the usual manner. After passing the finishing point, the subject fixed a mask over his face and lay down on a bed. Expired air was then collected in Douglas bags until ventilation had returned to the resting level. The percent of oxygen and carbon dioxide in expired gas was measured by a micro-Scholander apparatus.

The integrated electrical activity of rectus femoris, biceps femoris, tibialis anterior, and gastrocnemius was measured telemetrically from the right leg. The electrodes (10 mm diameter silver chloride, filled with electrode jelly) were placed 3 cm apart over the belly of the muscle and sealed to the skin with collodion. Electrode resistance was always between 5 and 10 k Ω and did not change over the day. The telemeter measured $25 \times 32 \times 16$ mm, weighed 18 g, and operated in the frequency band 88.2 to 93.9 MHz. The antennae of the receiver were stretched along the 100 m running course so that the distance between the antennae and runner was about 2 m throughout. No signal modification was observed.

The magnitude of the energy exerted during muscle contraction may be considered a function of the integrated EMG and muscle volume, as defined by the equation

$$VCM = iEMG \times MV$$

where VCM is the volume of activated muscle fibers, iEMG is the integrated electrical activity and MV is the volume of the muscle groups involved, as calculated by the equation

MV = Cross-sectional area of muscle expressed as a percent of the whole tissue area (%) × Volume of leg or thigh (g)

The percent cross-sectional area of the muscle was measured by roentgenography, and the leg or thigh volume was determined by water displacement plethsmography.

Results and discussion

SPEED AND OXYGEN DEBT RELATIONSHIP: The correlation coefficient relating maximal running speed and oxygen debt was significant (r = 0.913, p < 0.001). At the higher speeds, oxygen debt showed a relatively large augmentation for a small increase of speed, oxygen debt increasing as the 3.3rd power of the speed. This result is in good agreement with Sargent's study[7], where oxygen debt increased approximately as the 3.8th power of the speed. One possible reason for this result may be that because less external work is performed with increased speed of movement, a greater effort must be made at higher, rather than at lower, speeds in order to secure the same external work.[7]When oxygen debt per stride was related to running speed, the correlation increased to 0.943 (p<0.001), being defined by the equation

$$y = 0.449\,x - 1.795$$

   where y is the oxygen debt per stride and
         x is the running speed

The curvilinear increase of oxygen debt with running speed thus reflects increases in both oxygen debt per stride and stride frequency.

RELATIONSHIP OF SPEED AND INTEGRATED EMG ACTIVITY: Selected examples of the EMGs obtained from the rectus femoris, biceps femoris, tibialis anterior, and gastrocnemius while running 100 m at various speeds are shown in Figure 14-1. At the lower speeds, the EMG activity of each muscle group was smaller than at higher speeds, all subjects showing a similar pattern of response.

The integrated EMG activity increased curvilinearly with running speed; scores for rectus femoris, biceps femoris, and tibialis anterior increased as the 3.1st, 2.6th and 3.5th power of speed, respectively. However, a linear relationship between EMG and speed (r = 0.965, p<0.001) was observed for the gastrocnemius. The power relationship of EMG with speed was similar to the relationship between O_2 debt and speed, suggesting an interdependence of energetic and electrical changes.

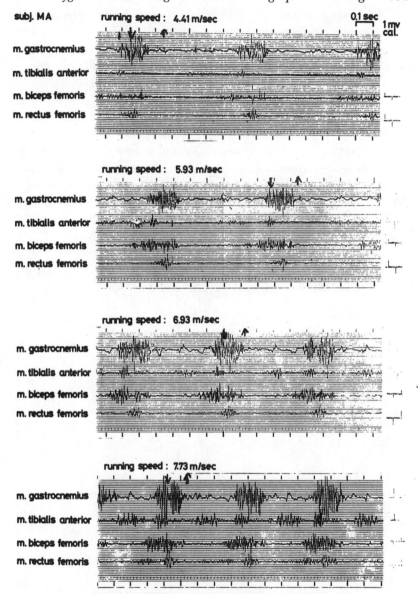

Figure 14-1. The EMG recording obtained from four muscle groups of the right lower extremity during sprint running at various speeds.

The speed at which a given subject runs is equal to the product of stride length and stride frequency. In the present study, running speed increased with stride frequency, regardless of stride length, at speeds above about 80 percent of maximum. The magnitude of integrated EMG per stride increased rectilinearly with increase of stride frequency (Fig. 14-2).

If the integrated EMG activity may be regarded as the summated electrical activity of all muscle fibers participating in a voluntary contraction, it may be deduced from the rectilinear increase of EMG activity with stride frequency that the number of contracting muscle fibers also increased linearly with stride

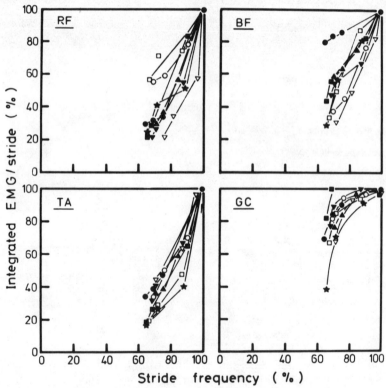

Figure 14-2. Relationship between integrated EMG activity per stride and stride frequency. RF: rectus femoris. BF: biceps femoris. TA: tibialis anterior. GC: gastrocnemius.

frequency. In contrast with our study, it has been reported that the relationship between integrated EMG activity and isometric strength was linear.[6] During dynamic contractions, Bigland and Lippold[1] also found a linear relationship between the integrated EMG and the velocity of shortening. In the present study, the augmentation of stride frequency implied an increased velocity of muscle contraction in the legs. Therefore, it may be considered that the velocity of muscle contraction in sprint running depends upon the electrical activity of the lower extremity muscles exerted per stride.

THE RELATIONSHIP OF O_2 DEBT AND INTEGRATED EMG ACTIVITY. The integrated EMG activity increased linearly with

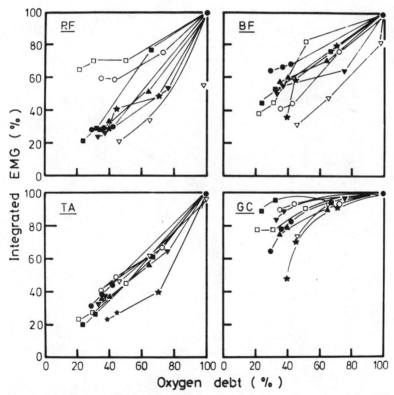

Figure 14-3. Integrated EMG activities as a function of oxygen debt. RF: rectus femoris. BF: biceps femoris. TA: tibialis anterior. GC: gastrocnemius.

oxygen debt (Fig. 14-3). Correlation coefficients for the O_2 debt per integrated EMG relationship were 0.856, p<0.001 (rectus femoris); 0.404, p<0.05 (biceps femoris); 0.969, p<0.001 (tibialis anterior); and 0.710, p<0.001 (gastrocnemius).

Henriksson and Peterson[5] showed a linear relationship between oxygen uptake and integrated EMG activity for the quadriceps muscle during bicycle exercise. Bigland and Woods[3] also found that during submaximal bicycling both integrated EMG and oxygen uptake were linearly related to the mean force exerted by the subjects. From these results one may conclude that the energy expenditure per active muscle fiber was not changed by work intensity.

The product of the integrated EMG and the volume of active muscle implies theoretically the volume of muscle fibers activated in voluntary contraction. It is meaningful, therefore, to add together the products obtained from the four muscle

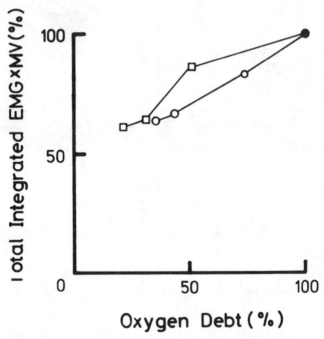

Figure 14-4. The product of integrated EMG and muscle volume in relation to oxygen debt.

groups. Figure 14-4 shows the relationship between the volume of activated muscle and oxygen debt. A linear relationship was observed in two subjects. These results support the hypothesis that the increase of oxygen debt at higher running speeds is due to an increment of activated muscle mass.

References

1. Bigland, B. and Lippold, O. C. J.: The relation between force, velocity and integrated electrical activity in human muscles. *J Physiol, 123:*214-224, 1954.
2. Bigland, B. and Lippold, O. C. J.: Motor unit activity in voluntary contraction of human muscle. *J Physiol, 125:*322-335, 1954.
3. Bigland, B. and Woods, J. J.: Integrated EMG and oxygen uptake during dynamic contractions of human muscles. *J Appl Physiol, 36:*475-479, 1974.
4. Cavagna, G. A., Saibene, F. P., and Margaria R.: Mechanical work in running. *J Appl Physiol, 19:*249-256, 1964.
5. Henriksson, J. and Petersen, F.: Integrated electromyography of quadriceps femoris muscle at different exercise intensities. *J Appl Physiol, 36:*218-220, 1974.
6. Lippold, O. C. J.: The relation between integrated action potentials in a human muscle and its isometric tension. *J Physiol, 117:*492-499, 1952.
7. Sargent, R. M.: The relation between oxygen requirement and speed in running. *Proc R Soc London (Ser B), 100:*10-22, 1926.

Chapter 15

THE INFLUENCE OF ENDURANCE TRAINING ON ROWING PERFORMANCE

P. L. Jooste, D. B. Read, and N. B. Strydom

Abstract

A university rowing team experienced doubts about fitness and certain aspects of preparation which appeared to be neglected in the training program. Accordingly, nine rowers (mean age 21.4 years) were tested twice at an altitude of 1,800 m. Measurements included their treadmill $\dot{V}O_2$ max (Douglas bag method) and their degree of fitness (lactic acid turnpoint test). Longer and more continuous high intensity exercise sessions (endurance training) were included in both rowing and running programs. The rowers were retested after seven weeks, when the mean $\dot{V}O_2$ max had increased slightly (from 4.42 to 4.50 l/min) and the mean lactic acid turnpoint had increased significantly (from 71.8 to 78 percent). The $\dot{V}O_2$, ventilation, and heart rate while running on the treadmill at 12 km/h had also decreased significantly, indicating a higher mechanical efficiency. The fact that they became national champions suggests that their rowing performance had also improved markedly.

Introduction

AFTER A DISAPPOINTING 1974 rowing season, the University of Witwatersrand Boat Club began to question why the youth, strength, and enthusiasm of student oarsmen could not place them in a dominant position in rowing, as in most European countries. It appeared from an analysis of eight teams racing over 2,000 meters that there was little difference between crews at the 1,000 meter mark, yet after this point the University crew would be completely outclassed. Times for the latter half of each course were 25 to 35 seconds slower than for the first part, the University crew fading relative to other crews. The problem now appeared fairly clear—how to beat the fade and maintain a constant racing pace.

Issues to be resolved included uncertainty about the physiological potential of the team members, along with doubts about the fitness of some of the rowers, and certain aspects of preparation which seemed to be neglected in the training program. One or two individuals who do not meet the requirements for rowing a 2,000 meter race in terms of gross oxygen uptake can cause a considerable decrease in the performance of an eights team even if the mean maximum aerobic power is high. Any team member with adequate power but no stamina also retards the team. In order to resolve these problems, team members were subjected to physiological tests before and after an endurance training program. The results form the basis of this chapter.

Subjects

Nine University rowers had a mean age of 21.4 (18 to 25) years. Their mean height and body mass were 178.4 cm and 78.4 kg respectively. All subjects were trained and accustomed to rowing but none were of national caliber at the time of the first series of tests. Physiological measurements were maximum oxygen intake ($\dot{V}o_2$ max) and the degree of fitness as estimated from the lactate "turnpoint;" all tests were conducted at an altitude of 1800 meters.

Methods and Procedures

Oxygen uptake ($\dot{V}o_2$) was measured by the conventional Douglas bag technique. The expired volume was measured in a chain compensated gasometer, the CO_2 concentration was determined on a medical gas infrared analyser (Beckman Model LB—1), and the O_2 concentration on two Beckman Model E 2 oxygen analysers according to the specifications of Strydom et al.[4]

The rowers ran intermittently on a motor-driven treadmill set at an inclination of 2.5 degrees, speeds being increased from 5 to approximately 17 km/h until the $\dot{V}O_2$ max was reached. Expired air was sampled between the 2nd and the 3rd minutes at each load. The heart rate was monitored during the last thirty seconds of each exercise bout, using chest electrodes and an electrocardiograph. Fingertip blood samples for the assessment of lactate concentrations were obtained from a pre-warmed finger at work loads through 13 km/h. Lactic acid was determined by an enzymatic spectrophotometric method (Boehringer-Mannheim GMBH).

Tests were repeated after seven weeks of training, during which period the rowers had been advised to concentrate more on endurance work. In order to achieve this aim, we added to their training program approximately twelve minutes of rowing at almost "racing pace," with good warm-up and warm-down exercises. This type of exercise was eventually converted into a series of 3,000 meter rows at a fast but constant speed (ten to eleven minutes duration), the number of repetitions being built up to six over an afternoon's rowing. The running distance was also increased from one to three miles per session, the initial time to cover one mile being multiplied by three to provide the target to achieve during running training.

Results

The "test" and "retest" means did not differ significantly with regard to body mass, $\dot{V}O_2$ max, maximum respiratory minute volume ($\dot{V}E$ max), or maximum heart rate (Table 15-I). While running at 12 km/h, however, there were significant decreases of $\dot{V}O_2$ (4.10 to 3.79 l-min^{-1}), $\dot{V}E$ (90.0 to 78.1 l-min^{-1}), and heart rate (176.6 to 168.6 beats-min^{-1}). The lactic acid "turnpoint" also increased significantly from 71.8 (test) to 78.0 (retest) percent of $\dot{V}O_2$ (max).

Curves of the form $\dot{V}O_2 = a_0 M + a_1 MV^2$ were fitted to test and retest data (where $a_0 + a_1$ are regression constants, M = body mass, and V = speed of running or walking). Separate

TABLE 15-I

MEAN RESULTS OBTAINED ON 9 ROWERS BEFORE AND AFTER 7 WEEKS OF
MODIFIED TRAINING

Variable	Test	Retest	Difference
Body mass (kg)	78.46	78.54	0.08
$\dot{V}O_2$ max (l-min^{-1})	4.42	4.50	0.08
(ml-kg^{-1}-min^{-1})	56.5	57.3	0.08
$\dot{V}O_2$ at 12 km/h (l-min^{-1})	4.10	3.79	−0.31*
$\dot{V}E$ max (l-min^{-1})	111.51	113.17	1.66
$\dot{V}E$ at 12 km/h (l-min^{-1})	90.04	78.11	−11.93*
Maximum heart rate (beats-min^{-1})	184.3	184.3	0
Heart rate at 12 km/h (beats-min^{-1})	176.6	168.6	−8.0*
Lactic acid turnpoint (%)	71.8	78.0	6.2

*Denotes a significant difference ($p < 0,05$)

curves were fitted for walking (5 to 8 km/h) and running (9 to 15 km/h); Figure 15-1 illustrates relationships for a mean body mass of 78 kg, the mean $\dot{V}O_2$ max being represented on this figure by horizontal lines. Running curves were extrapolated to these lines to estimate the speed at which $\dot{V}O_2$ max would be reached.

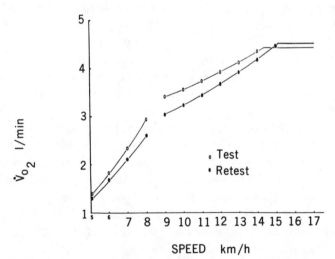

Figure 15-1. Relationship of oxygen consumption to speed of treadmill walking and running before and after training.

Discussion

The first important factor to be investigated was whether individual team members had the required physiological abilities to compete successfully locally and overseas. The mean $\dot{V}O_2$ max values on the two occasions were 4.42 and 4.50 l-min^{-1} respectively. These results are considerably higher than for other rowers previously tested in this country[5]; they also compare very favorably with the mean for seventeen rowers (4.4 l-min^{-1}) obtained by an indirect method at the Mexico City Olympic Games in 1968.[2] The mean sea level value for five Swedish champion rowers was 5.1 l-min^{-1},[3] 13.3 percent higher than the mean value for our second test. The difference in altitude above sea level could account for this discrepancy.

Rowing at 40 to 44 strokes per minute requires an oxygen uptake of 3.24 l-min^{-1}.[5] The stroke rate during a 2,000 meter race drops to about thirty-six strokes per minute, presumably with a proportionate decrease of oxygen consumption. The lowest individual $\dot{V}O_2$ max in the team was above 4 l-min^{-1}, well in excess of the requirement for rowing. Consequently, there was no doubt as to the physiological potential of the University senior rowing crew.

The remaining important factors of fitness (stamina, technique, and cooperation in the boat) were thus considered. The latter two factors were the responsibility of the coach and of the rowers themselves, but the scientific data provided a basis to assess and to enhance the degree of fitness.

The mean lactic acid "turnpoint," the only criterion used in this laboratory as a measure of fitness, was 71.8 percent during the first series of tests. In other words, the blood concentration of lactic acid started to increase markedly at a calculated oxygen uptake of 3.17 l-min^{-1}. The elevation of lactic acid levels in the blood leads to interference with muscle function and incoordination.[1] This phenomenon was apparently experienced by team members after they had completed 1,000 meters, as is evident from their slower times for the last half of the 2,000 meter course.

In the revised training program, endurance was emphasized, longer and more continuous high intensity exercise being included in both rowing and running sessions. After approximately seven weeks of this intensive training, there was no change in the average body mass, $\dot{V}_{O_2}$ max, $\dot{V}_E$ max, or maximum heart rate. However, the mean lactic acid "turnpoint" had increased significantly, from 71.8 to 78 percent. Endurance training leads to a fall in the lactic acid content of the blood during submaximum work, and this must be attributed to a more effective oxygen supply. This in turn enables the athlete to work both longer and closer to his maximum capacity, without producing excessive amounts of lactic acid.

Other significant differences after endurance training included decreases of $\dot{V}_{O_2}$, $\dot{V}_E$, and heart rate when running on the treadmill at 12 km/h. Figure 15-1 indicates that the retest $\dot{V}_{O_2}$ was lower at all levels of submaximal exercise. Better oxygen utilization would decrease the demands made on the circulatory and respiratory systems and lead to a greater mechanical efficiency.

The lack of a control group is a shortcoming of this study. However, the improved performance of the crew speaks for itself and compensates for this deficiency. The revised training program was put into action in February 1975. As the regatta season progressed, the eight showed a marked improvement, culminating with the establishment of a new course record for the 2,000 meter event in the National Championships.

The fading effect during the second half of a 2,000 meter race was reduced from 25 to 30 seconds (as experienced during the previous season) to 9.8 seconds in the 1975 National Championships. Thus the crew did not row much faster, but they were able to maintain their speed of rowing for a longer time.

As the rowing season developed, the crew became familiar with endurance training and racing pace, and once they appreciated the reduction in their pace over the second half of the course, they applied themselves more vigorously to training, achieving a higher level of success at each consecutive regatta.

References

1. Åstrand, P-O. and Rodahl, K.: *Textbook of Work Physiology.* New York, McGraw-Hill Book Company, 1970, pp. 300-303.
2. Di Prampero, P. E., Pinera Limas, F., and Sassi, G.: Maximal muscular power, aerobic and anaerobic, in 116 athletes performing at the XIXth Olympic Games in Mexico. *Ergonomics, 13*(6):665-674,1970.
3. Saltin, B. and Åstrand, P. O.: Maximal oxygen uptake in athletes. *J Appl Physiol, 23(3)*:353-358, 1967.
4. Strydom, N. D. et al.: Errors in respiratory gas analysis. A comparison of the Haldane and Pauling gas analysers. *Int Z Angew Physiol, 21:*13-26, 1965.
5. Strydom, N. B., Wyndham, C. H., and Greyson, J. S.: A scientific approach to the selection and training of oarsmen. *S Afr Med J, 41:*1100-1102, 1967.

Chapter 16

THE A.A.H.P.E.R. NATIONAL YOUTH FITNESS TEST: RESEARCHED, SLIGHTLY REVISED, AND REPUBLISHED, 1976

T. K. CURETON

Abstract

The National Fitness Test for United States Youth remains the same except for (1) an option to run 1½ miles (children >13 years) or 1 mile (children aged 10 to 12 years); (2) the use of bent-knee sit-ups; and (3) a recommendation of a reverse grip for chin-ups and flexed-arm hang. Evidence is presented that the test battery evaluates motor performance of a track and field nature, without cardiovascular interpretation or proven health relationships. Factors influencing the test scores include body density, body type and percentage fat, efficiency, effort tolerance, and trained neuromuscular responses. $\dot{V}o_2$ max bears little relationship to the results of any test except the longer runs. Factor analyses of the test battery fail to identify a cardiovascular factor but identify several muscular ability factors. One factor is related to endurance, but it has several loadings other than $\dot{V}o_2$ max. Research on 196 boys and girls shows density is more important than $\dot{V}o_2$ max; the latter contributes only 3 percent of net total variance in the 50-yard dash, 13 percent in the 600-yard run, and 21 percent in the mile run. Ability to run is an important factor. Running time does not identify known cardiovascular factors sufficiently to be of practical value for this purpose; after removing the density effect, age, height, and weight there is little variance left to analyze.

History of the A.A.H.P.E.R. Test

THE A.A.H.P.E.R. (American Alliance for Health, Physical Education and Recreation) *Youth Fitness Test Manual* (revised 1976) reports the results of the third random sample survey of

163

United States boys and girls aged 10 to 17 years. Testing was completed in 1975 under the supervision of P. A. Hunsicker. The first United States norms were established in 1957 through a survey of 8500 boys and girls from grades five through twelve. In 1965, when the second random sample was tested, there were moderate improvements in scores for boys, and slight improvements for girls (except in the 600-yard run where the girls scores were unchanged). This reflects the amount and type of programs conducted in the schools.*

The initial test battery comprised seven items: pull-ups, straight-leg sit-ups, shuttle run (4 × 30 feet, block test), standing broad jump, 50-yard dash, soft ball throw, and 600-yard run. Girls were permitted to substitute the flexed-arm hang for pull-ups. The softball throw was dropped after 1965. Other slight changes were made in the latest version of the test battery. The straight-leg sit-up was replaced by a bent-knee sit-up. The 600-yard run was retained, the *option* of running a mile (or a nine-minute run) was permitted for the 10 to 12 year age group, and the 1½ mile run became optional for the 13+ group. The reverse grip for pull-ups and bent-arm hang were also recommended.

There has been almost no improvement in scores for boys or girls from 1965 to 1975. This has caused concern, and some teachers now want to eliminate items in which pupils score poorly (such as the pull-ups), along with items in which there is a possibility of strain or more serious injury (softball throw, straight-leg sit-ups, backward extension of the back, and even a middle-distance run). Others have suggested the test should include items representative of basic physical ability or muscular fitness. Some have wanted to measure cardiovascular fitness and have demanded a 1½-mile run or a twelve-minute run for this reason. Most favor track-and-field-type tests, but some wish to include items more representative of gymnastic ability (including measurements of strength, flexibility, balance, and coordination). Many specialized coaches are not interested unless the test has meaning for their sport, be it aquatics,

---

*Possibly it may also reflect greater experience of test procedures by the children and their teachers—Ed.

soccer, football, tennis, golf, or diving. Medical and health professionals would like the test battery to examine nutritional status, blood pressure, stroke volume, and even eyesight and hearing. However, the A.A.H.P.E.R. test has never claimed to indicate long-range health, longevity, or cardiovascular status.

Research on the A.A.H.P.E.R. test battery

Individual test items are quite reliable, and the overall battery provides valid information on certain gross aspects of motor fitness: speed and power (50-yard dash and broad jump), dynamic strength of the arms and shoulders (pull-ups), strength and endurance of the thigh flexor and abdominal muscles (bent-knee sit-ups), agility (shuttle run), and running endurance (600-yard run or longer option).

The classification of scores is usually based simply on age, although the Cozens Age-Height-Weight Index has occasionally been used. Test results for the various distance runs are influenced by body density and a lack of body fat (Figs. 16-1 and -2). Such scores can be used to predict $\dot{V}o_2$ max with a fair degree of success, although predictions are not very good with girls, extremely heavy types, and untrained people generally.

Meaning of $\dot{V}o_2$ (max)

There is considerable disagreement as to the worth of predicting $\dot{V}o_2$ max, and in its usual format $(ml\text{-}kg^{-1}\text{-}min^{-1})$ the result is much influenced by body build (shape and density). The inadequate training of teachers in measuring pulse rates, blood pressures, and pulse waves precludes the possibility of making elaborate observations on cardiovascular fitness within the school system. Practical possibilities include the "drop-off" technique of McCloy et al., the progressive pulse ratio test, and the Harvard step test.

Improvements of $\dot{V}o_2$ max are heavily influenced by and generally parallel changes in growth and physiological maturity. There is much interest in what $\dot{V}o_2$ max measures, with

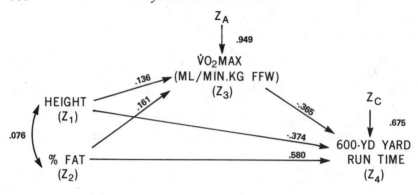

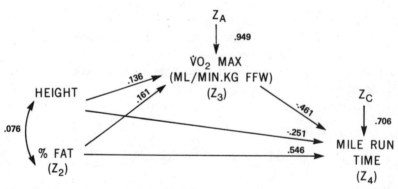

Figure 16-1. Path diagrams of 600-yard and mile run determinants. The upper diagram depicts the relationship of 600-yard run scores to percent body fat, standing height and $\dot{V}o_2$ (max) expressed per kg of fat-free weight. The lower diagram shows a similar relationship for the one-mile run.

warnings that factor analyses of performance data have failed to define a specific cardiovascular factor. There is now a growing interest in other simple laboratory procedures including the estimation of body fat by skinfold thicknesses, muscle force determinations by dynamometers and cable-tensiometers, and pulse wave analysis using instruments such as the "heartometer."

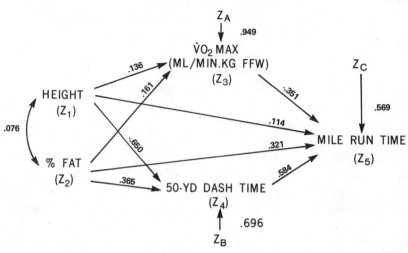

Figure 16-2. Path diagrams of 50-yard and mile run determinants, showing relationships to standing height, percent body fat, and $\dot{V}o_2$ (max) expressed per kg of fat-free weight.

Influence of body build

Kireilis and Cureton, and Costill, among others, have shown that fat is a definite detriment to endurance running. However, the speed of endurance running cannot be used as an indicator either of fat or of changes in body fat, since many other factors influence running: body size, bone mass, the ratio of muscle to bone, the style and efficiency of running, experience, and neuromuscular factors such as coordination and reaction speed.

C. T. M. Davies, Roy Shephard, and Gordon Cumming have all shown that the $\dot{V}o_2$ max has a correlation of up to 0.90 with running speed when the subjects are lean adults. Mayhew and Gifford have confirmed this for children, stressing that structure is always related to scores on the $\dot{V}o_2$ (max) test. Correlations are thus moderately good when a skeletal index is also related to $\dot{V}o_2$ max. A wave of anthropometric research has measured segmental volumes, density, and muscle strengths, sometimes including biopsy samples to determine the proportions of white and red muscle fibers. The researches of V.

Katch and F. Katch on young and middle-aged adults are interesting, but the work of K. J. Cureton et al. (1975) relates more directly to the youth fitness test of A.A.H.P.E.R.

Growth is a major factor in both motor test and $\dot{V}o_2$ max results. Neilson and Cozens have shown the marked effects of age, height, and weight on motor tests. Åstrand has shown the same for $\dot{V}o_2$ max. Over the age range of 7 to 24 years, the increase of height practically parallels the growth of $\dot{V}o_2$ max. Buskirk demonstrated the strong influence of weight on $\dot{V}o_2$ max. Several workers including Adams, Morse and Schultz, Cassels, Cumming, and Daniels have all shown that when $\dot{V}o_2$ is divided by weight, the result is not significantly correlated with performance. Cureton and Barry (1974) have shown that strength, endurance, power, and general motor ability scores increase from 7 to 11 years, hesitate briefly, and from 12 to 13 years accelerate markedly, enhancing general athletic ability. This last change is not paralleled by the growth curve of $\dot{V}o_2$ max.

Daniels and Oldridge (1971) found that boys engaged in an endurance running program made small gains of $\dot{V}o_2$ max but these changes were not proportionate to improvements in track times; rather, they mirrored changes in height, weight, and maturity.

Correlation of $\dot{V}o_2$ max with performance test scores

V. Corroll (unpublished Ph.D. thesis, University of Illinois, 1968) studied the relationship of all A.A.H.P.E.R. test items to the maximum O_2 intake, using forty-nine boys, 10.5 to 11.5 years of age.

By sampling over a narrow age range, he practically eliminated the effects of height and weight (as associated with growth). The multiple correlation between all motor test items and the $\dot{V}o_2$ criterion was 0.805. Specific relationships were as follows:

Test Item	Net Percent Contribution to Total Variance of Vo_2 (max)
600-yard run	59.2%
Push-ups	23.4%

Pull-ups	3.13%
Sit-ups	1.73%
Shuttle Run	.08%
Standing Broad Jump	.009%
50-Yard Dash	.049%
Softball Throw	.005%

Within the one year age span, longer duration events like the 600-yard run had a greater relationship to maximum oxygen intake than short duration events. This point has also been shown by others, including K. J. Cureton et al., who related $\dot{V}o_2$ max to scores for 50-yard, 600-yard and one mile runs.

Ikai and Kitagawa (1972) found that the $\dot{V}o_2$ max of boys (l/min) ran parallel with that of the girls until the age of 14; thereafter, the girls failed to improve their scores, but the $\dot{V}o_2$ max of the boys continued to improve until they reached 16 years of age. Cumming has shown that the $\dot{V}o_2$ max has a correlation of 0.90 with measurements of calf-width. This reflects the parallel between muscular development and growth of $\dot{V}o_2$ max.

Cardiovascular factors

Some studies, including those of Åstrand himself, have shown that if data is weight-adjusted, the presumed relationships of $\dot{V}o_2$ max to hemoglobin, stroke volume, and respiratory volume largely disappear. Cumming and Keynes found a very limited relationship between $\dot{V}o_2$ max and athletic fitness as measured by the motor items of the A.A.H.P.E.R. and C.A.H.P.E.R. tests. In the writer's opinion, the $\dot{V}o_2$ max test is not an adequate measure of cardiovascular-respiratory function because of its strong relationship to density, body shape, and size.

Orban trained seven young skaters for five months. The $\dot{V}o_2$ max (l/min) improved in three and retrogressed in the remainder. Those boys who gained weight increased their $\dot{V}o_2$ max (l/min), and those who lost weight showed a decrease.

Recent path analysis studies

K. J. Cureton et al. (1975-76) have applied net causal analysis (Path Coefficients) to performance data obtained on 196 boys and girls, 7 to 12 years of age. At the 50-yard distance, $\dot{V}O_2$ max contributed only 3 percent to the performance time; at 600-yards the net contribution was 13 percent and for the one mile run it was 21 percent (Figs. 16-1 and 16-2). The influence of body density was relatively greater than that of $\dot{V}O_2$ max. The influence of age, height, and weight was greater for the 50-yard than for the 600-yard or one-mile performances. If divided by lean body mass, the $\dot{V}O_2$ max made a somewhat larger contribution to the description of running time than when body weight was used. In fact, the greater the variation in soft tissue, the more the prediction was hurt relative to lean individuals. The difference in analysis for the 600-yard and one-mile runs was not enough to be of practical importance when predicting $\dot{V}O_2$ max. "Ability to run" probably accounted for a large part of the total variance in both the 600-yard and the 50-yard runs. Several factor analyses have shown an "ability to run" factor and a "muscular" factor. No strong factor indicating cardiovascular fitness has emerged from analysis of performance tests, and it should not yet be assumed with any confidence that the time required to run 600 yards or one mile indicates "cardiovascular fitness" (Cureton, 1945, 1947; Baumgartner-Zuidema, 1972). All-out treadmill run scores factor uniquely, and cardiovascular tests are not loaded on this axis (Cureton and Sterling, 1964). One major residual factor influencing running times is certainly the development of neuromuscular ability.

References

A.A.H.P.E.R.: *Youth Fitness Test Manual.* Washington, D.C., American Alliance for Health, Physical Education and Recreation, 1976 (revised).

Barry, A. J. and Cureton, T. K.: A factorial analysis of physique and performance in prepubescent boys. *Res Quart, 32*:283-300, 1960.

Berger, R. A.: Relationship of the AAHPER youth fitness test to total dynamic strength. *Res Quart, 38*:314-315, 1967.

Cureton, K. J. et al.: *Evaluation of Distance Running Times as Measures of Cardiovascular-Respiratory Capacity in Children.* Presented to the Research Section of AAHPER, April 4, 1976, Milwaukee, Wisconsin.

Cureton, K. J., Boileau, R. A., and Lohman, T. G.: Relationship between body composition measures and the AAHPER test performances in young boys. *Res Quart, 44*:218-229, 1975.

Cureton, T. K. et al.: Validity of the 28 items. In *Endurance of Young Men.* Washington, D.C., Society for Research in Child Development, Volume X, Serial No. 40, Number 1, 1945, pp. 156-172.

Cureton, T. K. and Barry, A.: Performance prediction and improvement in the all-out treadmill run and the 600-yard run. In *Improving the Fitness of Youth* (Society for Research in Child Development Monograph 95, Volume 29, Number 4). Chicago, University of Chicago Press, 1964, pp. 113-126.

Cureton, T. K. and Barry, A.: Summary of factors and conditions affecting improvement in the physical fitness of boys with recommendations. In *Improving the Fitness of Youth* (Society for Research in Child Development Monograph 95, Volume 29, Number 4). Chicago, University of Chicago Press, 1964, pp. 159-167.

Cureton, T. K. and Barry, A.: Standard score tables of physical fitness tests in preadolescent boys. In *Improving the Physical Fitness of Youth* (Society for Research in Child Development Monograph 95, Volume 29, Number 4). Chicago, University of Chicago Press, 1964, pp. 179-204.

Daniels, J. and Oldridge, N.: Changes in oxygen consumption of young boys during growth and running training. *Med Sci Sports, 3*:161-165, 1971.

Ikai, M. and Kitagawa, K.: Maximal oxygen intake of Japanese related to age and sex. *Med Sci Sports, 4*:127-131, 1972.

Kearney, J. T. and Byrnes, W. G.: Relationship between running performances and predicted maximal intake. *Res Quart, 49*:9-15, 1974.

Knuttgen, H. G.: Relationship of maximal oxygen consumption to height and weight (males and females, from Åstrand). *Med Sci Sports, 1*:1-8, 1967.

Mayhew, J. L. and Gifford, P. B.: Prediction of maximal oxygen intake in preadolescent boys from anthropometric parameters. *Res Quart, 46*:305-309, 1975.

Schwartz, E. et al.: Relationship of a kilometer run to aerobic capacity. *J Sports Med Phys Fitness, 13*:180-182, 1973.

Vodak, P. A. and Wilmore, J. H.: Validity of the 6-min. jog-walk and the 600-yards run-walk in estimating endurance capacity in boys 5-12 years of age. *Res Quart, 46*:230-234, 1975.

Welch, B. E. et al.: Relationship of maximal oxygen consumption to certain components of body composition. *J Appl Physiol, 12*:395-402, 1959.

Chapter 17

MAXIMAL AEROBIC POWER IN GIRLS AND BOYS AGED 9 TO 16 YEARS WHO PARTICIPATE REGULARLY IN SPORT

I. B. ILIEV

Abstract

A total of 760 subjects aged 9 through 16 years (330 girls and 430 boys) were tested spiroergometrically over a four-year period. All had been training for specific sports from one to five years. In the girls, the average maximal aerobic power increased from 1570 ml-min^{-1} STPD at 9 years to 2300 ml-min^{-1} at 16 years; in boys, the corresponding increase was from 1870 ml-min^{-1} to 3480 ml-min^{-1} . In boys, aerobic power was linearly related to age, while in girls the relationship was parabolic. Sport training increased maximal aerobic power, but did not alter sex-related differences of development.

DURING RECENT YEARS, more and more students have been included in systematic sports training, because of its potential contributions to social hygiene, good health, and physical development. On the other hand, the ambition for ever-increasing top sport achievements has led to changes in the sports training curriculum even for school children. Year by year, training loads have been increased. Such developments require careful medical control; in particular, one must guard against excessive loadings that would have adverse effects on health.

Material and methods

The medical examination of Bulgarian students undertaking systematic sports training has included maximum spiroergometric tests over the last four years. The "Zimmermann" GDR bicycle ergometer has been used, with step-wise increments of loading. Boys and girls both started pedalling at 60 watts, 60 rpm, and every ninety seconds the load was increased by 30 watts for the boys and 20 watts for the girls, until maximum effort was attained. Expired air was analysed with the Spyrolit II—Junkalor-Dessau—GDR apparatus.

We selected maximum testing not only for its virtues as an assessment of cardiovascular fitness, but also because ECG-control before, during, and after maximal physical work should reveal minimal, prepathologic disorders of cardiac function. Some authors[5, 7] have pointed out disadvantages when direct $\dot{V}o_2$ max measurements are used on a large scale; for example, almost maximal effort and considerable motivation are required of the subjects. The procedure is also time-consuming. Finally, the test is hard for obese subjects with some risk of acute incidents. However, we have now carried out more than 1850 maximum tests and have not found any difficulty in motivating athletic children to all-out effort, nor did our tests consume much more time than submaximal procedures. Andersen[2] indicated that a submaximal test would last about ten minutes. The maximal test which we used took only thirteen to fifteen minutes. There were no untoward medical incidents either during our investigations or in connection with them, and we think that fears of the maximal test are groundless, at least in this age group.

Our test subjects were aged 9 through 16 years; 330 were girls and 430 were boys. A total of 1850 observations were obtained. Individual students were training for one of several sports: light athletics, rowing, basketball, football, volleyball, swimming, or wrestling; each of those examined had one to five years of specific practice in their chosen discipline.

Results and discussion

Data on maximal aerobic power are presented in Table 17-I and Figure 17-1. Mean values ranged from 1870 ml-min^{-1} STPD for 9 year old boys to 3480 ml-min^{-1} for those aged 16

TABLE 17-I

MAXIMAL AEROBIC POWER OF ATHLETIC BOYS AND GIRLS FROM 9 TO 16

YEARS OF AGE ($\dot{V}O_2$ max, ml-min^{-1} STPD)

		9	10	11	12	13	14	15	16	years
Girls	$\bar{x}$	1570	1970	2080	2210	2400	2410	2500	2300	
	σ	249	213	165	156	185	170	250	114	
	Mx	40	49	18	15	20	21	45	26	
Boys	$\bar{x}$	1870	2220	2270	2490	2660	2890	3180	3480	
	σ	158	237	212	286	285	270	252	220	
	Mx	26	25	21	31	33	27	34	40	

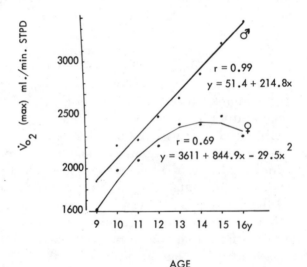

Figure 17-1. Maximal aerobic power of sports students, grouped by age.

years. In the girls, corresponding values ranged from 1570 ml-min^{-1} to 2300 ml-min^{-1}.

In the boys, maximal aerobic power developed as a linear function of age, as given by the formula $y = -51.4 + 214.8x$ (Fig. 17-1). In the girls, the diagram had a parabolic form, the regression equation being given by the formula $y = -3612 + 845x - 29.5x^2$. When the equation was differentiated, the theoretical maximum of the parabola was found to be at 14.3 years. Aerobic power increased significantly ($p < 0.01$) up to 13 years of age; between 13 and 14 years there was an insignificant increase, and after 14 the curve started falling again. The average increase was 240 ml/year for the boys and 190 ml/year for the girls.

The aerobic power of girls between 9 and 13 years of age was about 20 percent lower than that of the boys. After this age, the sex difference increased, and at 16 years of age it was about 40 percent.

The aerobic power of the young athletes was larger than that of the nonsporting male population (Figure 17-2). Differences were already apparent at 9 years of age, and mean values for the athletes increased more rapidly with growth. During the prepubertal and pubertal periods, maximal aerobic power increased under the influence of two main factors: growth/maturation and sports training.

The differing development of the girls may be related to their earlier maturation. While sports training increases aerobic power, it does not alter the sex-related trend of development for girls and boys between 9 and 16 years of age.

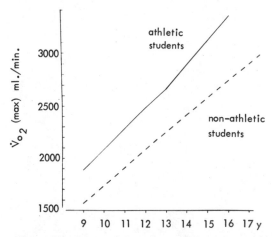

Figure 17-2. Maximal aerobic power for sports students and normal non-athletic students. Latter data from P. Kalaikova et al.: Characteristics in gas-exchange. *Hygiene and Health (Bulgaria),* 6:574-584, 1970.

References

1. Åstrand, P. O. and Rodahl, K.: *Text Book of Work Physiology.* New York, McGraw-Hill, 1970.
2. Andersen, K. L., Rutenfranz, J. and Seliger V.: *The Rate of Growth in Maximal Aerobic Power of Children in Norway.* VI Int. Symposium of Pediatric Group on Work Physiology, Prague, 1974.
3. Andersen, K. L. and Ghesquière, J.: Sex differences in the development of physiological performance capacity during the puberty growth spurt period in a population unit at the west coast of Norway. In Seliger, V. (Ed.): *Physical Fitness.* Prague, Charles University 1973, pp. 52-72.
4. Bengtsson, E.: The working capacity in normal children evaluated by submaximal exercise on the bicycle ergometer and compared with adults. *Acta Med Scand, 154*:91-109, 1956.
5. Hermansen L. and Oseid, S.: Direct and indirect estimation of maximal oxygen uptake in pre-pubertal boys. *Acta Paed Scand, suppl 217*:18-23, 1971.
6. Kalaikova P., Iordanov, T. and Mineva, T.: Characteristics in gas-exchange by maximal physical load for children and adolescents from 8 to 18 years of age. *Hygiene and Health (Bulgaria), 6*:574-584, 1970.
7. Mocellin R. et al.: Direct and indirect determination of maximal oxygen uptake in children and adolescents. In Seliger, V. (Ed.): *Physical Fitness.* Prague, Charles University 1973, pp. 282-288.

Chapter 18

PREDICTION OF ATHLETIC PERFORMANCE IN SWIMMERS AND RUNNERS BY MEASURES OF LACTIC ACID AFTER EXERCISE AT THE SPORTS GROUND*

A. MADER, H. HECK, AND W. HOLLMANN

Abstract

It is possible to predict the performance of endurance athletes in competition and to calculate the optimal intensity of training in the anaerobic range by measuring lactic acid after exercise at two different levels. This can be done by changing the speed over a given distance, yielding an individual equation relating anaerobic metabolism and exercise intensity. The evaluation is based on a model of anaerobic metabolism, which assumes the following:

(1) The total amount of lactic acid produced depends approximately on the energy demand (duration and speed of exercise) and the difference between this amount and the sum of aerobic and alactic-anaerobic energy release.

(2) The energy released in muscle by glycolysis is stopped by increasing acidosis if the intramuscular pH decreases by more than 0.6. The same drop of pH is seen in the blood. For exercise lasting one to three minutes, the amount of glycolytically released energy seems constant, depending only on body weight.

---

*Full text not available at time of publication.

Section Three

FITNESS TESTING IN THE ASSESSMENT OF SCHOOL PHYSICAL EDUCATION PROGRAMS

Chapter 19

FITNESS TESTING IN ASSESSING SCHOOL PHYSICAL EDUCATION PROGRAMS

J. SIMONS

GIVING AN OVERVIEW of "Fitness testing in assessment of physical education programs" is a fascinating, yet almost impossible task. We are dealing, on the one hand, with the problem of fitness testing and, on the other, with education through physical education programs. In order to situate both fields and underscore their mutual relationship, I would like to quote Barrow and McGee[6]:

> Evaluation is the art of judgment scientifically applied according to some predetermined standards. When it is applied to education, it is a distinct phase of a continuous, dynamic cycle. This cycle begins with the establishment of values and the formulation of goals growing out of philosophy, continues with the development of procedures to implement the goals, is related to the process of methodology and instruction, and culminates with the judgment and appraisal of results. Each of these phases is related to the other, although they follow each other in sequential pattern, starting with the statement of goals and ending in judgment. These judgments are made with reference to two things: the individual to be educated and the means of educating him. In the light of results from judgment, goals are appraised and restated, the procedures are replanned, and the whole cycle is repeated. Thus evaluation is a dynamic, never-ending process in education.

Physical education is one aspect of total education and, hence, has similar "educational objectives," although certain of these objectives are emphasized. The educational means used, physical activity, also places physical education in a special position, and physical education programs are developed on the basis of these chosen objectives. Although there is a general consensus on the educational objectives to be realized through physical education, very different educational means and very different physical education programs are employed in different countries.

In this context, measuring and evaluation techniques seem indispensable. Once objectives have been formulated and a program has been planned to produce the desired result, it is necessary to determine how well the objectives have been met, how efficiently the results have been achieved and how good the program is. One of the main objectives of physical education is to optimize fitness. Although I do not intend to define fitness precisely, I would stress this concept has several aspects. Therefore, both the curriculum and the students should be evaluated periodically to see how well the objectives are being met. This leads us to two essential fields—curriculum research and student evaluation.

Curriculum Research

Curriculum research involves the study of problems associated with the organization of the curriculum, such as (a) the grading of activities in terms of difficulty and anticipated student readiness, (b) the planning of a vertical sequence with respect to both individual activities and the sum of activities included in the program, (c) the distribution of time allotments, (d) provision for interindividual differences, and (e) decisions regarding required and elective activities. All of these aspects of curriculum may determine the fitness level obtained.

In general, there is a gulf of communication between curriculum builders and scientific research workers. In the past, widely differing physical education programs have been introduced, based on extremely vague or even erroneous theoretical considerations. Ling, for example, who had a great influence in many European countries, is strongly criticized by contemporary investigators. DuBois-Reymond, one of the masters of physiology during the nineteenth century, said of Ling:

> A mere glance at the writings of Ling is enough to show that they are a product of that miserable "natural philosophy" which for a quarter of a century made a laughing stock of German science. His arbitrary

constructions, his empty-sounding symbolism, his meaningless schematizations, and pedantic terminology no doubt impose on such semi-educated minds which, unable to detect the nonsense, accept a few scraps of anatomy and physiology as evidences of profound learning.[28]

Even now, the value of school physical education programs is rarely examined. An overview of methods, existing research, and major unsolved problems is found in Alley et al.[1] An excellent example of curriculum research is provided by the well-known "Vanves Experiment" in France.[29]

It seems necessary to determine the exact make-up of various school physical education programs, as was done recently in England by Kane.[21] Research to date has usually been limited to fragmentary studies, examining the influence of physical activity in general or participation in specific activities and programs. Examples of such studies include Reljic and Vukotic in Yugoslavia,[35] Davies in the U.S.A.,[11] Sprynarova[42] and Komadel et al.[24] in Czechoslovakia, Sterev in Bulgaria,[43] Bar-Or and Zwiren[5] and Weingarten and Bar-Or[45] in Israel.

In evaluating the school physical education programs, we can generally agree with Bailey's[3] conclusions regarding the unbalanced nature of education, with an insufficient allocation of time for physical education and poor preparation of physical education teachers at the elementary school level. Progression from grade to grade is also very unsatisfactory and programs are usually narrowly oriented, aimed at a minority of students and unhelpful to those who are less talented.

Student evaluation

The second major field is evaluation of results in the individual student. This provides information on the fitness levels attained in various countries, and thus allows an indirect comparison of school physical education programs. It is necessary to include assessment of all aspects of fitness. In addition to medical, anthropometric, motor, and physiological aspects, it is important to evaluate the psychomotor domain. This has rarely been done so far in physical education research.

Psychological aspects such as motivation, interest, personality development, psychosocial development, and attitudes have also been included relatively rarely in physical education research.

Nevertheless, some progress has been observed in recent years. Works by Oxendine,[33] Sage,[37] Cratty,[9, 10] Kane,[20] and Singer,[41] for example, show not only that psychological knowledge can be applied to physical education but also that a specific field of study here lies open for physical education investigators. Sociocultural aspects should also be included in research on fitness in schools, for they can either promote or limit the development of fitness.

Surveying research on fitness, we see two tendencies. There are many studies that investigate thoroughly physiological, neuro-physiological, anthropometric, motor, and other aspects of fitness. Such studies are indispensable and make valuable contributions to physical education science. Nevertheless, I wonder to what degree they have a practical influence on school physical education programs, since it is not the intention of the research to study such programs directly.

On the other hand, there are far fewer cross-sectional and longitudinal studies that make a *status questionis* of fitness for groups, nations, and races. Here, the relationship to physical education programs is much clearer. Having established growth curves and standards for simple but reliable and valid measurements, the physical educator can test and adapt his programs, evaluating and measuring his students. By repeating tests after a selected interval, progress can be examined and the efficiency of the programs can be tested indirectly. I will now cite a few such studies and try to evaluate them critically. My selection is obviously incomplete and intended only as an exemplary sample.

The first example of historical importance is the A.A.H.P.E.R. study. The immediate cause was a paper by Kraus and Hirschland[25] who, in 1954, had compared American and European children on the Kraus-Weber tests of muscular fitness. The authors had suggested that the poor American showing could be explained by a high degree of mechanization, and a consequent lack of physical activity. Since, in their experience, such low levels of fitness predisposed the children to orthopedic and emotional difficulties, the authors insisted on the need to increase the physical activity of the children—making physical activity scores a part of the child's school record—and giving tests of muscular performance at regular intervals. Despite its fundamental imperfections, the study of Kraus and Hirschland impressed the President of the United States, who was already aware of the inadequate fitness level of American young men reporting for military service. As a result, the President's Council for Physical Fitness was established. One of the first steps taken under its sponsorship was a pilot study on a nationwide sample, using a new test battery constructed by the A.A.H.P.E.R., in order to get reliable facts concerning the fitness of American boys and girls (Hunsicker[17]). At the same time a pamphlet was prepared emphasizing a basic and effective fitness program, with developmental and conditioning activities appropriate to student grade and maturation levels (Larson[26]).

The mass movement for the improvement of physical fitness levels in adults and children, unleashed by this action, was extremely impressive and was vigorously stimulated by the highest United States authorities. As for the practical results of the campaign, it can at least be said that eight years later when Hunsicker and Reiff[17] repeated the survey using the same tests, a general improvement of fitness scores was found.

Since its development, the A.A.H.P.E.R. test battery has been used systematically in many American schools. Representative standards have also been established in other countries such as Great Britain, South Africa, Japan, and Belgium. Such procedures allow national and international comparisons. However, there are some drawbacks. First of all, only a limited aspect of total fitness is measured. Some test items are culturally determined. Repeated use of the tests probably also has a training effect, so that the apparent progress observed may be due in part to this. Nevertheless, such studies are clear examples of how a testing program can influence physical education curricula.

A second example of historical importance is the Medford Boys Growth Study, directed by Clarke.[8] This more comprehensive longitudinal study began in 1956 and continued for twelve years. Besides motor and anthropometric measurements, it included data on the somatotype and maturity of 7- to 18-year-old boys. An important aspect of the study was its longitudinal approach. This permitted the drawing of growth curves and the observation of acceleration phenomena. Due to the wide range of measurements, interrelations could also be examined. Weak points were its poor test selection, the limited number of fitness aspects investigated and the nonrepresentativeness of the subjects examined. It is doubtful whether this research has had a direct influence on physical education programs.

Since 1925, when Burt[7] made the first factor analysis of motor variables, his example has been widely followed. It introduced some changes into physical education research, including an identification of basic dimensions and the more efficient selection of measuring methods. Fleishman[14] applied factor analysis to a large set of motor variables, isolating several basic factors. He then established a corresponding test battery and in 1962 published United States norms. It is regrettable that he did not determine the reliability of every test item and that he generalized the results obtained on male adults to much younger girls and boys. His test also has been used in various countries. McCaughan[31] used it to establish norms for New Zealand boys aged 13 to 17. This latter study clearly demonstrates that certain tests had insufficient reliability. Again, only one aspect of fitness was measured.

Many countries have tried to establish specific, adapted test batteries, as well as norms for their populations. A few examples can be given. Norms for the "Test d'éfficience physique de la C.A.H.P.E.R."[2] were established on 11,000 Canadian boys and girls aged 7 to 17, and the resultant test manual has been widely distributed. Trzesniowski[44] examined almost 80,000 Polish adolescents aged 7 to 19 years over a ten-year period. In Japan, Seto and his research team[38] between 1949 and 1959 performed motor tests on about 300,000 boys and girls aged 8 to 17 years. Under Pavek's[34] direction, anthropometric and motor characteristics have been measured on more than 63,000 Czechoslovakian boys and girls.

These few examples suffice to show that many countries have made considerable efforts to determine the immediate fitness status of their populations and to follow its subsequent evolution.

When surveying the literature, one has the impression that recently more and more extensive practice-oriented studies are being undertaken, with cross-sectional and longitudinal data being gathered from large test groups. The number of fitness aspects investigated is also being stepped up and selection of measuring methods is becoming more and more precise.

A first example of such studies is the Saskatchewan Child Growth and Development Study,[4] which began in 1964 and was completed in 1973. This study included a large number of variables, measuring the major aspects of boys' and girls' fitness. In addition to physiological, anthropometric, and motor measurements, the somatotype, skeletal age, personality aspects, "self-concept," and social behavior were examined. Information was also obtained on the socioeconomic level, physical activity, and sports participation. On the basis of such data, growth and acceleration curves can be established, and the interrelations between variables can be observed. The influence of physical activity and sports participation on various aspects of growth and development can also be studied. Such an all-inclusive project not only furthers our basic scientific knowledge but is also an example of an evaluation, by means of fitness measurements, of a physical education program. Although several articles have been published, the great bulk of the gathered information has yet to appear. I have no doubt that this study will make an extremely important contribution to the physical education sciences. Inherent in such a wide approach is a rather small number of subjects, reducing the generality of the results obtained. A somewhat different approach was used in the "Leuven Boys' Growth Study."[40] A mixed cross-sectional and longitudinal study was carried out on more than 21,000 boys aged 12 to 19, after a pilot study had been completed on a restricted number of students.

The study ran from 1969 to 1974, so that here too complete results are not available. The variables studied included anthropometric measures, motor tests, somatotyping, measurements of skeletal age, and examination of sociocultural factors. Besides norms and interrelations, longitudinal growth and acceleration curves will be studied, since more than 600 subjects have been examined annually over six years. Since we were informed about the school physical education programs (hours per week), about the sport facilities and about extra-curricular sports participation, the influence of physical activities on physical and motor development can also be studied. One early result of the study was very practical: On the initiative of the Ministry of Education, our test battery was placed at the disposal of all physical education teachers and it is now being used regularly to evaluate both programs and the progress of individual students.[32]

Our project also has its limitations. First of all, only a small age range has been examined. This shortcoming is met in part by the work of Hebbelinck and Borms,[15, 16] who studied the anthropometric and motor development of a representative sample of more than 13,000 boys and girls aged 6 to 13 on a cross-sectional basis. A further limitation is that only boys were examined. However, we are now planning a similar study of girls. A third limitation is the poor physiological information and a total lack of medical, psychomotor, psychological, and psychosocial data. Several other longitudinal projects are in progress or scheduled. The study at Trois-Rivières can be mentioned. This longitudinal research project started in 1970, after completion of a pilot study, and is being carried out in schools at Trois-Rivières and Pont-Rouge. The sample consists of both boys and girls. In all, a total of 250 variables are being studied, covering psychological, anthropometric, motor, medical, and social areas. The subjects are examined every six months, for example, with the C.A.P.H.E.R. motor test battery. Some aspects of this multidisciplinary study were presented at the 7th International Symposium on Paediatric Work Physiology by Jequier,[19] Lavallee,[27] Shephard,[39] and Marchand and Piché.[30] This study also will enable us to check the efficiency of school physical education programs and the influence of increased physical activities on different aspects of fitness.

Another project seeming of interest has been set up in the Netherlands by Kemper and co-workers.[22, 23] Through a multidisciplinary approach, they wish to verify the effect of physical education programs on the physical and psychological development of 12– to 19-year-old boys. In 1975 a pilot study was carried out to select test procedures. The last example I wish to cite is a project from the French research team of the "Ecole Nationale Supérieure d'Education Physique et de Sports,"[12] including a longitudinal multidisciplinary study on the role of physical education programs in the general development of young people.

From these various examples it is easy to see that several countries are aware that physical activities and school physical education programs have to be evaluated as completely and as accurately as possible in order to optimize their contributions to a well-balanced development of the individual. In this field, the International Committee on Standardization of Physical Fitness Tests should play an important role. Presided over by Larson, after several years of study it has delimited the field of physical fitness evaluation to include personal data, athletic history, a medical examination, physiological measurements data on physique and body composition, and basic physical performance tests. For all these aspects of fitness, well-adapted methods of evaluation have been selected. The publication of the book *Fitness health and work capacity*[26] is a tangible result of this intense international collaboration.

From this survey, it clearly appears that studies vary one from another. If one really wishes to achieve internationally comparable studies, one has to use identical tools and to follow a fixed research plan. These are the aims set by the I.C.P.F.R. committee. During the meeting at Jyväskylä the new name of "International Committee on Physical Fitness Research" was adopted with a view toward continuing sponsorship of international research. Since that time, data have been collected by Evans,[13] Ishiko,[18] Ruskin,[36] and probably several others. We are still in the phase of checking the measurement techniques proposed by the Committee. But in the near future, we should be able to use these methods in comparative studies on the physical fitness of different countries.

Despite such progress, I would like to stress the need for a yet broader approach to fitness evaluation, as expressed at the last meeting in Jerusalem. If one wishes to evaluate physical activities within the school physical education programs on an international basis, it is vital to use identical procedures to collect exact data on the physical education curriculum, including the volume and level of required physical activities and sports participation. I would like to express the hope that the gap between curriculum builders on the one hand and scientific investigators on the other will be bridged in the very near future and that fitness testing will assume its due role in curriculum planning and administration as well as in the evaluation of young people.

References

1. Alley, L. E. et al.: Research and the curriculum. In Scott, G. M. (Ed.): *Research Methods in Health, Physical Education, Recreation.* Washington, Am Assoc Health Phys Educ, Recreation, 1959, pp. 397-423.
2. L'Association Canadienne pour la Santé, L'éducation Physique et la Récréation. *Le manuel d'instruction du test d'éfficience physique de la C.A.P.H.E.R.* Toronto, C.A.P.H.E.R. 1966.
3. Bailey, D. A.: Exercise, fitness and physical education for the growing child—a concern. *Can J Publ Health, 54*:421-430, 1973.
4. Bailey, D. A.: *Saskatchewan Child Growth and Development Study. Final Report.* Saskatoon, College of Physical Education, University of Saskatchewan, 1976.
5. Bar-Or, O. and Zwiren, L. D.: Physiological effects of increased frequency of physical education classes and of endurance conditioning on 9 to 10 year old girls and boys. In Bar-Or, O. (Ed.): *Proceedings of the Fourth International Symposium on Paediatric Work Physiology, 1972.* Natanya, Israel, The Wingate Institute, 1973, pp. 183-198.
6. Barrow, H. M. and McGee, R.: *A Practical Approach to Measurement in Physical Education.* Philadelphia, Lea and Febiger, 1973.
7. Burt, C. L.: *Tests and Assessments of Physical Capacities.* London, London County Council, 1925.
8. Clarke, H.: *Physical and Motor Tests in the Medford Growth Study.* Englewood Cliffs, Prentice-Hall, 1971.
9. Cratty, B.: *Perceptual-motor Behavior and Educational Processes.* Springfield, Thomas, 1970.
10. Cratty, B.: *Movement Behavior and Motor Learning.* Philadelphia, Lea and Febiger, 1973.
11. Davies, B.: Effects of educational gymnastics on improvement of selected motor activities. *Br J Phys Educ. 2*:28-30, 1971.

12. Ecole Normale Supérieure d'Éducation Physique et Sportive: Valeur physique de la population française. *Annales E.N.S.E.P.S., 7*:1-50, 1975.

13. Evans, E. G.: *A Report of a Physical Performance Survey of Mid-Wales Secondary School Pupils.* Read before 10th meeting of I.C.S.P.F.T., Jyväskylä, 1973.

14. Fleishman, E. A.: *The Structure and Measurement of Physical Fitness.* London, Prentice-Hall, 1964.

15. Hebbelinck, M. and Borms, J.: *Tests en normenschalen van lichamelijke prestatie-geschiktheid, lengte en gewicht inbegrepen, voor jongens van 6 tot 13 jaar uit het lager onderwijs.* Brussels, Ministerie van Nationale Opvoeding en Nederlandse Cultuur, B.L.O.S.O., 1969.

16. Hebbelinck, M. and Borms, J.: *Tests en normemschalen van lichamelijke prestatie-geschiktheid, lengte en gewicht inbegrepen, voor meisjes van 6 tot 13 jaar uit het lager onderwijs.* Brussels, Ministerie van Nationale Opvoeding en Nederlandse Cultuur, B.L.O.S.O., 1973.

17. Hunsicker, P. and Reiff, G. G.: A survey and comparison of youth fitness, 1958-1965. *J Health, Phys Educ Recreation, 37*:23-25, 1966.

18. Ishiko, T.: Physical fitness of the Japanese. In Seliger, V. (Ed.): *Physical Fitness Proceedings of a Satellite Symposium,* XXV International Congress Physical Sciences, 1971. Praha, Universita Karlova, 1973, pp. 198-201.

19. Jéquier et al.: *History and Protocol of the Longitudinal Study of Trois-Rivières.* In Lavallée, H. and Shephard, R. J. (Eds.): *Frontiers of Physical Activity and Child Health.* Quebec City, Editions Pélican, 1977.

20. Kane, J.: *Psychological Aspects of Physical Education.* London, Routledge and Kegan, 1972.

21. Kane, J.: *Physical Education in Secondary Schools.* London, Macmillan, 1974.

22. Kemper, H. C. G. et al.: *Invloed van extra lichamelikje oefening.* Amsterdam, de Vrieseborch, 1974.

23. *Projekt Lichamelikje Oefening, fase 1: Ontwikkeling van meetinstrumenten; rapportage over het 2dc halfjaar 1975.* Amsterdam, U of Amsterdam, Jan Swammerdam Instituut, 1976.

24. Komadel, L., Havlicek, J., and Rehor, E.: The influence of four years sport training on the physical development of pupils aged eleven till fifteen years. In Grupe, O., Kurz, D. and Teipel, J. M. (Eds.): *Sport in the Modern World—Chances and Problems.* Berlin, Springer, 1973, pp. 213. Munchen, 1972.

25. Kraus, H. and Hirschland, R.: Muscular fitness and health. *J Health, Phys Educ Recreation, 24*:10-17, 1953.

26. Larson, L. (Ed.): *Fitness, Health and Work Capacity.* New York, Macmillan, 1974.

27. Lavallée, H. et al.: *Influence of a Primary School Physical Activity Program on Some Tests of Performance.* In Lavallée H. and Shephard, R. J. (Eds.): *Frontiers of Physical Activity and Child Health.* Quebec City, Editions Pélican, 1977.

28. Licht, S. and Johnson, C. W.: *Therapeutic Exercise*. New Haven, Elizabeth Licht Publisher, 1965, 449pp.
29. Mackenzie, J.: *The Vanves Experiment in Education*. Regina, Sask., Regina Board of Education, 1972.
30. Marchand, A. and Piché, D.: *Physical Education Program in Longitudinal Study of Children's Growth and Development*. In Lavallée, H. and Shephard, R. J. (Eds.): *Frontiers of Physical Activity and Child Health*. Quebec City, Editions Pélican, 1977.
31. McCaughan, L. R.: A physical ability test battery for New Zealand schools. *Capher J, 42*:8-17, 1975-1976.
32. Ostyn, M. et al.: Motorische vaardigheidstests voor jongens en meisjes uit het secundair onderwijs. Brussels, Ministerie van Nationale Opvoeding en Nederlandse Cultuur, B.L.O.S.O., 1975.
33. Oxendine, J.: *Psychology of Motor Learning*. Englewood Cliffs, Prentice Hall, 1968.
34. Pavek, F.: *The Motor Performance of 7-19 Years Youth in the Czechoslovak Socialist Republic*. Praha, Czechoslovak Sport Organisation, 1972.
35. Reljic, J. and Vukotic, E.: Quelques hypothèses sur l'influence des exercices physiques dans les écoles, sur les caractéristiques somatiques, motrices et conatives de la jeunesse. In Pieron, M. (Ed.): *Proceedings of the International Seminar on Research in Physical Education in Universities and Colleges, Paris, 1966*. Liège, 1968, pp. 57-67.
36. Ruskin, H. et al.: *Physical Performance of Elementary School Children in Israel*. Read before 11th meeting of I.C.P.F.R., Jerusalem, 1974.
37. Sage, G.: *Introduction to Motor Behavior*. Reading, Addison-Wesley, 1971.
38. Seto, S., Kawabata, A., and Oyama, Y.: The annual development of the motor ability of school boys and girls after the war. In Kato, K. (Ed.): *Proceedings of the International Congress of Sport Sciences, 1964*. Tokyo, The Japanese Union of Sport Sciences, 1966, pp. 468-471.
39. Shephard, R. J. et al.: *Influence of Added Activity Classes upon the Working Capacity of Quebec School Children*. In Lavallée, H. and Shephard, R. J. (Eds.): *Frontiers of Physical Activity and Child Health*. Quebec City, Editions Pélicans, 1977.
40. Simons, J., Beunen, G., and Renson, R.: *The Louvain Boys' Growth Study, Preliminary Report*. Leuven, Departement Lichamelikje Opvoeding, 1974.
41. Singer, R.: *Motor Learning and Human Performance*. New York, Macmillan, 1975.
42. Sprynarova, S.: Longitudinal study of the influence of different physical activity programs on functional capacity of the boys from 11 to 18 years. *Acta Paediatrica Belgica, Children and Exercise, 28* (suppl):204-213, 1974.
43. Sterev, P.: The effect of sport activities on physical development and physical fitness in teenagers. In Seliger, V. (Ed.): *XXV International Congress of Physical Sciences, 1971*. Praha, Universita Karlova, 1973, pp. 375-379.

44. Trzesniowski, R.: Stand der Körperlichen Entwicklung, der Körperlichen Leistungsfähigkeit und der Körperhaltung der Jugendlichen in Polen als Grundlage des Programs für die Körpererziehung in der Schule. Paper read at *International Congress of Physical Education, Liège, 1962.*

45. Weingarten, G. and Bar-Or, O.: The effects of frequency and content variation of physical education classes on social and athletic status in 4th grade children. In Bar-Or, O. (Ed.): *Proceedings of the Fourth International Symposium on Paediatric Work Physiology, 1972.* Natanya, Israel, The Wingate Institute, 1973, pp. 199-207.

Chapter 20

SEASONAL DIFFERENCES IN AEROBIC POWER

R. J. Shephard, H. Lavallée, J. C. Jéquier, R. LaBarre, M. Rajic,

and C. Beaucage

Abstract

Seasonal variations in fitness-related variables have been studied in a semilongitudinal sample of children from the Trois-Rivières region. Some 1600 measurements of maximum oxygen intake (direct treadmill measurements), P.W.C.$_{170}$, subcutaneous fat (nine skinfolds) and muscle strength (hand, back, knees) have been obtained on a population including equal numbers of boys and girls aged 6 to 12 years, drawn equally from an urban and a rural environment. Half of the group had received a normal single period of physical education per week, while the other half had been given five hours of additional training per week for one to three years. The maximal oxygen intake showed small (0.10 l/min) but highly significant (p<0.004) seasonal differences; irrespective of sex, milieu, or activity program, values were highest in November/December, with a decline throughout the remainder of the school year. The phenomenon cannot be explained in terms of seasonal variations in height, required activity, or the walk to school but may reflect voluntary participation in ice-hockey and figure skating from early November to mid-February. The bicycle ergometer data shows a disparate variation; urban children in particular have a high P.W.C.$_{170}$ during the summer months. It is suggested that in Quebec, unlike Europe, use of the bicycle is a seasonal event (mid-May to mid-October), and that local training of the quadriceps can have a favorable influence on the results of ergometer tests during the summer period. Muscle strengths and skinfold readings do not show any significant seasonal trends.

Seasonal Differences in Working Capacity

A RECENT STUDY FROM our laboratories[10] has shown a significant seasonal difference in the growth rate of French

194

Canadian schoolchildren. It was thus of interest to explore whether there were parallel variations in working capacity and other measures of physical fitness. Previous reports on this question have been conflicting. Adams et al.[1] examined Swedish children and found that physical working capacity at a pulse rate of 170 beats per minute (P.W.C.$_{170}$) was high during the summer months, seasonal discrepancies being particularly large in children who were initially unfit. In contrast Åstrand,[3] also in Sweden, and Knuttgen and Steėndahl[11] in Denmark found a low working capacity in the summer, with gradual recovery over the school year.

In reexamining this problem, we had several advantages over previous investigators. Our sample of children was large, and as each subject made several visits to the laboratory, problems of habituation and test learning[16] were minimized. The study participants were divided into equal sized groups, one (the "control") receiving only the standard program of physical education (one forty-minute period per week) and the other (the "experimental") having an additional nominal five hours of endurance training per week. There was thus a possibility of distinguishing true seasonal differences from the impact of the school training program. Students were also drawn in equal numbers from an urban area (Trois-Rivières) where the majority of students walked to school and from a rural region (Pont-Rouge) where they were transported by bus. This allowed consideration not only of activity required at school, but also of the possible training effect of a substantial daily walk during term time.[15, 18]

Methods

Subjects

The subjects were some 600 students recruited for the Trois-Rivières regional study of growth and development.[9] Three hundred of the group comprised entire classes from one of the twelve schools in Trois-Rivières, a medium-sized industrial city (population approximately 100,000); the remaining 300 were entire classes from the single school at Pont-Rouge, a fibre-board manufacturing village of some 4,000 people.

At each location, we examined approximately equal numbers of boys and girls, ranging in age from 6 to 12 years. The "experimental" group received an additional "hour" of endurance-type activities (running, vigorous ball games, and vigorous calisthenics) each school day, while the "control" group spent the corresponding period in academic pursuits.

When the present analysis was undertaken, students had participated in the special program for one to three years. Physiological measurements were made annually, within fifteen days of each child's birthday. Thus, three sets of annual data were available for most children, distributed throughout the year.

Physiological measurements

Physiological data were measured by standard techniques,[17] conforming closely with the recommendations of the International Biological Programme.[22]

MAXIMUM OXYGEN INTAKE: Maximum oxygen intake was determined directly during a progressive treadmill walk to exhaustion. After three-minutes warm-up at zero slope, 4 MPH (6.4 km/h) the same speed was sustained, and the slope was increased by 2.5 percent every two minutes until the child was exhausted. Oxygen consumption was determined by connecting a Collins-J valve to a gas analysis train (Capnograph® infrared CO_2 analyser, Servomex® O_2 analyser, and Parkinson-Cowan low resistance gas meter). Heart rates were measured from a continuously recorded chest electro-cardiogram. The test was necessarily self-limited at this age, although in view of frequent contacts with laboratory staff, the students were confident and well motivated. Average values for maximum oxygen intake, heart rates, and respiratory gas exchange ratios were thus well up to the values cited in most previous reports.

P.W.C.$_{170}$: P.W.C.$_{170}$ was determined by a three-stage progressive protocol.[8] The subjects pedalled a Monark bicycle ergometer at fifty pedal revolutions per minute, the load being increased at the end of the fourth and the eight minutes to produce a final effort of 75 to 85 percent aerobic power. Linear regressions were fitted to the data for individual subjects, and P.W.C$_{170}$ was obtained by interpolation or extrapolation.

MUSCLE FORCE: The handgrip force was measured for both right and left hands, using a handgrip dynamometer. Recorded values are the best of two definitive attempts. Back and leg strength were measured with a larger version of the dynamometer. For the back strength readings, the students tensed the arms against a horizontal bar with the back vertical. For the leg strength measurements, the subjects stood with their legs apart and flexed to about 120°, attempting to extend the knees against a harness passed around the hips.[12] The best of two definitive readings was again accepted for back and leg strength data.

SKINFOLD MEASUREMENTS: All readings were taken by a single experienced observer, using Harpenden skin calipers. Measurements sites included the chin, R. subscapular, R. triceps, R. biceps, R. midaxillary, abdomen, R. calf and R. chest. For the present purpose, only the average of these nine folds will be considered.

Statistical Analysis

For each of the variables studied, a linear regression was fitted, relating the measurement to age. From this line, predicted values were established for a given age, sex, milieu, and type of physical education program. Average discrepancies between observed and predicted values were then subjected to analyses of variance with respect to the season of measurement and age/season interactions.

A first series of analyses of variance was carried out separately on each age group (from 6 to 12 years old) to determine the effect of the time of the year on working capacity.

Further analyses made the assumptions that age was linearly correlated with physical performance, and that the time of year had no effect; appropriate statistical analyses were then carried out to detect any significant departures from the expected values.

The factor "time of year," computed in months, was also rearranged in groups of two, three, and six months, to assess more global trends.

The two independent covariables, age and time of the year, were utilized separately to adjust the observed values. The age by time of year interaction could not always be computed because there were unequal numbers of subjects in several categories.

Repeated measurements sampled annually on the same subject were treated as independent data, no specific provision being made to distinguish within from between-subject effects.

Results

Maximum oxygen intake

Data have been calculated both in absolute units (l/min) and relative to body weight (ml/kg-min). Formal statistical analysis (Table 20-I) shows deviations from the mean absolute maximum oxygen intake of 1.21 l/min ranging from -0.03 l/min in September and October to $+0.07$ l/min in November and December; although small, these trends have a chance probability <0.004. The high values of late fall are shown rather equally by boys ($p<0.026$) and girls ($p<0.014$); they are still apparent but less consistent when the data are divided into experimental ($p<0.12$) and control ($p<0.10$) groups and are found more uniformly in the rural ($p<0.018$) than in the urban ($p<0.16$) milieu.

The same phenomena are seen if maximum oxygen intake is expressed in relative units (ml/kg-min, Figs. 20-1 and 20-2). Values are lowest in the summer, with the highest values attained in the fall or winter. The maximum seasonal

Table 20-I. The effect of season on the directly measured maximum oxygen intake of children. Absolute values (l./min STPD), deviation from mean for all seasons, and significance of deviations after allowance for variation due to age and age/season covariance.

Season	All children Δ	Boys Δ	Girls Δ	Control Δ	Experi- mental Δ	Urban Δ	Rural Δ
Jan-Feb	-0.01	0.02	-0.02	-0.04	0.01	-0.03	-0.02
Mar-Apr	-0.01	-0.03	0.01	0.03	-0.04	0.00	-0.06
May-June	-0.01	0.06	-0.09	-0.02	0.01	-0.01	0.01
July-Aug	-0.01	-0.02	-0.02	0.00	-0.01	0.09	-0.01
Sept-Oct	-0.03	-0.08	0.03	-0.03	-0.04	-0.05	-0.05
Nov-Dec	0.07	0.08	0.07	0.06	0.08	0.07	0.09
Mean, all Season	1.31	1.36	1.25	1.29	1.32	1.43	1.22

Analysis of variance

	P	P	P	P	P	P	P
Age difference	0.190	0.999	0.999	0.001	0.033	0.117	0.999
Seasonal difference	0.004	0.026	0.014	0.119	0.100	0.157	0.018
Age/Season Interaction	.031	0.003	*	0.347	*	*	0.032

* Data insufficient for calculation

differential amounts to some 2.9 ml/kg-min (7%) in the girls and about 4 ml/kg-min (8%) in the boys. Statistical analysis (Table 20-II) with adjustment for age/season covariance again shows a peak during the months of November and December; this is largely sustained by the boys in January and February, but thereafter there is a progressive decline to a minimum in July and August. Curves for experimental and control groups move roughly in parallel (Fig. 20-1), and the phenomenon is seen in both urban and rural areas (Fig. 20-2).

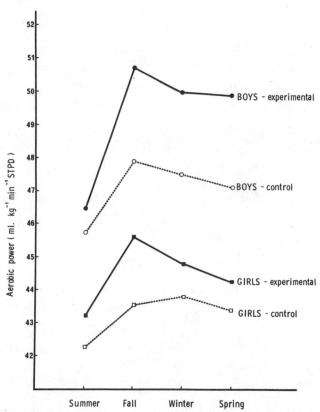

Figure 20-1. Aerobic power per kilo of body weight—seasonal differences for boys and for girls when divided into experimental and control groups.

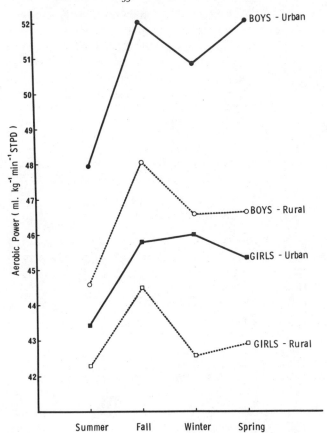

Figure 20-2. Aerobic power per kilo of body weight—seasonal differences for boys and for girls when divided into urban and rural groups.

Physical working capacity

The same type of analysis has been applied to the P.W.C.$_{170}$ data. Findings are similar for the absolute P.W.C.$_{170}$ and the values per unit body weight (kg-m/kg-min). In the boys (Fig. 20-3), both experimental and control groups show a high P.W.C.$_{170}$ in the spring and summer, with low results in the fall (October–December); the girls also show maxima in the summer (July–September) and minima in the fall.

Table 20-II.   The effect of season on the directly measured maximum oxygen intake of children. Relative values (ml./kg. min STPD) deviation from mean for all seasons, and significance of deviations after allowance for variation due to age and age/season convariance.

Season	All children	Boys	Girls	Control	Experimental	Urban	Rural
	Δ	Δ	Δ	Δ	Δ	Δ	Δ
Jan-Feb	0.16	1.51	0.02	1.24	-0.35	0.40	-0.37
Mar-Apr.	-0.23	-0.19	-0.05	-0.47	0.01	-0.19	-0.75
May-June	-0.01	-0.16	-0.16	-0.21	0.51	0.47	0.13
July-Aug.	-1.72	-2.08	-1.71	-1.84	-1.09	-1.47	1.14
Sept-Oct.	-0.49	-1.14	-0.27	-0.63	-0.57	-0.74	-0.76
Nov.-Dec.	1.57	1.80	1.22	1.96	1.13	1.22	2.04
Mean, all Season	46.4	48.3	44.2	45.3	47.2	48.3	45.0

Analysis of variance

	P	P	P	P	P	P	P
Age difference	0.297	0.999	0.318	0.121	0.008	0.056	0.999
Seasonal difference	0.003	0.007	0.130	0.024	0.155	0.289	0.004
Age/Season Interaction	0.021	0.051	*	0.012	*	*	0.999

* Data insufficient for calculation

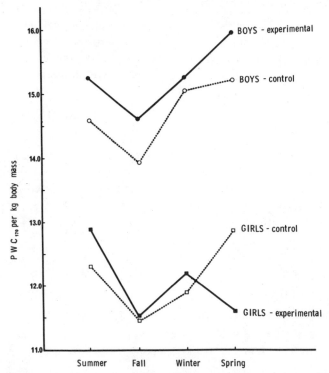

Figure 20-3. Physical working capacity (P.W.C.$_{170}$) per kg of body weight—seasonal differences for boys and for girls when divided into experimental and control groups.

The absolute P.W.C.$_{170}$ shows a fluctuation of 32.2 kg-m/min ($\approx$ 8%) about its mean value of 388 kg-m/min (Table 20-III). Low values are seen from November through February, with high values in the spring and summer. Results are less consistent than for maximum oxygen intake, and with the bimonthly grouping of data, the trend has a chance probability of 0.14. However, when the results are regrouped on a quarterly basis, the difference becomes significant ($p < 0.002$), with peak readings during the period July to September and a minimum from October to December. The relative P.W.C.$_{170}$ (kg-m/kg-min) shows a similar swing of 1.14 ($\approx$ 8%) about its mean value of 13.6 kg-m/kg-min, with the highest readings from July to September and the lowest from October to

Table 20-III. The effects of season on physical working capacity (P.W.C. $_{170}$) of children. Absolute values (kg-m/min), deviations from mean for all seasons, and significance of deviations after allowance for variation due to age and age/season covariance.

Season	All children Δ	Boys Δ	Girls Δ	Control Δ	Experimental Δ	Urban Δ	Rural Δ
Jan-Feb.	-18.1	-7.6	-7.3	-19-9	-16.9	-14.0	-21.2
Mar-Apr.	15.5	11.3	23.6	20.7	10.3	5.1	16.1
May-June	14.5	34.8	-7.4	17.2	12.4	12.8	20.9
July-Aug.	4.1	-1.5	-6.0	2.5	6.2	84.5	-16.4
Sept-Oct	4.0	-11.0	15.3	-7.4	10.3	0.2	0.1
Nov.-Dec.	-16.7	-23.6	-16.3	-19.6	-15.2	-23.9	-8.5
Mean, all Seasons	3.88	426	343	388	387	417	364

Analysis of variance

	P	P	P	P	P	P	P
Age difference	0.999	.254	.999	.108	.006	.999	.133
Seasonal difference	0.138	.117	.999	.999	.292	.075	.999
Age/Season Interaction	0.999	.390	*	.999	*	*	.064

* Data insufficient for calculation

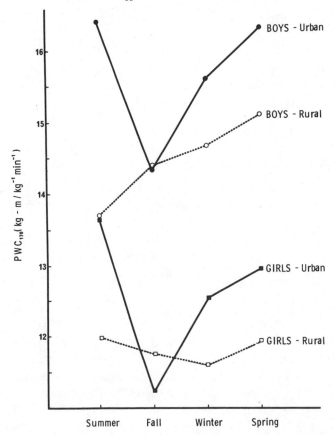

Figure 20-4. Physical working capacity (P.W.C.$_{170}$) per kg of body weight—seasonal differences for boys and for girls when divided into urban and rural groups.

December. Reasons for the less obvious seasonal trend in the bicycle ergometer data come from an analysis of subgroups. When data are divided by program, both experimental and control groups show a seasonal swing of 1.3 kg-m/kg-min, equally in the boys and the girls (fig. 20-4). However, when divided by milieu, seasonal differences are much larger in the urban environment (2.1 kg-m/kg-min in boys, 2.5 kg-m/kg-min in girls) than in the rural setting (1.4 kg-m/kg-min in boys, 0.4 kg-m/kg-min in girls).

Skinfold readings

None of the children studied were particularly obese, the average reading for the nine skinfolds amounting to 6.3 mm. Neither individual folds nor the summated readings for subcutaneous fat show seasonal differences significant at the 0.05 level of probability.

Muscle Strength

Average readings for hand-grip force and back and leg extension strength are all close to age-related norms, and no seasonal variations have been found.

Discussion

How far could the presently observed variations in fitness scores be attributable to the previously noted seasonal disparities of body size (10%)? The average height of the students was 129.3 cm, with a 0.5 cm deficit of height from April to June, and a 1.8 cm excess from July to September. Equally, with a mean weight of 27.6 kg, those tested in the spring were 0.4 kg lighter than predicted, while those seen in the summer and early fall were 0.7 kg heavier. The relationship between body size and physiological variables has been much discussed in recent years.[2, 18, 21] Theoretical considerations suggest power variables such as maximum oxygen intake and working capacity should be a quadratic function of height, but in practice both cross-sectional[4] and longitudinal[14] studies indicate an exponent of about 2.9. The seasonal variation in height could thus account for a 6 percent difference in working capacity, with a minimum in the spring and a maximum in the summer. While the bicycle ergometer results are thus at least partially explained, the variations of maximum oxygen intake, both absolute and relative, proceed in the opposite direction to what would be predicted from changes in body size.

A second possibility, advanced by Åstrand and Knuttgen and Steendahl,[11] is that required programs of physical education lead to a progressive increase of cardiorespiratory fitness over the school year. Several authors[5, 6, 13] have challenged this view, failing to find gains from either normal programs of physical activity or added physical education classes. Our data[20] do not support such a categoric indictment of physical education. Given a vigorous additional program of endurance activity, experimental students can develop a substantially higher aerobic power than control subjects. From Figure 20-1, this amounts to 2 to 4 ml/kg-min in boys, and about 1.5 ml/kg-min in girls. However, the advantage of the experimental group is present rather uniformly throughout the year. One must thus presume that the experimental students preserve a sufficient excess of physical activity during the summer vacation to maintain their advantage over the control group. Since parallel swings of aerobic power are shown by those receiving one and six periods of physical education per week, with both groups peaking in November and December and losing condition early in the calendar year, it seems impossible to attribute seasonal phenomena to the formal physical education classes.

A second common consequence of schooling is the need to walk a substantial daily journey to the place of instruction. Seliger[15] and the present authors[20] have both commented that the distance walked is greater for the urban child than for the rural student, since the latter usually has motor transport provided. The difference of required activity seems sufficient to produce slightly larger maximum oxygen intake readings in urban than in rural children.[15, 17, 20] However, it is not possible to explain seasonal variations of aerobic power on this basis—the winter journey is equally as long as in the fall, and in Quebec the work of the child is doubled or tripled[7] as he walks through deep snow. The weather is most conducive to additional voluntary outdoor activities in May and September; the pattern of variation in aerobic power that we have seen thus fails to match climatic changes.

It could be argued that hormonal factors regulating the growth of the cardiorespiratory system do not necessarily move in parallel with those regulating height. However, where separate development does occur (as at puberty), the sudden spurt of oxygen intake is accompanied by an increase of lean body mass. In the present experiments, total body weight and lean mass changed in phase with height. Another intriguing possibility is that we may be observing an inherent biorhythm, associated with winter migration. Nevertheless, before moving to such exotic concepts, it seems necessary to rule out more local environmental factors, such as the local ice-hockey and figure skating seasons, both of which extend from early November to mid-February.

It is now widely recognized[19] that, whereas the treadmill provides a measure of cardiorespiratory condition, responses to bicycle ergometer exercise are much more strongly influenced by local muscular training. The seasonal variation in $P.W.C._{170}$ may thus reflect the use of the bicycle as a means of transport. Because of weather conditions, children of the Trois-Rivières region use their bicycles only from mid-May to mid-October, a period that corresponds well with peak performance of the $P.W.C._{170}$ test. In rural Quebec, a combination of poorer socioeconomic conditions and an absence of sidewalks keeps many children from cycling even during the summer, so the different behavior of $P.W.C._{170}$ at Pont-Rouge is not unexpected. In Europe, conditions again differ, with children riding bicycles to school throughout the winter, an activity pattern that could well account for the progressive rise of P.W.C. readings over the school year, as reported by Åstrand and Knuttgen and Steendahl.[1]

In conclusion, we may note that there are significant seasonal differences in working capacity. These vary with the test modality and are of sufficient magnitude to require consideration when assessing responses both to physical education classes and to specific training programs.

References

1. Adams, F. H. et al.: The physical working capacity of normal school children. II. Swedish City and Country. *Pediatrics, 28*:243-257, 1961.
2. Asmussen, E. and Christensen, E. H.: *Kompendium i Legemsövelsernes*

Specielle Teori. Copenhagen, Kobenhavns Universitets Fond til Tilbejebringelse af Läremidler, 1967.

3. Åstrand, P. O.: *Fysiologiska synpunkter på skolungdomens fysika fostran; preliminär rapport till folksam.* Stockholm, Central Gymnastic Institute, 1961.

4. Åstrand, P. O.: The child in sport and physical activity—physiology. In Albinson, J. G. and Andrew, G. M. (Eds.): *The Child in Sport and Physical Activity.* Baltimore, University Park, 1976.

5. Bar-Or, O. and Zwiren, L. D.: Physiological effects of increased frequency of physical education classes and of endurance conditioning on 9 to 10 year old girls and boys. In Bar-Or, O. (Ed.): *Proceedings of the Fourth International Symposium on Paediatric Work Physiology, 1972.* Natanya, Israel, The Wingate Institute, 1973.

6. Cumming, G. R., Goulding, D., and Baggley, G.: Failure of school physical education to improve cardiorespiratory fitness. *Can Med Assoc J, 101*:69-73, 1969.

7. Henry, F. M.: Energy cost of progression. In Dittmer, D. S. and Grebe, R. M. (Eds.): *Handbook of Respiration.* Washington, D.C., American Physiological Society, 1958.

8. Howell, M. L. and MacNab, R. B. J.: *The Physical Work Capacity of Canadian Children Aged 7 to 17.* Toronto, Canadian Association for Health, Physical Education and Recreation, 1968.

9. Jéquier, J. C. et al.: History and Protocol of the Longitudinal Study of Trois-Rivières. In Lavallée, H. and Shephard, R. J. (Eds.): *Frontiers of Physical Activity and Child Health.* Québec City, Editions Pelican, 1977.

10. Jequier, J. C. et al.: *Seasonal variations in growth.* In preparation.

11. Knuttgen, H. G. and Steendahl, K.: Fitness of Danish school children during the course of one academic year. *Res Quart, 34*:34-40, 1963.

12. Mathews, D. K.: *Measurement in Physical Education.* Philadelphia, W. B. Saunders, 1963.

13. Mocellin, R. and Wasmund, U.: Investigations on the influence of a running-training programme on the cardiovascular and motor performance capacity in 53 boys and girls of a second and third primary school class. In Bar-Or, (Ed.): *Proceedings of the Fourth International Symposium on Paediatric Work Physiology, 1972.* Natanya, Israel, The Wingate Institute, 1973.

14. Ross, W. D. et al.: Maximal oxygen uptake and dimensional relationship in boys studied longitudinally. In *Proceedings, Pediatric Work Physiology Symposium.* Seč, Czechoslovakia, June 1974. To be published. Basel, Karger 1978.

15. Seliger, V.: Physical fitness of Czechoslovak children at 12 and 15 years of age. International Biological Programme. Results of investigations 1968-69. *Acta Univ Carol Gymnica (Prague), 5*:6-169, 1970.

16. Shephard, R. J.: Learning habituation, and training. *Int Z Angew Physiol, 28*:38-48, 1969.

17. Shephard, R. J. et al.: La capacité physique des enfants Canadiens: une

comparaison entre les enfants canadiens français, canadiens-anglais et esquimaux. I. Consommation maximale d'oxygène et debit cardiaque. *Union Méd, 103*:1767-1777, 1974.

18. Shephard, R. J.: Human Physiological Work Capacity: *I.B.P. Synthesis,* Volume IV. London, Cambridge University Press, 1978.

19. Shephard, R. J.: *Endurance Fitness,* 2nd ed. Toronto, University of Toronto Press, 1977.

20. Shephard, R. J. et al.: Influence of Added Physical Activity Classes Upon the Working Capacity of Quebec School Children. In Lavallée, H. and Shepard, R. J. (Eds.): *Frontiers of Physical Activity and Child Health.* Québec, City, Editions Pelican, 1977.

21. Von Döbeln, W.: Kroppsstorlek, Energiomsättning och Kondition. In Luthman G., Aberg, U., and Lundgren, N. (Eds.): *Handbook i. Ergonomi.* Stockholm, Almqvist and Wiksell, 1966.

22. Weiner, J. S. and Lourie, J. A.: *Human Biology. A guide to field methods.* Oxford, Blackwell, 1969.

Chapter 21

THE RELATIONSHIP BETWEEN SOMATIC DEVELOPMENT AND MOTOR ABILITY, AND THE THROWING VELOCITY IN HANDBALL FOR SECONDARY SCHOOL STUDENTS

J. Pauwels

Abstract

Correlations have been tested between handball throwing skill and physical fitness variables. Below the age of 16, strength is the most significant determinant, with some contribution from size. Speed and flexibility have little influence on scores. Over the age of 16, accumulated school instruction in handball apparently has a greater impact. Multiple correlations show that six variables account for 64 to 70 percent of variance at ages 13 to 15, 40 percent at age 16, and 50 percent at age 17.

HANDBALL IS A GAME which is becoming increasingly popular in Europe and, since Münich, has been included in the Olympic program. Throwing speed is a major skill; the faster the ball is thrown at the goal, the less time defense players and goal-keepers have for parrying the shot. We asked handball coaches from six countries what were the main determinants of the overarm throw. Their answers varied widely, referring to technical, somatic, and motor qualities. This made us decide to investigate the relationship between throwing speed and some aspects of physical fitness.

Methods

The test group consisted of 565 school boys between the ages of 12 and 19. The boys were asked to throw a regular leather

211

handball overarm at a target 0.5 m in diameter, positioned 9 meters from the throwing line. When the ball was released some photocells were obscured, thus starting a digital counter. The counter was stopped by the impact of the ball on the target. After a warm-up of five attempts, five maximum force throws were made. Of these throws, only those hitting the target were taken into account (Fig. 21-1).

We tested fifty-five experimental variables (see chapter Appendix), including anthropometric measurements and tests of strength, speed and flexibility. For the throwing test, a velocimeter was used.[20] The static strength was measured by cable tensiometry.[4] As for flexibility and speed, we included as-far-as-possible articulation, which plays an important part[2, 5, 12, 15, 18] in the throwing movement. Mindful of De Nayer's[7] statement that the choice of the measurement should be determined by the subject of the study undertaken, in addition to general somatic measurements we obtained specific data on the throwing arm. From these measurements, we derived various indices; because of the high growth rate between 12 and 16 years, such indices are preferable to gross

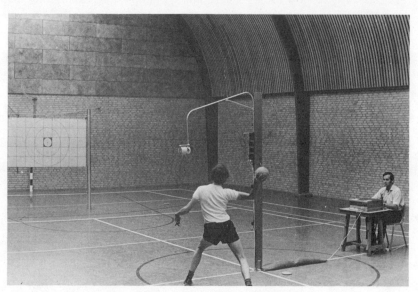

Figure 21-1. Test of throwing velocity.

measurements.[19, 29] We are well aware that other basic characteristics such as functional and explosive strength, running speed, body equilibrium, and eye-limb coordination[23] were not included in our test battery; however, these items seemed less interesting for our experiment.

The test group was given specific preparation for the throwing test. Their school physical education program included ball games as well as swimming and gymnastics. The time spent in developing the overarm throw was similar within a given age group, but as all classes had handball instruction, the older students were more experienced.

Both the throwing test (r = 0.95) and the flexibility and strength tests showed a very high reliability; the speed tests were also reliable, with coefficients of 0.70 to 0.85.

Results

For the throwing test, a remarkable increase of speed was observed from 12 to 16 years ($p < 0.01$), after which age the increase became less important. There are no other investigations of accurate throwing speed among a similar population. Nevertheless, if we compare our results with distance throws in motor performance tests,[1, 8, 9, 22] a striking difference emerges, since the most rapid increase of throwing speed took place between 15 and 16 years of age in our test. Whether this is because our throwing test is a specific skill or whether it reflects the composition of our test group is not clear.

The somatic data showed significant differences between successive age groups, except for the sixteen– and seventeen-year-olds. The averages for our group were somewhat lower than those observed by Twiesselman[25] and Vrijens,[27] but with the exception of the fourteen– and fifteen-year-olds, our results were somewhat higher than in the Leuven boy's growth study.[24]

The somatic indices generally remained constant, as the numerator and denominator both increased in a progressive and uniform way with age. However, some curves showed a rising or a falling line.

The static strength of the throwing arm increased constantly as a function of age up to 16 to 17 years. The largest increase was between 15 and 16 years. Handgrip force was very similar to that found in the Leuven boy's growth study.[24] Trunk strength also showed a consistent rise, performance more than doubling from 12 to 19 years, although coefficients of variation were large for these tests. Trunk indices did not differ between successive groups, except for the strength of abdominal and dorsal muscles. No general change of flexibility was observed. Speed of movement improved from 12 to 19 years, although to a much lesser degree than strength.

Relationships between throwing speed and physical fitness

SOMATIC DATA: Correlation coefficients suggest that this relationship was closest for the fourteen– and fifteen-year-olds, after which a sharp decline was seen. In the case of length measurements, the fall continued to eighteen– and nineteen-year-olds, whereas circumferences and weights showed a rise again after 16 years. Others have also found a decreasing influence of size and weight on throwing strength after 15 years.[8, 11] For subjects over the age of 15, Cozens,[6] Hooks,[13] and Watson[28] have reported low coefficients of correlation between throwing strength and anthropometric data. Several body indices showed maximum correlations at 14 and 15 and minimum correlations at 16, although, in general, differences were not so marked as for absolute measurements. In our study, absolute measurements correlated much better with motor throwing strength than did the indices (Fig. 21-5); we cannot support the preference for indices rather than simple measurements[19, 29] (see Fig. 21-2 and 21-3).

STATIC STRENGTH: As with the somatic data, large coefficients of static strength with arm throwing speed were observed for the fourteen– and fifteen-year-olds, with a sharp fall among sixteen-year-olds (Fig. 21-4). In the trunk (Fig. 21-5), the rise from 16 to 17 years continued through 18 and 19 years. Between 15 and 16 years, static strength increased, but there was a much larger increase of throwing speed. This may reflect improved throwing technique among the sixteen-year-olds.

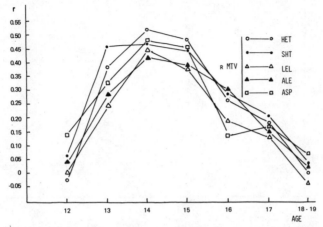

Figure 21-2. Correlation coefficients between throwing velocity and length measured as a function of age. See chapter appendix for key.

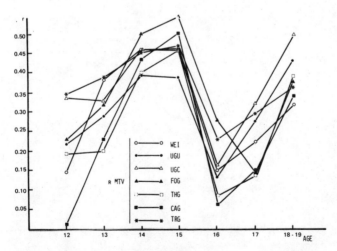

Figure 21-3. Correlation coefficients between throwing velocity and girths as a function of age. See chapter appendix for key.

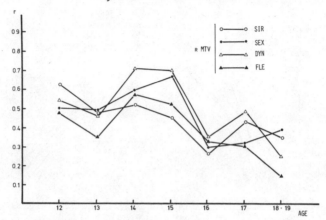

Figure 21-4. Correlation coefficients between throwing velocity and static strength of the arm as a function of age. See chapter appendix for key.

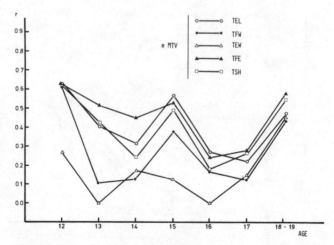

Figure 21-5. Correlation coefficients between throwing velocity and static strength of the trunk as a function of age. See chapter appendix for key.

The cross-sectional investigation cannot reveal whether the rate of increase of scores slows down during puberty with a rapid increase of the learning curve once puberty is over, since experience gathered in the fourteen– and fifteen-year-olds is "latent" and only exteriorized at the age of 16.[21]

FLEXIBILITY: Flexibility tests were poorly correlated, not only with throwing speed but also among themselves. Burley, Dobell, and Farell[3] also obtained low correlations.

LIMB SPEED: The relationship of limb speed to throwing speed was high in the fourteen-year-olds, and fell for the fifteen-year-olds rather than the sixteen-year-olds (Fig. 21-6). From the literature, it appears that the speed of a specific part of a movement does not necessarily imply an equal speed when performing the overall pattern. Motor variables have a limited correlation with throwing speed because of differences in throwing technique. Each subject makes maximum use of his specific motor qualities and disguises his weak points. Subjects who have not yet passed puberty seem to make more use of somatic and basic motor characteristics, whereas older and better trained subjects develop a greater throwing speed through better movement coordination.

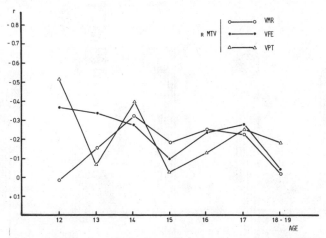

Figure 21-6. Correlation coefficients between throwing velocity and arm velocity as a function of age. See chapter appendix for key.

PREDICTION OF THROWING SPEED FROM SOMATIC AND MOTOR DATA: Multiple correlations show that for the thirteen–, fourteen–, and fifteen-year-olds, 64 to 70 percent of the variation in throwing speed can be explained by six variables. In sixteen-year-olds, the variance described drops to 40 percent, and for the seventeen-year-olds it is 50 percent. Strength has by far the best predictive value at all ages. The impact of somatic data is extremely variable, while flexibility and speed is—with a few exceptions—of little significance (Fig. 21-7). There is a great difference in the relative influence of somatic and motor data on throwing speed between the thirteen–, fourteen–, and fifteen-year-olds, and the sixteen– and seventeen-year-olds. Whether our hypothetical interpretation of this decrease in correlation is valid can only be shown by further large-scale longitudinal or cross-sectional research. However, our test does not reveal any decrease in throwing skill during puberty, as previously suggested by Gerdes,[10] Keeler,[17] and Meinel.[12] Our test group, in analogy with Knapp,[16] shows "no proof of loss in motor-coordination."

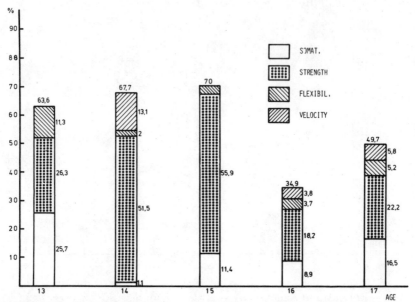

Figure 21-7. Multiple correlations, by age group. Ordinate shows percentage of total variance described.

APPENDIX: VARIABLES TESTED

A. Tests of Throwing Velocity

1. MTV : Maximal throwing velocity
2. ATV : Average throwing velocity

B. Static Strength of the Arm

3. SIR : Shoulder inward rotation
4. SEX : Shoulder extension
5. FLE : Elbow flexion
6. DYN : Handgrip dynamometer
7. TSA : Total strength of the arm
8. TSW : Total strength/weight

C. Static Strength of the Trunk

9. TFL : Trunk flexion
10. TEX : Trunk extension
11. TFW : Trunk flexion/weight
12. TEW : Trunk extension/weight
13. TFE : Trunk flexion + extension
14. TSH : Trunk flex. + ext./ sitting height
15. TEF : Trunk extension/trunk flexion

D. Flexibility

16. FLW : Flexibility of the wrist
17. FSI : Flexibility shoulder inward rotation
18. FSO : Flexibility shoulder outward rotation
19. TRO : Trunk rotation
20. SAR : Sit and reach

E. Velocity of the Arm

21. VMR : Velocity medial rotation
22. VFE : Velocity flexion-extension
23. VPT : Velocity plate tapping
24. TVE : Total velocity

F. Anthropometric measures

25. HET : Height
26. SHT : Sitting height
27. WEI : Weight
28. LEL : Leg length
29. ALE : Arm length
30. FOL : Forearm length
31. UPL : Upper-arm length
32. HAS : Hand span
33. HAH : Hand height
34. ASP : Arm span
35. SHW : Shoulder width
36. HWI : Hip width
37. UGU : Upper arm girth uncontracted
38. UGC : Upper arm girth contracted
39. FOG : Forearm girth
40. THG : Thigh girth
41. CAG : Calf girth
42. THG : Trunk girth
43. UUC : Upper arm circumference uncontracted-contracted

G. Anthropometric Indexes

44. TGW : Trunk girth/weight
45. STG : Shoulder width/trunk girth

46. TGTG : Thigh girth/trunk girth
47. UUTG : Upper arm girth uncontracted thigh girth
48. FGCG : Forearm girth/calf girth
49. SHH : Sitting height/height
50. ALH : Arm length/height
51. LLH : Leg length/height

52. SHLL : Sitting height/leg length
53. FGUA : Forearm girth + upper arm uncontracted/arm length
54. TGH : Trunk girth × height
55. WTCH : Weight + trunk girth × height

References

1. Anderson, C.: A method of data collection and processing for cinematographic analysis of human movement in three dimensions. Cited in *Completed Research in Health Phys. Ed. and Recreation,* Washington, D.C. A.A.H.P.E.R. 1970.
2. Broer, M. R. and Houtz, S. J.: *Patterns of Muscular Activity in Selected Sport Skills.* Springfield, Thomas, 1967.
3. Burley, L. R. et al: Relations of power, speed, flexibility and certain anthropometric measures of junior high school girls. *Res Quart, 32*:443-448, 1961.
4. Clarke, H. H.: Comparison of instruments for recording muscle strength. *Res Quart, 25*:398-411, 1954.
5. Cooper, J. M. and Glassow, R. B.: *Kinesiology.* St. Louis, The C. V. Mosby Company, 1963.
6. Cozens, F. W.: Strength tests as measures of general athletic ability in college men. *Res Quart, 11*:45-54, 1940.
7. De Nayer, P. P.: *Handleiding bij de cursus biometrie.* Leuven, Le Moniteur, 1956.
8. Espenschade, A. S.: Restudy of relationships between physical performances of school children and age, height and weight. *Res Quart, 34*:144-153, 1963.
9. Fleishman, E. A.: *The Dimension of Physical Fitness.* New Haven, Yale University, 1962.
10. Gerdes, O.: *Bezinning op de lichamelijke opvoeding.* Groningen, Wolters-Noordhoff & Stichting Onderwijs Oriëntatie, 1971.
11. Gross, E. A. and Casciani, J. A.: The value of age, height and weight as a classification device for secondary school students in the seven AAHPER Youth Fitness Tests. *Res Quart, 33*:49-58, 1962.
12. Hay, J.: *The Biomechanics of Sports Techniques.* Englewood Cliffs, Prentice-Hall Inc., 1973.
13. Hooks, G. E.: Prediction of baseball ability through an analysis of measures of strength and structure. *Res Quart, 30*:38-43, 1959.

14. Ismail, A. H., Christian, J. E., and Kessler, W. V.: Body composition relative to motor aptitude for preadolescent boys. *Res Quart, 34*:462-470, 1963.
15. Jankelic, J.: *Faktori koji dokazuju postojanje dvije tehnike sutiranja u rukometra.* Sarajewo, I. L. O., 1969.
16. Knapp, B.: *Skill in Sport.* London, Routledge & Kegan Paul, 1972.
17. Keeler, L. D.: The effect of maturation on physical skill as measured by the Johnson physical skill test. *Res Quart, 9*:54-58, 1938.
18. Lindner, E.: *Sprung und Wurf.* Schorndorf bei Stuttgart, Verlag Karl Hofmann, 1967.
19. Maglischo, W.: Bases of norms for cable-tension strength tests for upper elementary, junior high and senior high school girls. *Res Quart, 34*:595-596, 1968.
20. Malina, R. M. and Rarick, G. L.: A service for assessing the role of information feed-back in speed and accuracy of throwing performance. *Res Quart, 39*:220-223, 1968.
21. Meinel, K.: *Dewegungslehre.* Berlin, Volk und Wissen volkseigener Verlag, 1971.
22. Nys, G.: *De lichamelijke geschiktheid van de schoolgaande jeugd in België* (niet gepublic. doctoraatsthesis). K.U.L., Dept. L. O. Leuven, 1973.
23. Simons, J. et al.: Constructie van een motorische testbatterij van jongens van 12 tot 19 jaar, door middel van factor-analysen. *Sport, 13*:3-21, 1970.
24. Simons, J. et al.: *Studie van de physical fitness bij schoolgaande jongens van 12-tot 19 jarige leeftijd.* Leuven, I.L.O., Vol. I, 1971.
25. Twiesselmann, F., *Développement biométrique de l'enfant á l'adulte.* Bruxelles, Presses Universitaires, 1969.
26. Van Meerbeek, R.: Lichamelijke geschiktheidstests. *Sport, 12*:112-118, 1969.
27. Vrijens, J.: De huidige stand van de lichamelijke ontwikkeling bij de adolescenten. *Tijdschrift voor Lich Opvoed, 31*:22, 1969.
28. Watson, K. G.: A study of the relation of certain measurements of college women to throwing ability. *Res Quart, 8*:131-141, 1937.
29. Wutscherk, H.: Die Anthropometrie—eine Methode für die sportliche Praxis. *Theorie und Praxis der Körperkultur,* 648-660, 1969.

Chapter 22

PHYSICAL FITNESS AND SKELETAL MATURITY IN GIRLS AND BOYS 11 YEARS OF AGE

S. G. SAVOV

Abstract

Eleven-year-old boys attending sport schools have normal or late maturation, while girls at such schools are biologically advanced. Biological maturity
affects the total dimensions of the body and lengths but has less influence on
widths and diameters. Instances where biological maturity influences motor
performance are discussed with reference to strength, speed, and endurance.

WE EXAMINED 850 boys and 940 girls of chronological age 11
years who were attending Bulgarian sport schools. Biological maturation was determined from skeletal age and evaluation of genitalia. Physical development was determined from
twenty-seven anthropometric measurements of widths, lengths,
circumferences, and body proportions. A battery of fifteen
motor tests indicated certain motor abilities, including speed,
strength, endurance, and flexibility.

Methods

Skeletal age was determined according to Labitzke, Greulich,
and Pyle. We compared radiographic findings with an assessment of the genitalia as suggested by Tanner, checking the
reliability of the two methods and their correlation with other
data indicating the stage of maturation. Eight maturity groups
were established: three retarded groups (one, two and three

years respectively), one normal group, and four advanced groups (one, two, three, and four years respectively).

Results

Maturity

Evaluating subjects according to maturity, 41.2 percent of boys and 17.4 percent of girls belonged to the retarded groups (Fig. 22-1); on the other hand, 57.0 percent of girls and only 32.5 percent of boys fell into the advanced groups. The average chronological age of the boys was 11 years and 7 months, while their skeletal age was 12 years and 3 months; figures for the girls were 11 years and 9 months and 12 years and 11 months respectively. The development of the genitalia was found to vary as a function of the milieu, boys and girls from the cities being at a more advanced stage of development than those from small towns and villages. There was also a relationship between stature and genital maturity (Table 22-I), with coefficients of correlation of r = 0.64 and 0.73 for the two sexes.

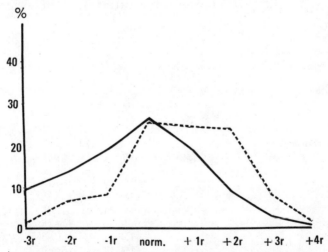

Figure 22-1. Percentage distribution of contigents by degree of maturity. Solid line: males. Broken line: females.

Table 22-I. Secondary sex characteristics of eleven-year-old girls and boys
in relation to the level of skeletal maturity.

Skeletal maturity	pubic hair		axillary hair		breast	facial hair	menarche
	boys	girls	boys	girls	girls	boys	girls
Normal	9.4%	37%	0.4%	18.4%	61%	–	0.21%
Advanced 1 year	14%	40%	0.7%	23.5%	66%	–	0.78%
Advanced 2 years	48%	71%	7.9%	54%	76%	–	12%
Advanced 3 years	55.6%	81%	20.0%	71.%	82%	2.5%	19%
Advanced 4 years	69.7%	94%	28.0%	79.0%	100%	6.4%	40%

Effects on body size

The average stature of the boys was 148.1 cm, and that of the girls 150.1 cm. There were significant differences of height ($p < 0.05$) between retarded, normal, and advanced groups of children (Table 22-II). We examined certain regional measurements. The most outstanding maturity-related differences were in length measurements, while diameters and widths showed only slight variations with biological age. These differences gradually disappeared with growth and by the age of 15 to 16 the girls showed only differences of weight and girth.

TABLE 22-II
STATURE OF ELEVEN-YEAR-OLD BOYS AND GIRLS AT DIFFERENT STAGES
OF BIOLOGICAL MATURITY.

Deviation of biological from chronological age.		Stature (cm)	
	(years)	Boys	Girls
	−3	134.95	133.10
	−2	138.97	137.18
	−1	142.02	145.88
	0	143.74	147.86
	+1	148.99	154.46
	+2	153.07	156.92
	+3	156.13	161.40
	+4	167.40	163.55

Effects on performance

There were differences of motor activity and coordination between boys and girls. The classification of biological maturity was also related to motor performance. We thus had to analyze details of the basic motor qualities (speed, strength, endurance, and flexibility) in our eight maturity groups, looking for effects of maturation on the evolution of motor activity.

Absolute speeds for 30 m and 60 m dashes were equal for boys and girls over the age range 8 to 12 years (Tables 22-III and IV). The scores of the boys were generally uninfluenced by maturity, although the most advanced scored better, probably because of puberty and associated development of body dimensions. In the girls, scores were unrelated to maturity.

Strength is determined largely by the total dimensions of the body. Thus biological maturity had a big influence on strength, as seen in such tests as the standing long jump, throwing a 1 kg ball with both hands, grip, and trunk power. The worst results were found in the retarded groups, although retarded groups fared better on the "chin up," probably because of the negative influence of body weight on performance of this test.

Endurance (as measured by an 800 m run for boys and a 600 m run for girls) was better in children with accelerated development, particularly in the boys. The maximal oxygen consumption (per kilogram of body weight) was maximal for girls of normal maturity, with decrements in both advanced and retarded groups.

Flexibility. Results of the flexibility tests were higher for girls one to two years advanced in development, while in more advanced groups (three to four years) there was a decrement. Score were also lower for retarded girls. In boys, values were higher only in those advanced by three to four years.

TABLE 22-III

PHYSICAL FITNESS IN RELATION TO SKELETAL AGE (BOYS WITH CHRONOLOGICAL AGE OF ELEVEN YEARS).

	Skeletal age						
	8y	9y	10y	11y	12y	13y	14y
30 m dash (sec)	4.55 ±0.04	4.41 ±0.02	4.38 ±0.05	4.36 ±0.04	4.34 ±0.03	4.28 ±0.02	4.18 ±0.03
60 m dash (sec)	10.41 ±0.88	10.01 ±0.84	10.21 ±0.89	10.18 ±0.78	9.79 ±0.70	9.57 ±0.82	9.34 ±0.79
standing broad jump	169.75 ±15	176.63 ±18	179.75 ±21	181.04 ±19	182.6 ±18	186.8 ±23	192.62 ±17
vertical jump	30.5 ±5	32.69 ±8	33.07 ±7	33.69 ±6	35.27 ±5	35.93 ±6	37.87 ±8
throwing 1 kg ball with two hands over the head	7.20 ±0.77	7.78 ±0.83	7.89 ±0.91	7.98 ±0.77	8.34 ±0.83	8.68 ±0.88	9.14 ±0.93
strength of left hand grip (kg)	20.77 ±8.11	22.12 ±9.17	27.79 ±41.21	28.51 ±10.13	29.47 ±9.77	31.15 ±8.97	34.12 ±12.11
strength of right hand grip (kg)	23.47 ±9.12	25.18 ±8.15	29.74 ±8.59	30.32 ±40.18	31.64 ±9.72	33.8 ±11.18	37.87 ±9.32
trunk power (units)	46.57 ±10.08	51.18 ±12.11	57.27 ±13.05	62.11 ±10.77	70.58 ±13.83	73.24 ±14.18	82.37 ±14.97
800 m run (min, sec)	3.29.2 ±0.11	3.28.4 ±0.10	3.26.4 ±0.08	3.20.2 ±0.13	3.18.6 ±0.14	3.18.5 ±0.10	3.14.8 ±0.12
$\dot{V}o_2$ (ml/kg-min)	53.9 ±4.7	51.37 ±3.8	51.20 ±4.0	52.99 ±3.9	52.09 ±4.5	50.13 ±4.3	50.40 ±4.4
flexibility (units)	9.28 ±4.8	8.47 ±7.2	9.39 ±6.4	9.57 ±8.1	11.37 ±6.2	17.71 ±4.9	16.78 ±5.8

TABLE 22-IV

PHYSICAL FITNESS IN RELATION TO SKELETAL AGE (GIRLS WITH CHRONOLOGICAL AGE OF 11 YEARS)

	Skeletal age							
	8y	9y	10y	11y	12y	13y	14y	15y
30 m dash (sec)	4.53	4.57	4.41	4.61	4.59	4.63	4.81	4.86
	±0.03	±0.02	±0.04	±0.04	±0.03	±0.04	±0.03	±0.02
60 m dash (sec)	9.78	9.80	9.83	9.81	9.84	9.88	9.84	9.79
	±0.78	±0.76	±0.91	±0.97	±0.87	±0.85	±0.98	±0.92
standing broad jump	167.92	170.57	178.9	182.21	183.83	185.33	186.27	186.97
	±18	±20	±21	±20	±23	±21	±17	±15
vertical jump	30.17	32.02	32.99	33.17	34.8	38.55	36.80	36.97
	±5	±6	±7	±7	±5	±7	±6	±9
throwing 1 kg ball with two hands over the head	6.73	7.07	7.44	7.59	7.92	8.01	8.44	8.89
	±0.75	±0.80	±0.73	±0.92	±0.77	±0.94	±0.87	±0.99
strength of left hand grip (kg)	14.37	15.83	17.42	18.51	20.28	23.79	25.01	26.32
	±7.32	±8.15	±7.77	±9.75	±8.44	±9.1	±12.1	±11.77
strength of right hand grip (kg)	15.12	16.38	18.52	19.17	22.47	24.88	27.31	28.58
	±7.15	±8.31	±9.25	±10.48	±13.15	±10.72	±9.15	±10.28
trunk power (units)	37.21	43.01	52.72	56.96	63.61	65.09	67.38	68.28
	±11.77	±12.15	±10.47	±13.72	±14.28	±13.52	±12.38	±13.73
800 m run (min/sec)	2.23.5	2.23.9	2.25.7	2.22.1	2.23.3	2.22.6	2.23.1	2.23.9
	±0.11	±0.10	±0.08	±0.07	±0.08	±0.13	±0.11	±0.09
$\dot{V}o_2$ (ml/kg·min)	46.52	46.87	47.24	50.24	49.37	49.13	48.29	46.79
	±3.4	±3.6	±3.9	±4.2	±3.8	±3.7	±3.4	±3.3
flexibility (units)	9.97	10.21	10.82	14.19	15.68	13.17	12.33	13.25
	±5.8	±6.7	±4.9	±8.3	±5.7	±6.5	±7.4	±8.1

References

Greulich, W. W. & Pyle, S. I.: *Radiographic Atlas of Skeletal Development of Hand and Wrist. 2nd Ed.* California, Stanford University Press, 1959.

Tanner, J. M., Whitehouse, R. H. & Healy, M. J. R.: *A new system for estimating skeletal maturity from the hand and wrist, with standards derived from a study of 2600 healthy British children.* Paris, Centre Internationale de l'Enfance, 1962.

Chapter 23

MOTOR PERFORMANCE AS RELATED TO CHRONOLOGICAL AGE AND MATURATION

G. Beunen, M. Ostyn, R. Renson, J. Simons, and D. Van Gerven

Abstract

Relationships of chronological age (CA) and skeletal age (SA) (Tanner et al., 1959, 1962) to motor performance (Simons et al., 1969) have been analysed in 2162 boys with CA 13y and 1574 boys with SA 13y (Louvain Boys' Growth Study). First order partial correlations between SA and the measurements were calculated with CA held constant, and between CA and the measurements with SA held constant. The evolution of mean values for different SA– and CA-levels was also studied. Partial correlations between SA and height, weight, and static strength were highly significant. They were lower, but still significant, for speed of limb movement and explosive strength. A negative correlation was found between trunk and functional strength. Partial correlations between CA and height or weight were zero or negative. Positive relationships were found for all motor tests. The results indicate that correlations are higher in tests where complex and repeated movement is required, e.g. speed of limb movement ($r = .265$), than for static strength ($r = .054$); CA has a greater influence on complex than on simple tests.

Several authors have stressed the importance of physical maturation to the development of physical fitness during preadolescent and adolescent years (Beunen, 1974). Attempts have been made to determine to what degree the better performance of older boys depends on their greater height, larger muscular cross sections and masses, larger lung volumes, etc. (Asmussen and Heebøll-Nielsen, 1955, 1956; Åstrand, 1970; Asmussen, 1973; Carron and Bailey, 1974, 1975). Such studies suggest that the performance of older boys improves more than would be expected from their increase of size. In the present study we have analyzed relationships between motor fitness and chronological and skeletal age, taking groups that were homogenous for skeletal and chronological age respectively.

Methods and material

Data are taken from a longitudinal and cross sectional study of Belgian school boys (The Louvain Growth Study,* Simons, Beunen, and Renson, 1974). The present paper concerns results on 8165 boys of 12 through 15 years chronological age and 7454 boys of 12 through 15 years skeletal age. All subjects were tested during the months of January through March, 1969–1972. Height and weight were measured, along with eight motor tests (Simons et al., 1969). Skeletal age was determined according to the method of Tanner, Whitehouse, and Healy (1959, 1962), all assessments being by the same observer. Pearson product-moment correlations were calculated between dependent variables. Within each chronological age group, first order partial correlations were also calculated between skeletal age and the independent variables, with adjustment for chronological age within each skeletal age group; first order partial correlations were also calculated between chronological age and the independent variables, skeletal age being held constant. Finally, one year skeletal age categories were formed in every chronological age group and one year chronological age categories were formed in every skeletal age group.

Results

Differences in the relationships between skeletal age and the measurements and between chronological age and the same

*Grants have been received from the Ministries of Dutch and French Culture; Administrations of Physical Education, Sports and Open Air Activities; and the Ministry of Public Health and Welfare.

measurements are similar at all ages. We will thus report only the data obtained for thirteen-year-old boys (chronological or skeletal age).†

In Table 23-I the first order partial correlations between the two dependent variables and the independent variables are given. Height, weight, and static strength (arm pull) are highly related to skeletal age. Relationships with other motor fitness components are fairly low but differ significantly from zero, except for eye-hand coordination (stick balance) and running speed (shuttle run). Trunk strength (leg lifts) and functional strength (flexed arm hang) are negatively correlated with skeletal age at this age, although at 14 or 15 a positive relationship is found.

Chronological age has a slight negative relationship to weight and no correlation with height. Of the motor fitness items, the lowest partial correlation is for static strength. For other tests, the correlations are larger, especially for speed of limb movement (plate tapping). The figures show mean data for

TABLE 23-I

FIRST ORDER PARTIAL CORRELATIONS BETWEEN SKELETAL AGE (SA), CHRONOLOGICAL (CA), AND PHYSICAL FITNESS COMPONENTS. DATA FOR THIRTEEN-YEAR-OLD BOYS.

	$r_{SA\text{-}Var.\ CA}$	$r_{CA\text{-}Var.\ SA}$
Height	.663	−.012*
Weight	.604	−.086
Stick balance	−.016*	.126
Plate tapping	.096	.265
Sit and reach	.027*	.063
Vertical jump	.155	.101
Arm pull	.526	.054
Leg lifts	−.122	.100
Flexed arm hang	−.134	.137
Shuttle run	.004*	−.079
N	2162	1574

*partial correlation not significantly different from zero.

---

†Data for the other groups studied can be obtained from the senior author. For the evolution of relationships between skeletal age and physical fitness, see Beunen et al., 1976.

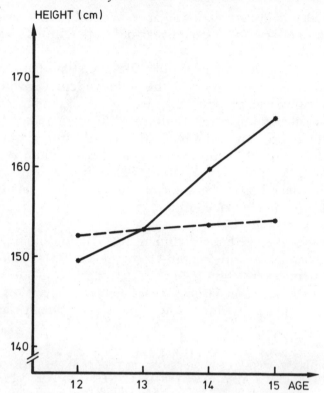

Figure 23-1. Evolution of height as a function of chronological and skeletal age. Solid line: skeletal age, with chronological age held constant at thirteen years. Broken line: Chronological age, with skeletal age held constant at thirteen years.

thirteen-year-old boys of differing skeletal age categories (12 through 15) and mean data for boys with a skeletal age of 13 years, chronological age varying from 12 through 15.

The increase of height as a function of chronological age at a given skeletal maturity is rather small (Fig. 23-1). On the other hand, the increase of height as a function of skeletal age at a given chronological age is fairly large. Almost the same trends are found for static strength, although the increase as a

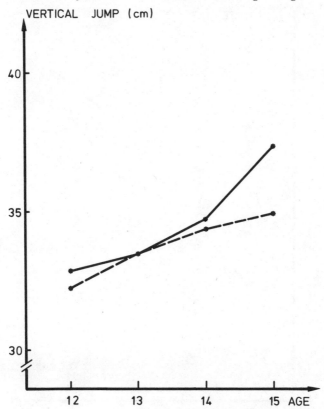

Figure 23-2. Evolution of vertical jump scores as a function of chronological and skeletal age. Solid line: skeletal age, with chronological age held constant at thirteen years. Broken line: Chronological age, with skeletal age held constant at thirteen years.

function of chronological age is a little larger than for standing height. The evolution of explosive strength (vertical jump, Fig. 23-2) is similar whether expressed as a function of skeletal age or of chronological age. For plate tapping (speed of limb movement), a still more complex motor test, the increase of score depends more on chronological age than on skeletal age (Fig. 23-3).

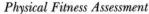

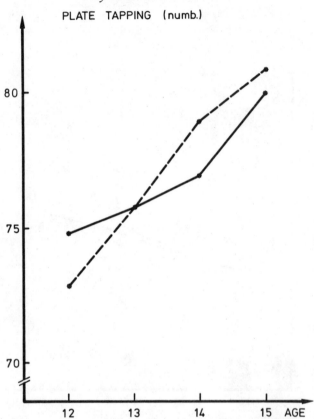

Figure 23-3. Evolution of plate tapping scores as a function of chronological and skeletal age. Solid line: skeletal age, with chronological age held constant at thirteen years. Broken line: Chronological age, with skeletal age held constant at thirteen years.

Discussion

The height trend reported in this study is in agreement with Tanner (1969) who stated that "children who are slow to reach a given bone age are eventually taller than those who reach it earlier." Skeletal maturity is related to static strength over the whole age range studied. For most other components, a positive relationship occurs at a chronological age of 14 and 15 years

(Beunen, 1976). If adjustment is made for skeletal age, the relationship between chronological age and static strength is slight but significantly different from zero at 12 and 13 years; at 14 and 15 years the relationship vanishes. More complex tests such as the vertical jump and plate tapping have higher partial correlations, indicating that age per se contributed to such performance. This confirms the findings of Asmussen and Heebøll-Nielsen (1955, 1956), Åstrand (1970), Asmussen (1973), and Carron and Bailey (1974-1975). All of these authors found increases of performance larger than anticipated from the increase in size; all concluded that performance was related to chronological age.

Some possible explanations can be suggested on the basis of previous work. Cheek (1968) has proven that there is a remarkable increase of cell number during adolescence. In boys, the population of muscle cells doubles during the period 10 to 16 years of age. Cheek suggested that androgens may act with growth hormone to ensure multiplication of muscle nuclei. He also noted that, in the first instance, cell number should be related to chronological age, since the number of mitoses is time-dependent. The low partial correlations between chronological age and static and functional strength could possibly be explained through this phenomenon.

Åstrand and Rodahl (1970) suggested a possible sexual maturity factor. However, skeletal maturity and sexual maturity are interrelated, and relationships with chronological age must be attributed to other factors.

Asmussen and Heebøll-Nielsen (1955, 1956) and Carron and Bailey (1974, 1975) suggested the possibility of qualitative changes in the muscle or the neuromuscular system. This seems plausible, since higher correlations are found for more complex motor fitness components. In support of this hypothesis, Åstrand and Rodahl (1970) state that the pyramidal system only attains full functional maturity at puberty. Fine coordinated movements depend on integration of nervous activity from various levels of the CNS and from peripheral receptors. Ungerer (1973) reported that only from age 15 were boys able to execute some of the peripheral movements by which the different movement entities are dynamically connected.

Fomin and Filin (1975) also commented that the precision of movement developed markedly from 11 through 13 years of age; from 13 through 15, children were less susceptible to negative influences from the external environment, due to better inhibition and regulation of movement under the influence of the cerebral cortex. Zaciorskij (1972) has stated that the more motor connections a child possesses, the more motor skills he can control and the easier new movements are executed. It is reasonable to assume that with increasing age, a child builds up additional motor connections from the experiences of daily physical activity.

As a final remark, the findings of Connolly are worth mentioning; he showed that gains in speed of muscular movement were a linear function of age to 16 years. Three types of variable may account for the observed increases in speed of performance:

1. Hardware changes, i.e. neurological, neurophysiological and mechanical changes. Overall functioning develops with improvement in the different parts.
2. Software changes, i.e. the use made of existing functions. A child cuts out unnecessary operations and develops more effective filtering mechanisms.
3. Interactions of hardware and software changes: with the progressive establishment of organized neural networks and enriched experience, the effective functional size of the brain is increased and the capacity for central processing is enlarged.

As a final conclusion, we would agree with Carron and Bailey (1975) that those who are involved in the evaluation of physical performance must be aware of the influence of maturation upon this performance. Nevertheless, they should also be aware that during growth, age per se influences performance. Both maturation and chronological age should be taken into account when the physical educator evaluates the performance of growing children.

References

Asmussen, E. and Heebøll-Nielsen, Kr.: A dimensional analysis of physical performance and growth in boys. *J Appl Physiol,* 7:593-603, 1955.

Asmussen, E. and Heebøll-Nielsen, Kr.: Physical performance and growth in children. Influence of age, sex and intelligence. *J Appl Physiol, 8*:371-380, 1956.

Asmussen, E.: Growth in muscular strength and power. In Rarick, G. L. (Ed.): *Physical Activity. Human Growth and Development.* New York, Academic Press, 1973, pp. 60-79.

Åstrand, P. O. and Rodahl, K.: *Textbook of Work Physiology,* New York, McGraw Hill, 1970.

Beunen, G. et al.: Skeletal maturity and physical fitness in 12– to 15-year old boys. In Borms, J. and Hebbelinck, M. (Eds.) *Children and Exercise. Proceedings of the Vth International Symposium, Acta Paed. belg., 28,* suppl.:221-232, 1974.

Beunen, G. et al.: *A Correlational Analysis of Skeletal Maturity, Structural Measures and Motor Fitness of Boys 12 through 16.* Read before International Congress of Physical Activity Sciences, Quebec, 1976.

Carron, A. V. and Bailey, D. A.: Growth and development in strength. *J. C.A.H.P.E.R., 41*:8-11, 1975.

Cheek, D. B.: *Human Growth—Body Composition, Cell Growth, Energy and Intelligence.* Philadelphia, Lea & Febiger, 1968.

Connolly, K.: Skill development: Problems and plans. In Connolly, K. (Ed.): *Mechanisms of Motor Skill Development.* London, Blackwell, 1970, pp. 3-17.

Fomin, N. A. and Filin, W. P.: *Altersspezifische Grundlagen der körperlichen Erziehung,* Schorndorf, Hofman, 1975.

Simons, J. et al.: Construction d'une batterie de tests d'aptitude motrice pour garçons de 12 à 19 ans, par la méthode de l'analyse factorielle. *Kinanthropologie, 1*:323-362, 1969.

Simons, J., Beunen, G., and Renson, R.: *The Louvain Boys' Growth Study. Preliminary report,* Leuven, Dept Physical Education, K. U. Leuven, 1974.

Tanner, J. M. and Whitehouse, R. H.: *Standards for Skeletal Maturity, Part I.* Paris, International Children's Centre, 1959.

Tanner, J. M., Whitehouse, R. H., and Healy, M. J. R.: *A New System for Estimating Skeletal Maturity from the Hand and Wrist, With Standards Derived from a Study of 2,600 Healthy British Children. Part II; The scoring system.* Paris, International Children's Centre, 1962.

Tanner, J. M.: *Growth at Adolescence.* Oxford, Blackwell, 1969.

Ungerer, D.: *Leistungs- und Belastungsfähigkeit im Kindes- und Jugendalter.* Schorndorf, Hofmann, 1973.

Zaciorskij, V. M.: *Die Körperlichen Eigenschaften des Sportlers.* Berlin, Bartels & Wernitz, 1972.

Chapter 24

THE IMPACT OF ECOLOGICAL FACTORS AND PHYSICAL ACTIVITY ON THE SOMATIC AND MOTOR DEVELOPMENT OF PRESCHOOL CHILDREN

J. Pařízková

Abstract

In a representative sample of 6.4-year-old Czech children (n = 5631), boys were significantly taller and heavier than girls, with higher values for most somatic variables except thigh circumference and skinfold thicknesses. Performance in the 20 m dash, broad jump, and cricket ball throw were better in boys, while the results in skill and sensori-motor tests tended to be better in girls. Children from Prague were taller and heavier and had worse physical performance than children from small villages. The same applied to children from families with a high per capita income and first born children. Regularly exercised children had greater heights and weights, and also better performance, than those not taking regular exercise. In Prague, 246 children were followed from 3 to 6 years of age. Results showed improving performance, better step test scores, larger body dimensions, unchanged or decreasing subcutaneous fat, and deteriorating posture.

THERE IS LITTLE comprehensive data on the somatic, functional and motor development of preschool children, particularly in reference to their economic, ecologic, hygienic, and familial background. Optimal motor stimulation results not only from spontaneous physical activity (which is at a very high level at this period of life)[4] but also from physical education specific to this age period. The latter may be very important for desirable development of the child, not only immediately but also in later life. In some sports (figure skating, gymnastics, swimming), a certain amount of training has already started at this age. However, we do not know the effect of intensive training at an early age; it may have either positive or negative immediate and delayed manifestations. On the other hand, marked restriction of physical activity is becoming characteristic of the way of life in industrially developed countries, and this may interfere with the development of the child with regard to functional capacity, fitness, posture, and body composition.

Six-year-old Children

Our first study examined 2866 boys and 2765 girls from Bohemia and Moravia; forty-five variables were measured just before the children entered the first class of primary school. Their mean age was 6.4 years.

SEX DIFFERENCES: The boys were taller, heavier, and had larger chest and abdominal circumferences; their performance in the 20 m dash, standing broad jump, and cricket ball throw were also significantly better than in the girls. On the other hand, the girls had greater arm and thigh circumferences, better posture, more success in skill tests (walking on a beam, forward roll, catching a ball in different situations) and a higher level of sensori-motor development as evaluated by the "open-close hands test"[3] especially in its more complicated items.

ECONOMIC FACTORS: Children from the capital were taller and heavier than children from communities with less than 1000 inhabitants, but in spite of better results in sensori-motor tests, they had a poorer performance for the 20 m dash and (in the cases of the boys) for the cricket ball throw (Fig. 24-1). With regard to economic level (per capita income) mean values of height and weight were always within the national standards (±0.5 SD), but nevertheless children from families with a higher income were taller and heavier. This did not guarantee them a higher level of performance; indeed it was usually poorer, or at best the same (Fig. 24-2).

SOCIOCULTURAL FACTORS: Children from happy families displayed better development than children from broken homes, and a similar situation was found in children brought

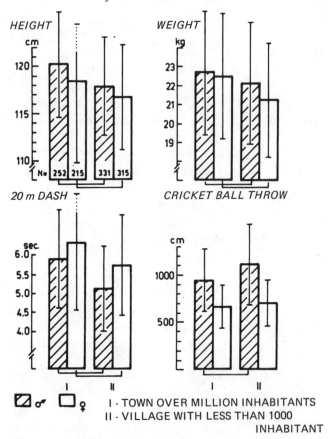

Figure 24-1. Somatic development and performance of preschool children (6.4 years) from communities with differing numbers of inhabitants.

up in kindergartens. First born children were taller and heavier than children born as fourth to fifteenth members of a family. Again, greater somatic dimensions did not lead to better physical performance; indeed the results of the 20 m dash and the cricket ball throw were significantly worse, especially in girls.

PHYSICAL EDUCATION: Children who had already participated in preschool age physical education had a higher level of physical performance on such items as broad jump and cricket

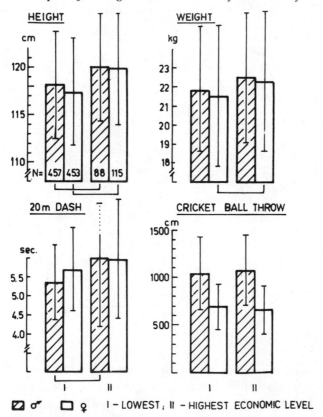

Figure 24-2. Somatic development and performance of preschool children (6.4 years) from families with differing per capita income.

ball throw, and also showed larger body dimensions (Table 24-I).[6-8]

Children Aged 3 to 6 Years

A further sample of children aged 3 to 6 years was drawn from four kindergartens in different parts of Prague (boys n = 127, girls n = 112). The children had a relatively constant daily regimen of activity and diet and came from a homogeneous

Physical Fitness Assessment

Table 24-I. Characteristics of six-year-old children.

Physical education (years of duration)		0		1		2-3	
		X̄	SD	X̄	SD	X̄	SD
Weight (kg)	♂	22.19	3.20	22.26	2.71	23.60	2.30
	♀	21.60	3.30	22.30	3.40	22.10	3.60
Height circumf (cm)	♂	118.6	5.3	119.4	5.3	120.8	5.1
	♀	117.6	5.2	118.6	5.3	119.0	5.5
Chest (cm)	♂	59.2	3.3	59.6	2.9	61.0	3.4
	♀	57.9	3.7	58.5	3.6	58.2	4.1
20 m dash (sec)	♂	5.4	1.1	5.6	1.3	5.5	1.2
	♀	5.7	1.2	5.7	1.3	5.7	1.2
Broad jump (cm)	♂	108.0	20.9	109.9	17.9	119.9	22.3
	♀	100.7	20.4	105.0	20.1	110.6	18.4
Cricket ball throw (cm) (right hand)	♂	1060	391	1075	421	1081	419
	♀	676	220	722	235	717	240
Cricket ball throw (cm) (left hand)	♂	672	240	683	278	752	302
	♀	519	163	549	166	551	168

familial and socioeconomic environment. A broad selection of morphological variables was examined. Skinfold thicknesses were measured by both Best and Harpenden calipers, and a modified step test was used (height 25 cm, rate of mounting 30/min).[1] As the children were not yet able to keep time, a technician ascended the steps with two children, holding their hands lightly. From the pulse rate during the step test, we calculated Brouha's step index and the cardiac efficiency index:[1]

$$CE = \frac{\text{total amount of work}}{\text{sum of pulses during work and recovery}}$$

total amount of work = number of mounts × height of the step

The performance in selected disciplines, skill tests, and hand grip strength (using a special tensiometric dynamometer[10]) brought the total variables measured to 145.

DEVELOPMENT OF BODY BUILD: Dimensions were greater in boys than in girls, except in the four-year-old boys where we happened to select slightly smaller subjects (Table 24-II). The skeleton was more robust, with greater circumferences of the head, neck, etc. With advancing age, different variables increased at a differing pace. Growth of the lower extremities contribute more to height than growth of the trunk (especially the iliospinal-tibial length). Weight increased much more than height. Breadths and circumferential measurements increased less than linear dimensions. The skeleton, as judged from wrist

Table 24-II. Development of six-year-old children.

		♂	♀	♂	♀	♂	♀	♂	♀
Age (years)	X̄	3.52	3.42	4.44	4.47	5.55	5.46	6.36	6.33
	SD	0.28	0.32	0.27	0.33	0.27	0.30	0.24	0.22
Height (cm)	X̄	101.1	99.5	105.3	107.7	113.5	112.8	119.2	118.7
	SD	4.2	5.0	5.1	5.9	5.8	4.8	4.1	4.9
Weight (kg)	X̄	16.62	15.69	17.44	18.34	20.85	19.65	22.10	21.59
	SD	1.97	2.24	2.40	3.47	2.76	2.52	2.68	2.81
Length of lower extre-	X̄	42.5	40.9	43.5	44.9	48.9	46.8	51.2	50.0
mities (cm)	SD	2.0	2.5	2.8	2.5	3.2	2.6	2.0	2.5
Biacromial	X̄	23.1	22.8	23.9	24.4	25.6	25.6	26.2	26.1
diameter (cm)	SD	1.0	1.2	1.2	1.4	1.4	0.9	1.0	1.1
Biiliocrist	X̄	16.8	16.5	17.4	17.7	18.6	18.0	19.4	19.2
diameter (cm)	SD	0.8	1.0	1.0	1.1	0.9	1.5	0.9	1.1
Bicondylar	X̄	7.1	6.6	6.9	6.9	7.4	7.0	7.5	6.9
femur (cm)	SD	0.3	0.4	0.3	0.4	0.3	0.3	0.3	0.5
Chest circum-	X̄	54.2	52.6	54.4	54.3	57.3	55.4	58.2	57.2
ference (cm)	SD	2.4	2.6	2.8	2.8	2.7	2.6	3.1	3.4
Thigh circum-	X̄	31.9	32.2	31.7	34.1	34.8	35.2	35.4	36.4
ference (cm)	SD	2.3	2.5	1.8	3.2	2.7	3.2	2.5	2.2
Sum of ten skinfolds	X̄	41.7	53.3	41.6	50.1	43.1	46.6	38.3	49.3
(Best; mm)	SD	17.5	18.8	9.6	11.9	17.0	15.0	10.1	18.1
20 m dash	X̄	6.8	7.4	5.9	6.2	5.0	5.1	4.9	5.1
(sec)	SD	0.8	0.8	0.8	0.7	0.4	0.2	0.9	0.2
Broad jump	X̄	60.7	59.0	75.5	71.6	95.8	90.9	103.4	96.2
(cm)	SD	15.3	18.6	12.8	15.6	14.4	17.7	18.7	16.4
Cricket ball	X̄	419.4	326.5	562.5	438.3	813.1	601.2	1028.0	695.6
throw (cm)	SD	142.3	101.4	199.9	131.9	209.3	126.9	404.7	135.2
Step test	X̄	87.0	82.8	91.4	90.6	92.2	92.7	99.9	98.3
index	SD	8.0	6.5	9.2	7.4	10.2	10.3	9.9	10.8
Cardiac effi-	X̄	0.469	0.426	0.508	0.525	0.604	0.551	0.653	0.643
ciency index	SD	0.079	0.076	0.080	0.115	0.113	0.093	0.078	0.112
Hand grip	X̄	7.6	5.6	7.6	7.5	12.0	9.6	13.7	11.3
strength (kp)	SD	1.5	1.4	2.2	2.4	2.5	2.4	2.4	2.2

breadth, bicondylar humerus, femur and ankle breadths, and the circumferences of the neck and head increased the least. This development is reflected in various relative dimensions, e.g. a decrease of sitting height relative to total height and a decrease in shoulder breadth relative to total height.

The only morphological variables which did not increase from 3 to 6 years were the skinfold thicknesses. In boys, the sum of ten or eleven skinfolds actually decreased, while in girls the changes were insignificant. Thus, the increase of body weight reflected development of lean body mass. Such changes may be related to the increasing level of physical activity in this period of life,[4] which has been called "the golden age of motrice."[11, 12] After mastering basic motor skills, the child improves its motor abilities further and enjoys activity and exercise very much.

POSTURE: Body posture was evaluated simply,[2] making a three-grade classification of the back, neck, and abdomen (observed from the profile) and shoulders, shoulder blades, and vertebral column (observed from the back). Girls tended to have a better posture than boys. The worst postures were found in the back and abdomen. With advancing age, the situation deteriorated, presumably due to insufficient physical activity in the urban environment.

FITNESS INDICES: The step test results improved from 3 to 6 years, both in boys and girls. Although the older children performed more work, increments of pulse rate during exercise were smaller.

SPORTS PERFORMANCE: The taller and older the child, the better the efficiency of work on the step test. Practically all age groups showed significant correlations between somatic development and the cardiac efficiency index (CE); sometimes, there were also correlations with Brouha's step test index. Taller children have their center of gravity situated slightly higher and this can play an important role during the step test. Correlations among breadth and circumferential measurements on the one hand and the cardiovascular indices on the other again showed that larger and more robust children had a greater efficiency of work. Sex differences were apparent even at the age of 3 years. The performance of boys in running, jumping, and throwing was better than that of the girls, while the latter were better in some skill tests such as forward roll and standing on one foot. Achievements in all the disciplines mentioned improved with advancing age.

SENSORI-MOTOR SKILLS: Scores for the "open-close hands test" did not display any marked sexual differences, although such had been seen in the larger sample of 6.4-year-old children. The same applied to laterality tests. Improvements with age were obvious in both boys and girls, although even in the oldest children tested perfection had not been reached relative to reported data for United States children.[3]

STRENGTH: The hand grip force (right and left) was significantly greater in boys than in girls. In both sexes, it practically doubled from 3 to 6 years. However, in the youngest age group, the sex difference was relatively greater (30%) than in the oldest age group (20%).

GENETIC FACTORS: Significant correlations were found between the height of the child and the height of mother or father. The same indicators were related to the linear dimensions of the trunk and extremities in the children. There were also relationships between the height or weight of the parents and selected breadth measurements (biiliocristal diameters, bicondylar humeral and femoral diameters etc.) or circumferential measurements in the children. No relationships were apparent between the height or weight of the parents and the development of subcutaneous fat in children.

OVER-NUTRITION: Only two children were obese. Severe obesity is very rare at this age period; it seems that over-nutrition results in a general increase of all body dimensions rather than in the deposition of excess fat.[5, 6] Nevertheless, children with more subcutaneous fat had poor results in running, jumping, and throwing, while children with large dimensions displayed better performance. There were also significant positive correlations between hand grip force and performance in running, jumping, and throwing. Correlations between the step test results (especially when expressed as indices) and performance suggested that cardiovascular development predisposed to a better performance in running, jumping, and muscle strength tests.

Conclusions

Both studies indicate marked sexual differentiation of morphological and motor development among preschool boys and girls. Only step test scores displayed no sex differences. In motor performance, primary sexual differentiation was apparently involved, since physical education was identical for both sexes. Urban life, family income, a happy home, and birth order all modified the morphological and motor development of preschool children. Regular exercise accelerated both somatic and motor development even at this period of life.

References

1. Čermák, J. et al.: Reaction of the circulatory system of preschool children to a work-load of medium intensity as related to the degree of somatic development. *Physiol Bohemoslov, 22*:377-8, 1974.
2. Jaroš, M. and Lomíček, K.: Posture in children in school age. *Čs Hygiena, 1*:342-7, 1956 (in Czech).
3. Keogh, J. F.: *Developmental Evaluation of Limb Movement Tasks.* Technical Report 1-68 (USPHS Grant HD 01059). Los Angeles, U California, 1968, p. 31.
4. Ledovskaya, H. M.: Physical activity in preschool children in Novosibirsk. In Slonim, A.D. and Smirnov, K. M. (Eds.): *Physical Activity of Man and Hypokinesia.* Novosibirsk, Acad Sci USSR, Siberian Dept, Inst Physiology, 1972, pp. 22-29 (in Russian).
5. Pařízková, J.: Body composition and lipid metabolism. (Proceedings of European Nutrition Conference, Cambridge, July 1973.) *Proc Nutr Soc, 32*:181-6, 1973.
6. Pařízková, J.: Body composition, lipid metabolism and physical activity. Stenfert, H. E. and Kroese, N.V. (Eds.). Leiden, Holland, Leiden Univ. Press, 1976.
7. Pařízková, J. and Berdychová J.: The impact of ecological factors on somatic and motor development in preschool children. *Teor Praxe těl Vých, 24*:58-62, 1976 (in Czech).
8. Pařízková, J. and Berdychová J.: The impact of physical education and kindergarten on the development of preschool children. (International Conference Spartakiade, Prague, 1975.) *In Proceedings,* Metod. Bull. ČSTV, Prague, 1976.
9. Pařízková, J., Čermák, J., and Horná, J.: Nutritional requirements, somatic and functional development of preschool children. In Débry G. & Blayer R. (Ed.) *Proceedings 2nd International Symposium "Alimentation et travail," Vitell, France,* Paris, Masson & Cie, 1974.

10. Sukop, J.: The development of muscle strength and sport performance as related to age and different physical education regime. In: *Proceedings Scientific Committee of Czechoslovak Sport Organization (ČSTV), Prague,* 127-41, *1966* (in Czech).

11. Wolaňski, N.: Methods of control and norms of the development of children and adolescents. *Panstwowy zaklad wydawnictw lekarskich.* Warsaw, Polish Acad. Sciences, 1975 (in Polish).

12. Wolaňski N. and Pařízková, J.: Physical fitness and the development of man. *Sport i Turystyka.* Warszaw, 1976 (in Polish).

Chapter 25

SOCIAL DIFFERENTIATION OF PHYSICAL FITNESS OF PREADOLESCENT BELGIAN BOYS

R. Renson, G. Beunen, M. Ostyn, J. Simons, P. Swalus, and D. Van Gerven

Abstract

This chapter investigates the extent to which the somatic development, the motor ability, and the sport behavior of Belgian preadolescent boys are differentiated by sociocultural factors. Data were analyzed from 5,336 twelve- to fourteen-year-old boys, stemming from a representative sample of the Belgian lower secondary school system. The following sociocultural factors were operationalized as independent variables: educational level of the parents, socioprofessional and sociogeographic origin, family size and birth order, grade point average, type of schooling, school affiliation, language group, and parents' sports involvement. Boys of the lower social strata, rural youth, boys from larger families, and pupils in vocational schools were somewhat retarded in physical development and general motor ability and were less active in particular sports.

IN ATTEMPTING TO outline the conceptual background of the social approach to physical fitness, one may call upon the sociological theory of action (Parsons, 1961). As for "the sport group" (Lüschen, 1969), so also "physical fitness" is part of the general social action system, which consists of (1) culture— values and norms, (2) the social system—all types of social groups and structures, (3) the personality system, and (4) the behavioral organism. These four systems are arranged in a hierarchy of *control* ranging from culture to behavioral organism and a hierarchy of *conditioning* in the reverse direction. The general action system is related most directly to the physical and organic environment through the behavioral organism. Furthermore . . . "factors such as age, sex, social class and skill are partly environmental, but they may be the focuses of rules of the sport group, arising in part from the overall concern for such broad values as competitive achievement, (physical fitness)*, and fair play" (Lüschen, 1969). This chapter investigates the extent to which somatic development, motor ability, and sport behavior of twelve– to fourteen-year-old Belgian boys are differentiated by sociocultural factors. Special attention is paid to methodological aspects of the social approach to physical fitness.

Methods

Results were analyzed from 5,341 twelve– to fourteen-year-old Belgian school boys, taken from the Leuven-Louvain Boy's Growth Study (Simons et al. 1974). Data were collected in fifty-eight schools across Belgium from 1969 to 1971. The *physical fitness evaluation* consisted of nineteen anthropometric measures, determination of the body type and skeletal maturity, eight motor ability tests, and a one minute step test (Table 1).

A questionnaire completed by the boys' parents gave information on sociocultural background. A detailed survey of sports participation by both the boys and their parents was also made. Missing data, response errors, and falsifications were detected by interviewing each student. Of the questionnaires delivered, 89 percent were returned properly completed. An overview of the *sociocultural variables* is presented in Table 25-I.

In addition to factor analyses and reliability studies on the various physical fitness items (Simons, 1969; Van Gerven, 1972; Beunen, 1973), a reliability and an objectivity study was undertaken on the questionnaire data (Renson, 1973).

Methodological Design

One of the aims of data analysis was to distinguish sociocultural variables primordial to the differentiation of the

---

*Author's insertion.

TABLE 25-I
LIST OF THE DEPENDENT AND INDEPENDENT VARIABLES

Independent Variables:
Sociocultural Determinants
• Educational level of father (9 levels)
• Educational level of mother (9)
• Socioprofessional status, father (9)
• Degree of urbanization (9)
• Family size
• Birth order
• Sports participation of father (7)
• Sports participation of mother (7)
• School point averages
• Type of schooling
• School affiliation
• Language group (Renson, 1973)

Dependent Variables: Physical Fitness Items

Age
—Chronological age
—Skeletal age (Tanner, Whitehouse, and Healy, 1962)

Somatic
—Body weight
—Body length (3 measures)
—Body width (4 measures)
—Perimeters (6 measures)
—Skinfolds (5 measures) (Van Gerven, 1972)
—Endomorphy
—Mesomorphy
—Ectomorphy
—Ponderal index (Sheldon, Stevens, and Tucker, 1963)

Motor
—Stick balance
—Plate tapping
—Sit and reach
—Vertical jump
—Arm pull
—Leg lifts
—Flexed arm hang
—Shuttle run (50 m)
—Sum T-scores (Simons et al., 1969)
—One minute step test (40 cm bench) (Ostyn and Van Gerven 1967-68)

Sport
—Soccer
—Volleyball
—Basketball
—Handball
—Swimming
—Track & field
—Gymnastics
—Tennis
—Judo
—Rugby
—Badminton
—"Other sports"
—"Other watersports"
—"Other ballgames"
—Number of sports practised
—Number of hours per week (Renson, 1973)

various aspects of physical fitness from secondary or pseudo-relationships. This was not easy, since sociocultural variables coincide to a certain degree, and one also has to consider the reciprocal influences between physical, motor, and sports items. However, in addition to studying the relationship between each separate sociocultural variable on the one hand and the various physical fitness items on the other, an attempt was made to unravel the network of interdependent physical, motor, and sport-behavioral factors. This social approach to physical fitness can be presented as a conceptual model.

Results

The Interrelationship Between Sociocultural Variables (Independent Variables)

In order to assess the degree of interdependence between the sociocultural variables, *Pearson-correlations* as well as *multiple correlations* were calculated. These indicated, for instance, a high correlation between the educational level of the father and his socioprofessional status (r = 0.80). There was also a correspondence between the educational and the socioprofessional level of the father and the educational level of the mother (r = 0.69 and 0.60 respectively). The relationship between the other sociocultural determinants was smaller, with the exception of the anticipated correspondence between family size and birth order (r = 0.74).

A sociographic analysis concerning the socioprofessional and sociogeographic constitution of all categories of each sociocultural variable is reported elsewhere (Renson, 1973).

The Relationship Between Somatic Development, Motor Fitness, and Sports Participation (Dependent Variables)

SOMATIC DEVELOPMENT AND MOTOR FITNESS: The relationship between anthropometric characteristics and skeletal maturity on the one hand and the results of motor tests on the other has been investigated using *Pearson r's* (Swalus, 1970; Renson, Beunen, and Van Gerven, 1972; Beunen, 1973; Renson, 1973).

Striking positive correlation were seen between body weight and arm pull test results in thirteen-year-old boys (r = 0.70). There was also a significant negative correlation between skinfold measurements and scores on the flexed arm hang test (r = 0.47). These correlations have to be taken into account when comparing the physical fitness of different social groups. The fact that one category (for example, the sons of independent tradesmen and craftsmen) is characterized by a relatively heavy body weight might explain their high arm pull results relative to other social groups (Renson, 1973).

SOMATIC DEVELOPMENT AND SPORTS PARTICIPATION: In the Leuven-Louvain Boy's Growth Study, comparisons have been made between athletes and nonathletes, boys with varying amounts of sports participation, and boys from different sport disciplines (Renson, 1971; 1973; 1974-75). However, somatic development cannot be viewed seperately from motor development.

MOTOR FITNESS AND SPORTS PARTICIPATION: Most studies of the relationship between sports participation and motor fitness take into consideration physical as well as motor aspects of the individuals studied. Athletes and nonathletes are much more differentiated for motor fitness variables than for anthropometric characteristics, but the mesomorphic component is clearly higher for sports participants than for nonparticipants (Renson, 1973).

The Relationship Between Sociocultural Variables (Independent) and the Physical Fitness Items (Dependent)

Although many correlation coefficients between the sociocultural variables and the physical fitness items were statistically significant, their actual dependence was small, the highest correlation coefficient between an anthropobiological variable and a sociocultural variable (between family size and the mesomorhpic component among twelve-year-old boys) amounting to only r = 0.18.

Among motor tests, the highest correlation was found between the flexed arm hang results and family size (r = 0.16) while for sports participation the largest r was between the practice of swimming and the mother's sports participation (r = 0.26), both for twelve-year-old subjects.

Table 25-II lists the highest correlation coefficient between each sociocultural variable and somatic motor and sports behavioral variables for twelve–, thirteen–, and fourteen-year-old boys.

Discussion

The nature of individual correlation coefficients was fairly similar for the three preadolescent age groups. From the low correlations observed, multiple and partial correlations would have little application in detecting primary and secondary sociocultural determinants: Moreover, the relationship between sociocultural variables and physical fitness variables was generally nonlinear. This implied that Pearson correlation coefficients were not particularly appropriate methods of data analysis. Therefore, the rather cumbrous calculations involved in t and F tests were applied.

Of the three status determinants (*father's and mother's educational level and father's socioprofessional status*), the socioprofessional background produced the greatest differentiation of anthropobiological and motor variables. The positive correlation of socioprofessional background with ectomorphic component and ponderal index (see Table 25-II) indicated that the relatively greater body height of the higher social groups was not associated with a parallel development of breadth. The preadolescent boys of the higher intellectual and socioprofessional strata were in fact characterized by more body linearity. On the whole, there was a positive relationship between the status determinants and explosive strength (vertical jump, see Table 25-II), functional strength, and running speed. On the contrary, the step test pulse rates were inversely related to sociocultural background. In respect to sports participation, identical differentiation patterns were found for the three social status determinants, proving that a social stratification of sports already existed among preadolescent Belgian boys.

The differentiation of physical fitness as a function of

TABLE 25-II
HIGHEST CORRELATION COEFFICIENTS BETWEEN SOCIOCULTURAL VARIABLES AND THE SOMATIC, MOTOR, AND SPORT BEHAVIORAL DATA FROM 12 TO 14 YEAR OLD BOYS.

Sociocultural Variables*	Physical Fitness Variables — Somatic, motor and sport behavioral aspects					
	12 year old boys N = 528		**13 year old boys** N = 2,131		**14 year old boys** N = 2,682	
Educational Level of Father (9 levels)	Ponderal Index	.154	Ponderal Index	.145	Ponderal Index	.150
	Vertical Jump	.095	Vertical Jump	.127	Step test	−.115
	Swimming	.207	Swimming	.186	Swimming	.166
Educational Level of Mother (9 levels)	Ponderal Index	.136	Ponderal Index	.130	Ponderal Index	.117
	Vertical Jump	.125	Vertical Jump	.086	Step test	−.100
	Tennis	.217	Swimming	.170	Tennis	.166
Socioprofessional Status of Father (9 strata)	Ponderal Index	.151	Ponderal Index	.125	Ponderal Index	.121
	Vertical Jump	.125	Vertical Jump	.069	Step test	−.094
	Tennis	.174	Swimming	.134	Swimming	.150
Degree of Urbanization (9 levels)	Suprailiac fold	.158	Height	.110	Ponderal Index	.102
	Step test	−.140	Vertical Jump	.126	Vertical Jump	.095
	Swimming	.207	Swimming	.179	Swimming	.149
Family Size (N of children)	Mesomorphy	.176	Height	−.141	Thigh circumf.	−.141
	Flexed Arm Hang	.162	Vertical Jump	−.106	Step test	−.100
	Track & field	.129	Swimming	−.078	Soccer	.066
Birth Order	Mesomorphy	.166	Height	−.115	Mesomorphy	.124
	Flexed Arm Hang	.145	Step test	.086	Flexed Arm Hang	.081
	Volleyball	.144	Swimming	−.056	Soccer	.073
Sports Participation of Father (7 categories)	Skinf. upp. arm	.105	Ponderal Index	.081	Ponderal Index	.084
	Plate Tapping	.075	Vertical Jump	.123	Leg lifts	.106
	Swimming	.215	Swimming	.218	Number of sports	.205
Sports Participation of Mother (7 categories)	Skinf. upp. arm	.155	Mesomorphy	−.062	Ponderal Index	.082
	Arm pull	.085	Leg lifts	.063	Vertical Jump	.083
	Swimming	.257	Swimming	.214	Number of sports	.211
.05 level of significance		.086		.040		.038
.01 level of significance		.112		.053		.050

*Only those sociocultural variables were included which contained an hierarchical order.

urbanization presented several points in common with differentiation according to socioprofessional origin. The sociographic analysis of the sample had shown that certain socioprofessional layers were associated with specific sociogeographic environments. Vertical jump results were positively related to the degree of urbanization, whereas step test results showed an inverse relationship (as was the case for the socioprofessional group of farmers' sons).

The average skeletal age decreased as a function of *family size* and *birth order*. All anthropometric measures demonstrated a negative relationship to family size and birth order. Endomorphy was highest among only children and first borns and it decreased with an increase of family size or birth order. For the mesomorphic component, the opposite was true. Only children differed significantly in their somatic development not only from children of larger families, but also from other first borns of families with several children. With regard to motor fitness, boys of smaller families and first born boys obtained better results for explosive strength (vertical jump), whereas the boys of larger families and those with a higher birth order exhibited greater functional strength (flexed arm hang), faster running speed, and better step test results. There was no significant difference of sports behavior between boys from different types of family, nor were there differences related to birth order.

The breaking down of *parental sports participation* into seven categories based on the age limit of their sports participation and on their club membership did not appear relevant to the somatic and motor differentiation of their preadolescent sons. A dichotomous distinction between sporting and nonsporting categories, however, revealed some differences. The sons of nonathletic fathers exhibited a poorer general motor fitness but had better step test results. Boys with athletic parents showed a greater sports participation, practiced a greater number of sports (Table 25-II), and were overrepresented in the "higher social status sports." The last observation must be related to the fact that the sports participation of adult Belgians is determined by their social status and the degree of urbanization of their dwelling area (Renson and Vermeulen, 1972).

References

Beunen, G.: *Skeletale ontwikkeling en physical fitness.* Doctor's thesis Physical Education, Leuven, Dept Phys Ed, K.U. Leuven, 1973.

Lüschen, G.: Small group research and the group in sport. In Kenyon, G. S. (Ed.): *Aspects of Contemporary Sport Sociology.* Chicago, Athletic Institute, 1969, pp. 57-66.

Ostyn, M. and Van Gerven, D.: Application d'un steptest de 1 minute au contrôle médico-sportif. *Trav Soc Med Belg Ed Phys Sports, 20*:133-139, 1967-68.

Parsons, T.: An outline of the social system. In Parsons, T. et al. (Eds.): *Theories of Society.* pp. 30-84, New York, Free Press, 1965.

Renson, R.: Comparison of athletes versus nonathletes among Belgian secondary school boys aged 12 to 19. *J Sports Med Phys Fitness, 11*:213-221, 1971.

Renson, R., Beunen, G., and Van Gerven, D.; Relations entre des mesures somatiques et les résultats de certains tests de souplesse. *Kinanthropologie, 4*:131-145, 1972.

Renson, R. and Vermeulen, A.: Sociale determinanten van de sportpraktijk bij Belgische volwassenen. *Sport* (Brussel), *15*:25-39, 1972.

Renson, R.: *Sociokulturele determinanten van de somatische ontwikkeling, de motorische vaardigheid en het sportgedrag van 13-jarige Belgische jongens.* Doctor's thesis Physical Education, Leuven, Dept Phys Ed, K.U. Leuven, 1973.

Renson, R. et al.: Physical fitness van 13-jarige Belgische jongens in funktie van hum sportparticipatie. *Werk Belg Gen Veren Lich Opvoed Sport, 24*:138-147, 1974-75.

Sheldon, W. Stevens, S. S., and Tucker, W. B.: *The Varieties of Human Physique.* Darien, Conn., Hafner, 1970.

Simons, J. et al.: Construction terie de tests d' aptitude motrice pour garçons de 12 á 19 ans, par la méthode de l'analyse factorielle. *Kinanthropologie, 1*:323-362, 1969.

Simons, J. Beunen, G., and Renson, R.: *The Louvain Boys' Growth Study, a preliminary report.* Leuven, Dept Phys Ed, K.U. Leuven, 1974.

Swalus, P. et al.: Comparaison des méthodes de Sheldon, Parnell et Heath-Carter pour la détermination du somatotype ou du phénotype. *Kinanthropologie, 2*:31-42, 1970.

Tanner, J. M., Whitehouse, R. H., and Healy, M. J. R.: *A new system for estimating skeletal maturity from hand and wrist.* Paris, Intern. Children's Centre, 1962.

Van Gerven, D.: *De dimensies van de physical fitness bij mannelijke pre-adolescenten en adolescenten.* Doctor's thesis Physical Education, Leuven, Dept Phys Ed, K.U. Leuven, 1972.

Chapter 26

ANTHROPOMETRIC AND PHOTOSCOPIC SOMATOTYPING OF CHILDREN*

W. D. Ross, J. E. L. Carter, R. L. Rasmussen, and J. Taylor

Abstract

Criterion photoscopic ratings of somatotype in children are compared with anthropometrically derived ratings with and without height correction of the endomorphy component. The height correction increased endomorphy by one half unit; however, even after application of this correction the endomorphy component still tended to be underestimated and mesomorphy overestimated. It is suggested that photoscopic raters with an adult orientation to the shape gestalt interpret relative fatness in children as muscularity.

SINCE THE INTRODUCTION of the concept of somatotype by Sheldon et al. (1940), a number of modifications have been proposed, such as those by Cureton (1951), Parnell (1958), Heath (1963), and Heath and Carter (1967). The last method retains the Sheldonian concept of describing human shape by a three numeral rating of the primary components present in every individual in differing relative amounts: endomorphy (relative fatness), mesomorphy (relative musculoskeletal robustness), and ectomorphy (relative linearity or "stretched-outness").

Unlike the conceptually stable Sheldonian somatotype, the Heath-Carter somatotype is strictly a phenotype or rating of the

---

*The authors recognize the assistance of D. McKim and J. A. Day and the cooperation of Rossland and Nelson Nancy Greene Ski Leagues for data assembly. Basic support was supplied by a Simon Fraser University President's Research Grant and a National Research Council of Canada Operational Grant for Kinanthropometric Research (number A9402).

present morphology. It also differs from the Sheldonian system in the following ways: (a) ratings for each component are not limited to a seven-point scale and thus can accommodate extreme physiques, (b) there is no restriction on the magnitude of the sum of the three components, (c) the somatotypes are ascribed systematically to a height-weight ratio, and (d) no extrapolations or adjustments are made for age or sex of the subjects. These modifications stemmed from the criticism of the Sheldonian system by Heath (1963) and Heath and Carter (1966). Later (Heath and Carter, 1967), the new system was made more objective by incorporating anthropometic procedures.

In the Heath-Carter anthropometric somatotype, the second and third component scales are adjusted for body size by the use of stature (height). The second (mesomorphic) component is based on the deviation of elbow and knee widths and fat-corrected flexed upper arm and standing calf girths from height specific values that would indicate a score of 4 in that component. The third (ectomorphic) component is based on the geometrically dimensionless ratio of height to the cube root of body weight.

The purpose of this chapter is to compare criterion photoscopic ratings and anthropometrically derived ratings with and without the proposed height correction for the first component.

Mehods and Materials

Somatotype photographs and Heath-Carter anthropometric data (Carter, 1972) were obtained on two groups of downhill skiers under the age of 14.0 years (Table 26-I). The photographs were rated by one investigator (JELC) independent of all anthropometric data except the ratio (ht/ $\sqrt[3]{\text{wt}}$) which was needed to complete the rating procedure.

Results and Discussion

In both groups of boys and girls, use of the height correction increased the anthropometric first component rating by

TABLE 26-I
AGE, HEIGHT AND WEIGHT OF STUDY PARTICIPANTS (MEAN, S.D.).

Item	Group One		Group Two	
	Boys (26)	Girls (14)	Boys (30)	Girls (22)
Age	10.9 (1.7)	10.7 (2.2)	11.7 (1.9)	11.5 (1.7)
Height	143.0 (13.2)	139.7 (13.9)	147.7 (13.0)	146.2 (9.4)
Weight	34.6 (9.9)	32.7 (8.8)	39.9 (9.4)	37.1 (9.3)

approximately one-half unit (Table 26-II). However, while the correction was in the right direction, it still underestimated the criterion rating for endomorphy. Compared to the criterion, 92 percent of uncorrected anthropometric ratings were lower, 6 percent were the same, and 2 percent were higher; 76 percent of the corrected ratings were lower, 19 percent were the same, and 5 percent were higher. In both groups of boys and girls the anthropometric procedure overestimated the criterion rating of mesomorphy by approximately one-half unit (Table 26-III). When compared to the criterion, 54 percent of the anthropometric ratings were higher, 28 percent were the same, and 13 percent were lower. There appeared to be no difference in either group between photoscopic and anthropometric ratings of ectomorphy.

Longitudinal studies of boys (Ross et al., 1975) have shown that up to the age of 14, girths over fleshy body parts increase proportionally and girths over boney parts decrease proportionally while proportional skinfold values are reasonably stable. Thus, a photoscopic rater with an adult orientation to the shape gestalt may, as suggested in this data, be rating relative fatness as muscularity.

The first component (endomorphy) is found from the sum of three skinfolds. Height is not considered, since it is often not significantly related to fatness in adult samples. Multiple regression equations to predict the body density or percent fat of adults exclude height (Brozek and Keys, 1951; Pascale, 1956; Pařízková, 1959; Sloan, 1967; Durnin and Rahaman, 1967; Katch and Michaels, 1969; and Wilmore and Behnke, 1970). However, a simple example suggests that size and skinfold readings are related in humans. A sum of three skinfolds of 63

TABLE 26-II

DIFFERENCE OF UNCORRECTED AND HEIGHT CORRECTED ANTHRO-
POMETRIC ENDORMOPHY RATINGS FROM PHOTOSCOPIC CRITERION

| | Group 1* | | | | Group 2* | | | |
| | Boys (26) | | Girls (14) | | Boys (30) | | Girls (22) | |
Diff.	U	C	U	C	U	C	U	C
1.5								1
1.0							1	
0.5	1	3				1		
0.0	3	7		2	2	6		2
−0.5	7	6	2	2	8	7	2	9
−1.0	4	6	3	6	9	13	11	9
−1.5	7	4	2	3	8	1	7	1
−2.0	4		6	1	1	1	1	
−2.5			1		1			
−3.0								
−3.5						1		
−4.0					1			
Mean Δ	−.98	−.52	−1.54	−.96	−1.12	−.77	−1.07	−.61

u = uncorrected
c = corrected to standard height of 170.18 cm.
* numbers of subjects falling in each category

TABLE 26-III

DIFFERENCE BETWEEN PHOTOSCOPIC CRITERION AND ANTHROPOMET-
RIC RATING OF MESOMORPHY

| | Group 1* | | Group 2* | |
Diff.	Boys (26)	Girls (14)	Boys (30)	Girls (22)
2.5			2	1
2.0	1		1	1
1.5	1	2	2	1
1.0	2	2	4	5
0.5	8	7	8	6
0.0	11	2	9	4
−0.5	2	1	3	1
−1.0	1		1	3
Mean Δ	+.29	+.57	+.52	+.47

* numbers of subjects falling in each category

mm would not indicate the same relative fatness in a 120 cm stature six-year-old child and a 190 cm basketball player. Logically, as the linear distance between the pressure plates of a caliper, a skinfold should be geometrically proportional to any other linear measure.

Hebbelinck, Duquet, and Ross (1972) thus suggested that the anthropometric endomorphy rating should be corrected to some standard height, such as the 170.18 cm specified for a unisex reference human (Ross and Wilson, 1974):

$$\text{Height adjusted endomorphy} = 3 \text{ skinfolds} \times \frac{170.18 \text{ cm}}{\text{Stature in cm}}$$

Carter (1975) pointed out that while this kind of correction is theoretically appropriate, it has not yet been validated. Nevertheless, limited empirical application of the correction to children's data indicated the correction was basically sound. In an unpublished study of seventy eleven-year-old boys, Clarys and Carter found that anthropometric endomorphy ratings averaged one-half unit lower than photoscopic ratings. Typically, this discrepancy would be overcome by the proposed correction.

Example: Given that the sum of three skinfolds equals 33.5 mm, endomorphy is 3.5. Also given that height is 151.0 cm.
Corrected skinfolds = 33.5 (170.18/150.0) = 37.8 mm
=rating of 4

References

1. Brozek, J. and Keys, A.: The evaluation of leanness-fatness in man: Norms and interrelationships. *Br J Nutr, 5*:194-206, 1951.
2. Carter, J. E. L.: *The Heath-Carter Somatotype Method,* 1st ed. San Diego, San Diego State University, 1972.
3. Carter, J. E. L.: *The Heath-Carter Somatotype Method,* 2nd ed. San Diego, San Diego State University, 1975.
4. Cureton, T. K.: *Physical Fitness of Champion Athletes.* Urbana, University of Illinois Press, 1951.
5. Durnin, J. V. G. A. and Rahaman, M. M.: The assessment of the amount of fat in the human body from measurements of skinfold thickness. *Br J Nutr, 21*:681-89, 1967.

6. Heath, B. H.: Need for modification of somatyping methodology. *Am J Phys Anthropol, 21*:227-233, 1963.
7. Heath, B. H. and Carter, J. E. L.: A comparison of somatotype method. *Am J Phys Anthropol, 24*:87-99, 1966.
8. Heath, B. H. and Carter, J. E. L.: A modified somatotype method. *Am J Phys Anthropol, 27*:57-74, 1967.
9. Hebbelinck, M., Duquet, W., and Ross, W. D.: A practical outline for the Heath-Carter somatotyping method applied to children. In Bar-Or, O. (Ed.): *Proceedings of the Fourth International Symposium on Paediatric Work Physiology, 1972.* Natanya, Israel, The Wingate Institute, 1973.
10. Katch, F. I. and Michael, E. D.: Densitometric validation of six skinfold formulas to predict body density and percent body fat of 17-year-old boys. *Res Quart, 44*:712-16, 1969.
11. Pařízková, J.: The development of subcutaneous fat in adolescents and the effect of physical training and sport. *Physiol Bohem 8*:112-17, 1959.
12. Parnell, R. W.: *Behavior and Physique.* London Edward Arnold Ltd., 1958.
13. Pascale, L. R., Grossman, M. J., and Stone, H.: Correlations between thickness of skinfolds and body density in 88 soldiers. *Human Biol 28*:165-75, 1956.
14. Ross, W. D. and Wilson, N. C.: A strategem for proportional growth assessment. *Acta Paed Belg, 28* (Suppl.): 169-182, 1974.
15. Ross, W. D., McKim, D. R., and Wilson, B. D.: Kinanthropometry and Young Skiers. In Taylor, A. W. (Ed.): *Application of Science and Medicine in Sport.* Springfield, Thomas, 1975, pp. 257-277.
16. Sheldon, W. H., Stevens, S. S. and Tucker, W. B.: *The Varieties of Human Physique.* New York, Harper and Bros, 1940.
17. Sloan, A. W.: Estimation of body fat in young men. *J Appl Physiol, 23*:311-312, 1967.
18. Wilmore, J. H. and Behnke, A. R.: An anthropometric estimation of body density and lean body weight in young women. *Am J Clin Nutr, 23*:267-274, 1970.

Chapter 27

CHANGES IN THE BODY TYPE OF JAPANESE PUPILS FROM 1955 TO 1975

KIN-ITSU HIRATA

Abstract

The height, weight, and chest-girth of Japanese pupils aged 6 to 17 years were collected; the sample size was 420,000 in 1955, 50,000 in 1967, and 130,000 in 1975. Changes in body type were calculated in terms of the Ponderal Index:

$$\text{P.I.} = \frac{\sqrt[3]{\text{weight (kg)}}}{\text{height(cm)}} \times 1000$$

During the period of study, most Japanese pupils became leaner, but the proportion of obese pupils (P.I. above 25.0) increased very much, especially in the preadolescent group. The numbers in the middle group (P.I. from 25.0 to 21.5) decreased and the frequency distribution curve for the P.I. thus became distorted to the left. Changes of life style, especially more abundant food and lack of exercise owing to increased use of the automobile, are probably responsible for these changes of body type.

F OR ABOUT ten years, there has been a gradual increase in the proportion of obese boys and girls in Japan. In 1955, 1967, and 1975, the Hirata Institute of Health collected data on height, weight, chest-girth, 50 m run, standing broad jump, and softball throw for Japanese pupils aged 3 to 18, developing a chart to distinguish obese from lean boys and girls. This chapter concerns a secular change in the proportions of stout and lean boys and girls, as indicated by both the ponderal index and the evaluation chart for physique and physical fitness.

263

Materials and Methods

Subjects

1. Average values of height and weight of Japanese pupils aged 6 to 18 from 1900 to 1975, as collected by the Japanese Ministry of Education.
2. Measurements on about 420,000 Japanese pupils aged 6 to 18, collected by our colleagues in 1955.
3. Measurements obtained annually on about 200,000 pupils aged 6 to 18, drawn from all over Japan.
4. Measurements on about 80,000 pupils in Japan and Gifu prefectures made in 1967.
5. Measurements of standard and supplementary items on 131,789 pupils selected by excluding questionable data (children aged 3 to 18, all Japan, 1975).

Measurements

1. *Standard items*
   Height, weight, chest-girth, 50 m run, standing broad jump, and softball throw.
2. *Supplementary items*
   - Endurance running: (1500 m for males aged 12 years and older, 1000 m for females aged 12 years and older, 600 m for pupils aged 11 years and younger).
   - Pull-ups for males aged 12 years and older, flexed arm hang for females aged 12 years and older and all pupils aged 11 years and younger.
   - Grip-strength.

Selection

PONDERAL INDEX: The Ponderal Index was calculated as follows:

$$\frac{\sqrt[3]{\text{Weight (kg)}}}{\text{Height(cm)}} \times 1000$$

Body type was classified as follows:

larger than 25.0	obese
25.0 to 21.5	average
smaller than 21.5	lean

SYNTHETIC EVALUATION CHART: This was based on Japanese standards of physique and physical fitness for 1967 and 1975. By this method, body type was classified as follows:

Stout figure	Weight +2 and Chest-girth +2	
Muscular	Physical fitness score	+3 or over
Intermediate		+2 to −2
Obese		−3 or below
Lean figure	Weight −2 and Chest-girth −2	

The synthetic evaluation chart of 1967 was used for values obtained from 1970 to 1975, while for the 1975 data the 1975 chart was used.

Results

Ponderal Index (P.I.)

AVERAGE VALUES: Average values were calculated for pupils aged 3 to 18 in 1900, 1955, 1967, and 1975 (Table 27-I). The PI was largest for infants, becoming smaller until age 14 in the male and 11 to 12 in the female. Thereafter, it became a little larger in the male and much larger in the female, this change of body type being almost equal in 1900, 1955, 1967, and 1975. Average values of PI at every age were largest in 1900, and those of 1967 or 1975 were smallest. Thus the average body type of Japanese pupils was stoutest in 1900 and became leaner until 1967; the change of body type from 1967 to 1975 was less distinct.

PERCENTAGE OF STOUT FIGURES: The percentage of stout figures was calculated for pupils aged 3 to 18 years in 1955, 1967, and 1975 (Table 27-II, Figure 27-1). In 1955, the percentage of stout subjects was largest in infancy and became gradually smaller through childhood, that of the female subjects increasing again in junior and senior high schools. In

Table 27-I. Average values for Ponderal Index
classified by age and sex.
Data for 1900, 1955, 1967, and 1975.

		Male				Female			
		1900	1955	1967	1975	1900	1955	1967	1975
Infant	3				25.1				25.1
	4				24.6				24.5
	5				24.1				24.1
Primary School	6	24.6	24.0	23.7	23.7	24.6	24.0	23.7	23.7
	7	24.4	23.7	23.4	23.4	24.3	23.6	23.3	23.4
	8	23.9	23.5	23.3	23.3	23.8	23.4	23.1	23.2
	9	23.6	23.3	23.1	23.1	23.5	23.3	23.1	23.1
	10	23.5	23.2	23.0	23.0	23.5	23.2	22.9	22.9
	11	23.4	23.1	22.9	22.9	23.4	23.0	22.9	22.9
Jun.HS.	12	22.9	23.0	22.8	22.8	23.3	23.1	23.0	23.0
	13	22.8	22.9	22.8	22.8	23.3	23.3	23.2	23.2
	14	22.7	22.9	22.8	22.7	23.7	23.6	23.3	23.5
Sen.HS.	15	23.0	23.0	22.8	22.8	24.0	23.7	23.6	23.7
	16	23.2	23.1	22.9	23.0	24.3	23.9	23.8	23.7
	17	23.3	23.1	23.0	23.0	24.5	24.0	23.9	23.8
Univ.	18	23.3	23.1		23.0	24.5	23.9		23.6

Table 27-II. Percentage of stout and lean pupils by
sex and age in 1955, 1967, and 1975

		Male						Female					
		stout figure (25.0–larger)			lean figure (21.5–smaller)			stout figure (25.0–larger)			lean figure (21.5–smaller)		
		1955	1967	1975	1955	1967	1975	1955	1967	1975	1955	1967	1975
Infant G	3			67.7			0.0			66.1			0.0
	4			20.7			0.0			23.4			0.0
	5			7.0			0.2			8.3			0.1
Primary S.	6	7.2	2.6	3.9	0.3	0.2	0.2	6.9	4.0	4.7	0.7	0.5	0.1
	7	3.6	2.0	2.3	0.4	0.2	0.2	3.3	1.7	2.6	0.6	0.7	0.2
	8	2.2	1.4	2.5	0.3	0.4	0.2	1.8	1.1	2.2	0.4	0.4	0.3
	9	1.4	0.8	2.6	0.8	0.5	0.4	1.4	1.1	2.4	0.6	0.5	0.9
	10	0.7	1.1	3.1	0.9	1.3	0.7	1.0	0.8	2.2	1.2	2.1	1.4
	11	0.7	1.1	2.3	1.2	1.6	1.3	0.9	1.1	2.0	1.4	2.2	2.2
Jun.H.S.	12	0.6	0.9	2.3	1.5	1.6	1.9	1.4	1.1	3.1	1.4	2.3	2.0
	13	0.4	0.5	1.4	1.5	2.2	2.4	2.3	2.7	3.9	1.0	2.1	1.1
	14	0.5	0.6	1.8	1.8	2.7	2.6	4.5	4.7	6.1	0.6	1.3	0.5
Sen.HS.	15	0.4	0.8	1.9	1.7	2.0	2.4	5.3	5.8	7.4	0.3	0.3	0.4
	16	0.4	0.6	1.7	0.6	1.0	1.8	8.5	9.1	8.1	0.1	0.1	0.3
	17	0.3	0.6	2.4	0.6	1.0	1.4	10.6	9.7	10.6	0.1	0.2	0.1
Univ	18			2.6			0.9			4.6			0.2

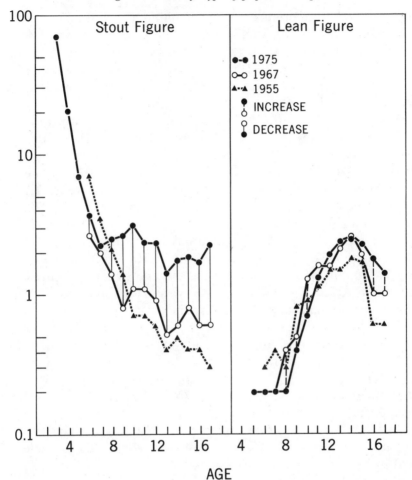

Figure 27-1. Percentage of stout and lean pupils in 1955, 1967, and 1975 (male).

1967, the percentage was smaller than in 1955 for those aged 6 to 9 years, but then became larger in the males. In 1975, the percentage was very much larger than in 1955 and 1967, particularly in the case of males aged 8 to 17 and females aged 8 to 14.

PERCENTAGE OF LEAN FIGURES: The percentage of lean figures was smallest in infancy, increasing to age 14 in the male and 11 or 12 in the female, then becoming a little smaller in the male and very much smaller in the female. This trend was shown almost equally in 1955, 1967, and 1975, but a small difference was found: in 1967 and 1975 the percentage of lean figures was larger than in 1955 for males aged 11 years and over, and for females aged 10 years and over.

FREQUENCY DISTRIBUTION CURVE: Logarithmic coordinates have been used (Figure 27-2). The frequency distribution curve for 1975 is not normal, the mode being located to the left (lean figure); however, the curves for 1955 and 1967 are near normal. The mode of the frequency distribution curve for 1955 lies between 23.0 and 23.5, with an average value of 23.2. That of 1967 is similar, but the average value is 23.0. That of 1975 lies between 22.5 and 23.0, with an average value of 23.0. The percentage of lean figures is largest in 1967 and smallest in 1975. On the other hand, the percentage of stout figures is largest in 1975. These phenomena are shown almost equally by males and females aged 9 to 14 years.

The characteristics of the frequency distribution curve have been distinguished further by calculating skewness and kurtosis ($\sqrt{B_1}$, B_2). If $\sqrt{B_1} = 0$ and $B_2 = 3.0$, the curve has a normal distribution. Calculations were completed at all ages for the data of 1943, 1955, 1967, and 1975. Table 27-III shows the results for ages 11 and 15.

In 1943 and 1955 the frequency distribution was close to a normal curve, but in 1967 it was displaced somewhat to the left and in 1975 this tendency was distinct.

Synthetic evaluation chart

This method has been applied annually from 1970 to 1975, the subjects being some 200,000 boys and girls aged 6 to 18 years, drawn from all over Japan. The relative percentages of stout and lean figures are shown in Table 27-IV.

The percentage of muscular, intermediate, and lean figures has remained almost constant every year, but the proportion of obese stout figures has gradually increased.

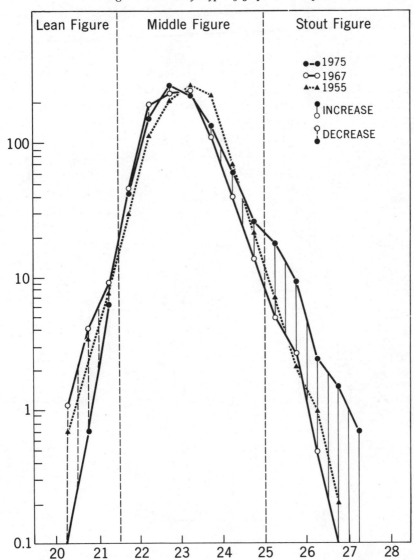

Figure 27-2. Frequency distribution curve for ponderal index (log coordinates, males aged ten).

Physical Fitness Assessment

Table 27-III.

age	era	male $\sqrt{\beta_1}$	β_2	female $\sqrt{\beta_1}$	β_2
	1955	0.143	4.331	0.202	4.694
age	1967	0.758	5.470	0.534	4.655
11	1975	1.062	5.474	0.734	4.260
	1943	0.126	3.125		
age	1955	0.142	4.516	0.236	4.251
15	1967	0.407	4.176	0.440	3.501
	1975	1.185	8.089	0.566	4.564

Table 27-IV.

	Year	stout figure muscular	intermediate	obese	lean figure
Primary School	1970	0.8	1.2	2.0	3.9
	1971	0.7	1.0	2.2	3.3
	1972	0.5	1.1	3.1	3.8
	1973	0.6	1.3	4.0	4.1
	1974	0.5	1.1	3.8	3.7
	1975	0.4	1.0	3.6	3.6
Junior HS.	1970	1.2	1.2	2.0	5.8
	1971	1.2	1.5	2.8	5.9
	1972	1.0	1.5	3.6	6.0
	1973	1.0	1.6	3.9	5.7
	1974	1.3	1.6	4.0	5.2
	1975	0.8	1.3	4.1	6.0

Discussion

This investigation confirms that the number of stout boys and girls has increased greatly in recent years. However, the number of lean boys and girls has also increased, so that the mode of the frequency distribution curve has been shifted leftward (lean tendency), while the average PI has not changed greatly. While obese stout figures have increased, the proportion of muscular stout figures has remained constant or even diminished.

It has been generally believed that such phenomena are due to an overabundance of food and a lack of physical exercise. The author agrees with this opinion, but would suggest that the largest cause is lack of physical exercise due to a remarkable increase in the use of motor-cars. The number of motor vehicles registered in Gifu prefecture (population 1,900,000) has been as follows:

1970	367,972
1971	420,995
1972	472,007
1973	527,137
1974	565,266
1975	616,523

Infants and pupils can no longer play on the road or nearby open space and they travel by car instead of walking. Physical exercise in daily life is thus extremely limited.

Japanese male champions at the Tokyo Olympic Games had a muscular stout figure because of hard physical training but the female champions had a lean figure because their bodies contained little fat (Table 27-V).

TABLE 27-V

	Ponderal Index	
	male	*female*
Japanese pupils aged 20	23.4	24.4
Japanese Olympic Champions	23.7	23.5

With training, a stout figure with much fat becomes leaner because of a decrease in fatty tissue. On the other hand, an individual classed as having a lean or intermediate figure without excess fat may become stouter because of an increase in muscle. Lack of physical exercise associated with increasing use of motor cars may thus be responsible for the increase in both obese/stout individuals and lean subjects with little muscle.

References

Asher, P.: Fat Babies and Fat Children. The Prognosis of Obesity in the Very Young. *Arch Dis Child, 41*:672, 1966.

Correnti, V.: Il Metodo Degli Auxogrammi. *Riv Anthropol, 37*:46-89, 1949.

Hirata, K.: The new theory for the physical judgment and its practical application. *Jap Med J 2*:318, 1949.

Hirata, K. et al.: The standard physique of Japanese pupils for 1955 and the newest synthetic method of physical states and strength and its practical application. *J Nagoya Med Assoc, 74*:4, 1957.

Hirata, K.: Age and physique of Tokyo Olympic Champion. *J Sports Med Phys Fitness* (Torino) *6*:207-228, 1966.

Hirata, K. et al.: Stout and lean boys and girls in Gifu prefecture. Report of Gifu Medical Association. *Japanese Congress of School Health,* pp. 77-131, 1968.

Hirata, K. and Kaku, K.: *The Evaluating Method of Physique and Physical Fitness and its Practical Application.* Mino-shi, Japan, Hirata Institute of Health, 1968.

Hirata, K.: Ponderal Index. *Res J Phys Educ, 17*:395-421, 1973

Hirata, K.: Appearance percentage of stout and lean figure of Japanese pupils. *Educ Med, 19*:6-13, 1974

Hirata, K. et al.: The standard physique and physical fitness and newest synthetic evaluating chart of physique and physical fitness. *Educ Med, 21*:3-91, 1975

Kaku, K.: Standard of growth of babies and preschool children in Japan, based on national survey in spring. *Educ Med, 56*:285, 1952

Larson, L. A. et al.: *Fitness, Health, and Work Capacity. International Committee for the Standardization of Physical fitness Tests.* New York, McMillan, 1974.

Livi: *Anthropometrica.* Italy, 1886. Cited by Hirata, K. & Kaku K., 1968.

Ranke: Grosse und Gewicht und ihre Korrelation bei 17-18 Jahrigen. *Z f mens Verch Konst* 1944. Cited by Hirata, K. & Kaku K., 1968.

Sato, R.: *Mathematical Statistics.* Tokyo, Baifukan, 1943.

Tanner, J. M.: *Growth at Adolescence.* Oxford, Oxford University Press, 1962.

Tomonari, H.: The evaluation of physique by sum of index number. *Educ Med, 9*:1, 1963.

Wetzel, N. C.: Physical fitness in terms of physical development and basal metabolism with a guide to individual progress from infancy to maturity. JAMA, 116:1187, 1941.

Wolanski, N.: A new graphic method for the evaluation of tempo and harmony of physical growth of children. The method of developmental channels and steps. *Hum Bicl, 33*:283, 1961.

Chapter 28

PHYSICAL PERFORMANCE OF SCHOOL CHILDREN IN ISRAEL

H. Ruskin

Abstract

The physical performance levels of school children were assessed according to I.C.P.F.R. standard tests.* The subjects were Israeli children aged 6 to 18 years, 1279 girls and 1239 boys. The development of physical performance was almost equal for boys and girls from 6 to 13 years of age, and increased significantly on all performance variables for ages 14 to 18. The largest positive intercorrelations were between height-weight and hand grip variables, and between sprint-run-standing broad jump and shuttle run. The lowest correlations related hand grip and forward trunk flexion to all other test variables. Relative to findings in other countries, Israeli boys and girls had a higher level of physical performance on muscular strength variables and a lower level of performance on items involving speed, muscular power, flexibility, and endurance.

The Development of Physical Performance of Boys and Girls Between Ages 6 to 17

Figures 28-1 through 28-10 illustrate the development of physical performance for boys and girls, from age 6 to 17.
1. There was a considerable increase of achievement commencing at age 13, this being shown by both boys and girls. In pull-ups, the boys initiated this sharp increase from the age of 12 years.

---

*L. A. Larson (Ed.): *Fitness, Health and Work Capacity,* International Committee for the Standardization of Physical Fitness Tests, New York, Macmillan, 1974.

273

2. Significant differences of achievements between boys and girls were seen from age 13. This was true of all test variables, but particularly weight, height, sprint speed, hand grip (force), standing broad jump, sit-ups, and shuttle-run. Only on forward flexion of the trunk did the girls achieve a greater increase than the boys.

3. Between the ages of 6 and 13, gains were similar for boys and girls, the increases being relatively small from one year to another. However
   (a) Boys scored a little higher than the girls on most test variables.
   (b) The girls scored higher than the boys for forward trunk flexion.

4. There was a significant deterioration of the long distance run times between the ages of 16 and 18. This can be attributed mainly to lack of motivation and lack of an appropriate physical education program before the final matriculation examinations of the high schools.

Relationships Between Physical Performance Variables

Correlation matrixes (Tables 28-I and 28-II) for ages 6 to 13 show that the highest correlations were between the following items:

a. height and weight (0.70 boys, 0.65 girls)
b. height and hand grip (0.49 boys, 0.38 girls)
c. weight and hand grip (0.52 boys, 0.41 girls)
d. 50 m sprint and shuttle run (0.40 boys, 0.39 girls)
e. 50 m sprint and standing broad jump (0.43 boys, 0.47 girls)
f. standing broad jump and shuttle run (0.43 boys, 0.41 girls)

Several correlations of less than 0.3, mainly negative, were seen, including those between

a. height and weight and pull-ups (boys) and flexed arm hang (girls),
b. height and forward flexion,

TABLE 28-I
CORRELATION MATRIX OF TEST VARIABLES COLLECTED ON GIRLS AGED 6-13 YRS.

	Age	Weight	50 m Run	Jump	Dist. Run	Flexed Arm Hang	Shuttle Run	Sit-ups	Forward Flexion	Hand Grip
Height	6	.59	.12	.08	.11	.02	.07	.20	-.49	.33
	7	.63	.21	.13	-.08	-.08	.07	.10	.07	.46
	8	.74	-.07	-.01	.01	-.09	-.28	.02	-.07	.32
	9	.69	-.08	.04	.10	-.09	-.03	-.10	.06	.32
	10	.74	.15	.02	.13	-.24	-.11	-.14	-.06	.43
	11	.64	.20	.24	.13	.01	.22	.11	-.02	.49
	12	.65	.16	.08	.04	-.27	-.03	-.16	.06	.40
	13	.53	.15	-.03	.27	-.01	-.04	.07	.11	.33
Weight	6		.03	-.05	.03	-.24	-.01	.05	.00	.23
	7		.01	.04	.02	-.12	.03	-.07	.08	.39
	8		-.17	-.02	-.15	-.19	-.19	-.06	.07	.38
	9		-.25	-.13	-.00	-.30	-.14	-.03	-.02	.35
	10		.02	-.18	-.16	-.33	-.16	-.10	-.20	.50
	11		.06	.01	.12	-.22	.03	.07	.08	.55
	12		.05	-.12	-.18	-.39	-.01	-.22	.00	.51
	13		-.05	-.11	-.03	-.22	.06	.06	.24	.38
50 m Run	6			.21	.34	.20	.23	.29	.03	.20
	7			.27	-.03	.03	.19	.19	.09	.31
	8			.47	.20	.35	.45	.38	.22	.32
	9			.64	.41	.29	.63	.56	.24	.36
	10			.41	.27	.30	.44	.35	.22	.41
	11			.66	.26	.21	.53	.42	.31	.32
	12			.53	.51	.27	.31	.24	-.07	.27
	13			.58	.44	.38	.37	.44	.25	.39

Jump

Age						
6	.10	.18	.20	.37	.33	.08
7	.16	.31	.36	.28	.12	.08
8	.33	.31	.31	.35	.19	.14
9	.28	.42	.37	.48	.34	.30
10	.12	.39	.26	.39	.45	.38
11	.25	.30	.42	.61	.29	.18
12	.19	.34	.55	.37	.38	.44
13	.19	.18	.41	.49	.47	.30

Distance Run
Ages 6-11—600m
Ages 12-13—800m

Age					
6	.16	.01	.24	.01	.13
7	.01	-.04	-.07	.06	.11
8	-.00	.09	.05	.24	.29
9	.27	-.01	.16	.51	.28
10	.13	.29	.24	.27	.28
11	.21	.07	.14	.18	.19
12	.05	.04	.25	.14	.26
13	.11	.17	.51	.07	.33

Flexed Arm Hang

Age				
6	.01	-.03	.25	.30
7	-.07	.12	.23	.15
8	.11	.07	.28	.42
9	.15	.12	.36	.43
10	-.01	.38	.31	.25
11	.06	.26	.44	.34
12	-.01	.15	.35	.17
13	.14	.10	.52	.31

Shuttle Run

Age			
6	-.08	.06	.08
7	-.04	.25	.26
8	.20	.19	.16
9	.25	.14	.29

Sit-ups

10	.10	.08	.18
11	.47	.38	.18
12	.34	.05	.31
13	.17	-.02	.30

6	.03	.04
7	.27	.09
8	.19	.24
9	.17	.05
10	.31	.23
11	.30	.06
12	.44	.04
13	.25	.08

Forward Flexion

6	-.02
7	.21
8	.25
9	-.03
10	.12
11	.06
12	-.11
13	.24

TABLE 28-II

CORRELATION MATRIX OF TEST VARIABLES COLLECTED ON BOYS AGED 6-13 YRS.

	Age	Weight	50 m Run	Jump	Dist. Run	Flexed Arm Hang	Shuttle Run	Sit-UPS	Forward Flexion	Hand Grip
Height	6	.70	.08	-.18	-.05	-.19	-.10	.03	-.10	.40
	7	.71	.03	.07	-.01	-.18	.05	-.12	.11	.44
	8	.70	.13	.11	.03	.13	.01	.03	-.25	.49
	9	.63	.10	.10	-.04	-.13	.09	.00	.13	.39
	10	.77	.13	.07	-.02	-.16	-.02	.02	-.17	.56
	11	.66	.07	.15	.11	.00	.06	.02	.05	.48
	12	.72	.20	.20	.00	.05	-.00	-.00	-.05	.60
	13	.73	.47	.33	.14	.20	.08	.10	.24	.58
Weight	6		.02	-.18	-.03	-.09	-.12	.12	-.11	.33
	7		-.14	-.09	-.10	-.26	-.08	-.15	-.03	.40
	8		.11	-.02	-.24	-.10	-.11	-.00	-.14	.60
	9		-.02	-.03	-.03	-.19	-.12	.12	-.00	.51
	10		.03	.07	-.09	-.23	-.08	-.07	-.13	.58
	11		-.19	-.10	-.09	-.13	-.06	-.26	-.05	.43
	12		.11	.10	-.19	-.06	-.07	-.06	.00	.67
	13		.29	.02	-.13	-.01	-.18	-.08	.16	.67
50 m Run	6			.32	.33	.20	.22	.14	.13	.34
	7			.51	.14	.32	.44	.28	.30	.09
	8			.31	.26	.18	.15	.45	.23	.36
	9			.48	.29	.33	.59	.24	.01	.23
	10			.32	.54	.31	.53	.37	.09	.22
	11			.62	.16	.29	.27	.46	.07	.27
	12			.63	.49	.42	.54	.28	.14	.39
	13			.65	.43	.54	.53	.40	.42	.56

Jump	Age						
	6	.04	.27	.24	.49	.17	.14
	7	.24	.29	.27	.46	.36	.17
	8	.11	.24	.12	.37	.08	.25
	9	.21	.33	.29	.37	.37	.24
	10	.16	.19	.24	.36	.35	.31
	11	.36	.37	.47	.33	.38	.16
	12	.29	.30	.36	.47	.47	.42
	13	.39	.45	.47	.59	.41	.50

Distance Run Ages 6-11—600m Ages 12-13—1000m	Age					
	6	.24	.05	-.09	-.02	.20
	7	-.00	.05	.17	.19	.10
	8	-.04	.11	.26	.39	.12
	9	.23	-.02	.39	.23	.29
	10	-.08	.22	.37	.33	.40
	11	.13	-.08	.20	.15	.16
	12	.02	.00	.49	.42	.34
	13	.10	.16	.37	.37	.41

Pull-Ups	Age				
	6	.26	.11	.14	-.02
	7	.03	.05	.13	.14
	8	.20	.07	.10	.16
	9	.08	.11	.18	.32
	10	.05	.28	.45	.28
	11	.27	.12	.27	.14
	12	.24	.11	.30	.36
	13	.36	.25	.52	.33

Shuttle Run	Age			
	6	-.23	.15	.30
	7	-.02	.35	.09
	8	.07	.12	.11
	9	.17	.03	.25

10	.15	−.01	.13
11	.34	.11	.31
12	.22	−.02	.26
13	.28	.22	.35

Sit-ups

6	.14	.31
7	.11	.08
8	.19	.16
9	−.20	−.03
10	−.01	.21
11	.23	.21
12	.06	.23
13	.17	.43

Forward Flexion

6	.06
7	−.03
8	−.01
9	−.06
10	−.09
11	.09
12	.00
13	.27

c. height of boys and sit-ups, forward flexion, long distance run, and standing broad jump.

The lack of correlation between various variables strengthens the assumption that each test measures a different component of physical fitness. This in turn justifies the inclusion of many individual tests in the overall battery.

Smallest Space Analysis of Physical Performance Variables

To investigate the relationships between the various tests, Schlesinger-Guttman's Smallest Space Analysis (SSA) method of two-dimensional mapping was used. According to this method, distances between variables are ordered on the basis of the measure of association between them.[1] The advantage of the two-dimensional SSA map over the correlation matrix is that with its aid it is possible to study the structure of relationship between all variables.

Analysis of such maps (Figs. 28-11 through 28-26) shows that:

1. Height and weight are situated relatively close to each other and to hand grip in all groups. The taller or heavier subjects perform better in activities which require strength of the arm muscles.
2. Trunk flexion and hand grip variables are relatively distant from the remaining variables and are also far apart from each other. Flexibility seems to be independent of all other variables.
3. For most of the tested groups, the sprint run, shuttle run, and standing broad jump cluster together.
4. The long distance variables which test mainly cardiovascular endurance are relatively distant from other variables, not being associated with achievements in other tests that require running.
5. Variables which test muscle strength of the shoulders and trunk (pull ups, flexed arm hang, sit-ups) cluster together in most age groups.
6. Although some variables are situated relatively close to each other, these relationships do not necessarily

suggest physical performance could be determined with a smaller number of tests.

7. The relationships mentioned above are quite stable, being seen in both boys and girls at all ages.

The pattern appears to concur with that observed previously for children aged 15 to 18.[2]

Comparison of Physical Performance in Israel and Other Countries

In comparing test findings with data* collected by I.C.P.F.R. methodology in other countries, the following limitations should be taken into consideration.

a. Some of the comparative studies did not test the entire population aged 6 to 18 years.

b. Some of the comparative studies examined very specific populations, such as particular socioeconomic groups or rural communities.

c. The size of samples differed between countries like Taiwan (400 boys and girls in each age) and other nations where data were reported for samples of only twenty boys and girls.

d. Although I.C.P.F.R. has tried to standardize methods, the recommended methodology was not followed in all reported studies.

e. Comparison is thus limited to data which appeared legitimately comparable.

Figures 28-27 through 28-46 compare means and standard deviations in Israel and other countries.

---

*This data was gathered from reports submitted to annual meetings of I.C.P.F.R. since 1968, in which some reported findings of studies since 1961. The researchers are Hung (S. Vietnam) 1971; Tsuruta et al. (Japan) 1967; Bartolome (Philippines) 1968; Hebbelinck and Borms (Belgium) 1968; Great Britain (cited by Pavek, 1972) 1965; Tsai (Taiwan) 1968; Pavek (Czechoslovakia) 1966; Kirsh and Kunze (West Germany) 1972.

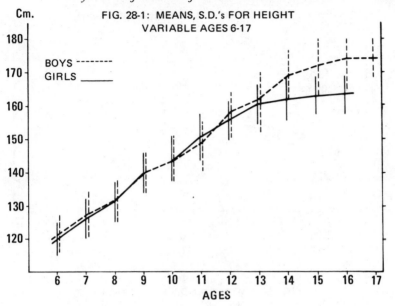

FIG. 28-1: MEANS, S.D.'s FOR HEIGHT
VARIABLE AGES 6-17

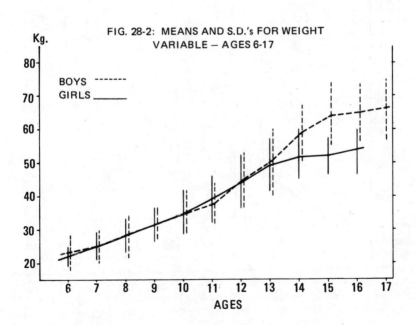

FIG. 28-2: MEANS AND S.D.'s FOR WEIGHT
VARIABLE — AGES 6-17

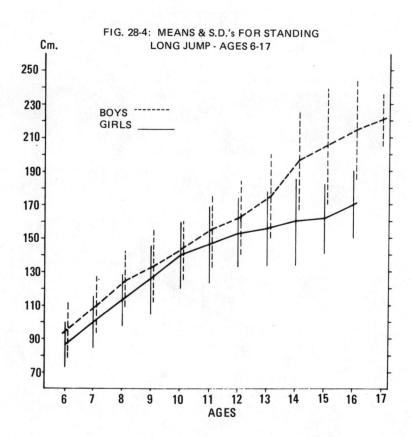

FIG. 28-3: MEANS & S.D.'s FOR 50m SPRINT AGES 6-17

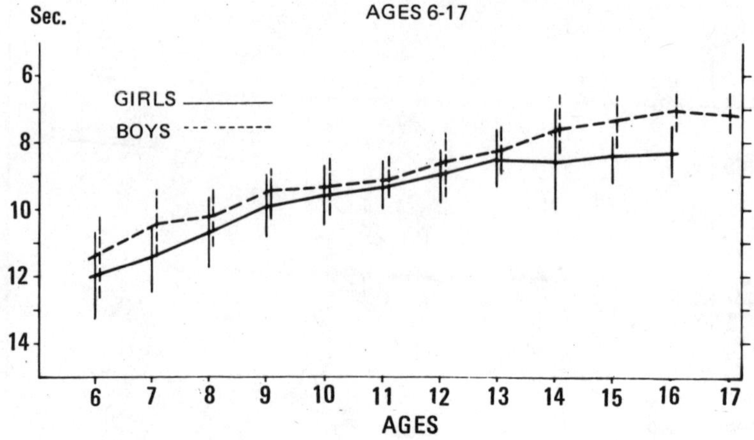

FIG. 28-4: MEANS & S.D.'s FOR STANDING LONG JUMP - AGES 6-17

FIG. 28-5: MEANS S.D.'s FOR 800m RUN GIRLS
AGES 11-17

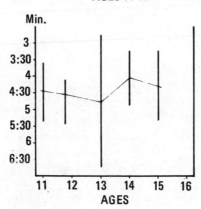

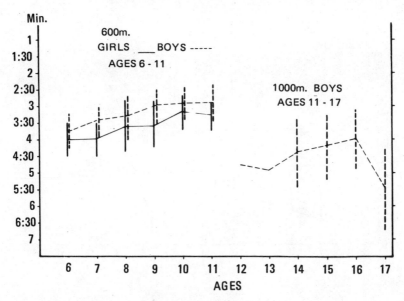

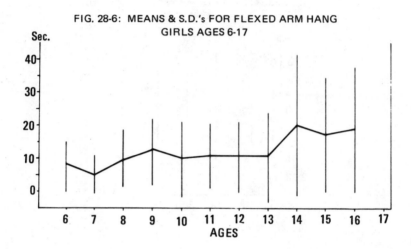

FIG. 28-6: MEANS & S.D.'s FOR FLEXED ARM HANG
GIRLS AGES 6-17

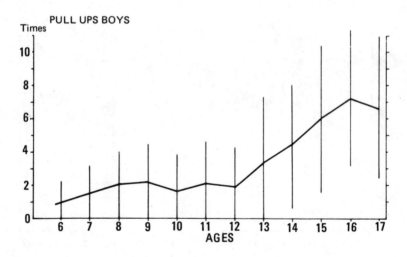

PULL UPS BOYS

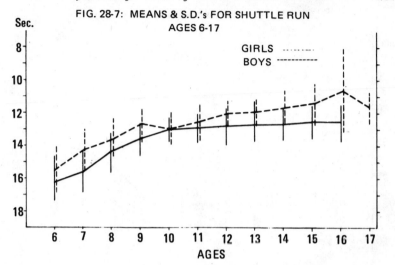

FIG. 28-7: MEANS & S.D.'s FOR SHUTTLE RUN
AGES 6-17

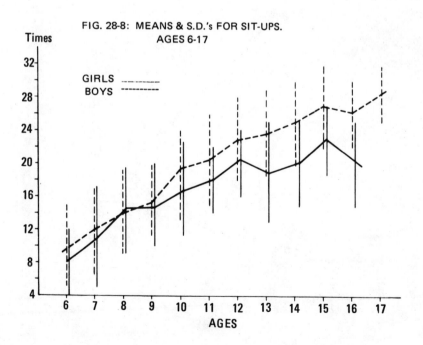

FIG. 28-8: MEANS & S.D.'s FOR SIT-UPS.
AGES 6-17

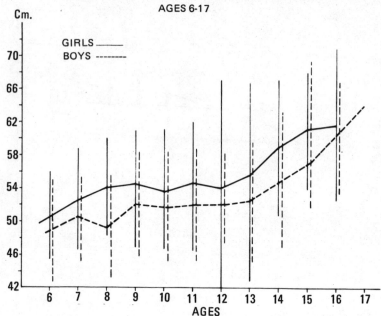

FIG. 28-9: MEANS & S.D.'s FOR FORWARD FLEXION
AGES 6-17

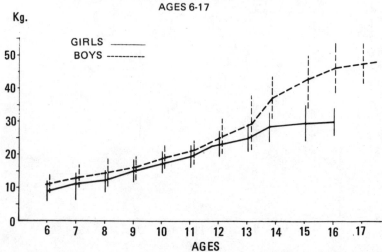

FIG. 28-10: MEANS & S.D.'s FOR ARM GRIP
AGES 6-17

FIG. 28-11: SPACE DIAGRAM MAP 1: SSA, GIRLS, AGE 6

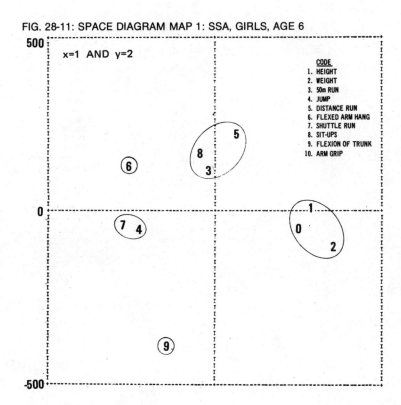

FIG. 28-12: SPACE DIAGRAM MAP 2: SSA, GIRLS, AGE 7

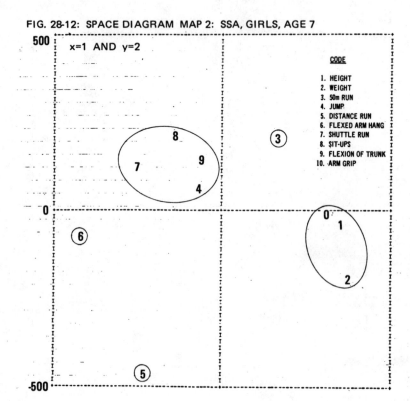

x=1 AND y=2

CODE

1. HEIGHT
2. WEIGHT
3. 50m RUN
4. JUMP
5. DISTANCE RUN
6. FLEXED ARM HANG
7. SHUTTLE RUN
8. SIT-UPS
9. FLEXION OF TRUNK
10. ARM GRIP

FIG. 28-13: SPACE DIAGRAM MAP 3: SSA, GIRLS, AGE 8

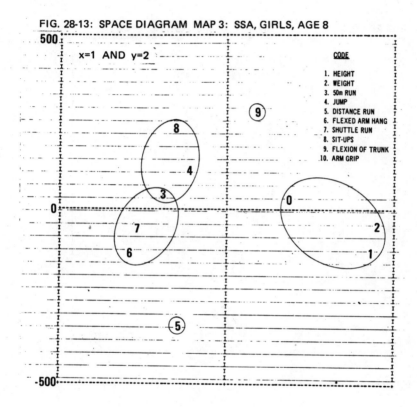

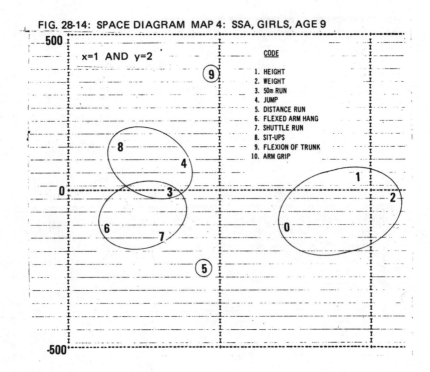

FIG. 28-14: SPACE DIAGRAM MAP 4: SSA, GIRLS, AGE 9

x=1 AND y=2

CODE

1. HEIGHT
2. WEIGHT
3. 50m RUN
4. JUMP
5. DISTANCE RUN
6. FLEXED ARM HANG
7. SHUTTLE RUN
8. SIT-UPS
9. FLEXION OF TRUNK
10. ARM GRIP

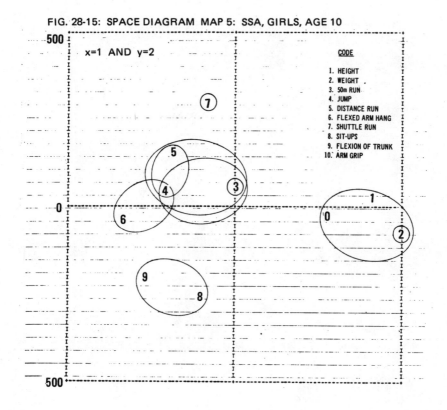

FIG. 28-15: SPACE DIAGRAM MAP 5: SSA, GIRLS, AGE 10

x=1 AND y=2

CODE

1. HEIGHT
2. WEIGHT
3. 50m RUN
4. JUMP
5. DISTANCE RUN
6. FLEXED ARM HANG
7. SHUTTLE RUN
8. SIT-UPS
9. FLEXION OF TRUNK
10. ARM GRIP

FIG. 28-16: SPACE DIAGRAM MAP 6: SSA, GIRLS, AGE 11

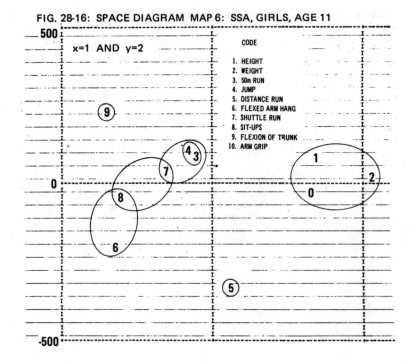

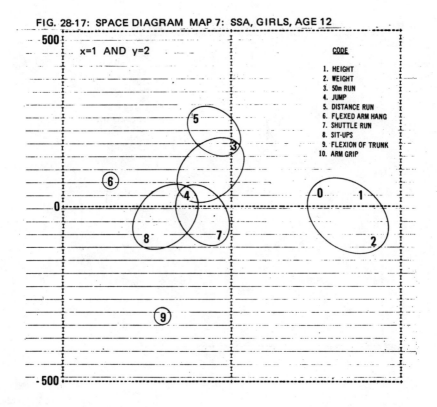

FIG. 28-17: SPACE DIAGRAM MAP 7: SSA, GIRLS, AGE 12

x=1 AND y=2

CODE

1. HEIGHT
2. WEIGHT
3. 50m RUN
4. JUMP
5. DISTANCE RUN
6. FLEXED ARM HANG
7. SHUTTLE RUN
8. SIT-UPS
9. FLEXION OF TRUNK
10. ARM GRIP

FIG. 28-18: SPACE DIAGRAM MAP 8: SSA, GIRLS, AGE 13

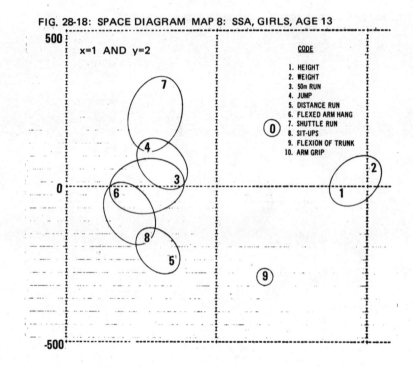

FIG. 28-19: SPACE DIAGRAM MAP 9: SSA, BOYS, AGE 6

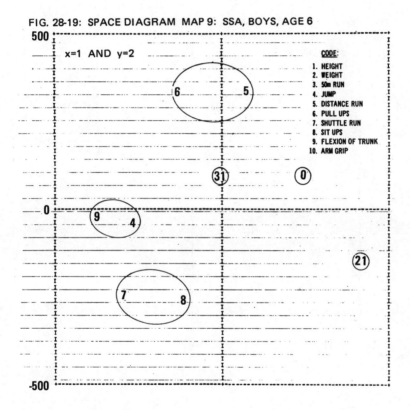

FIG. 28-20: SPACE DIAGRAM MAP 10: SSA, BOYS, AGE 7

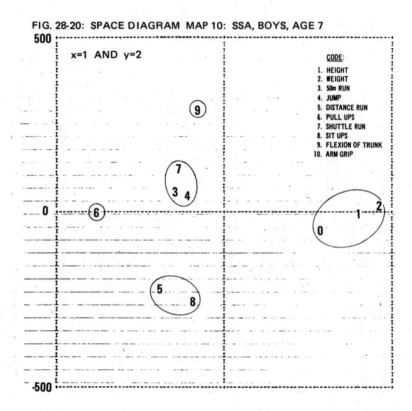

FIG. 28-21: SPACE DIAGRAM MAP 11: SSA, BOYS, AGE 8

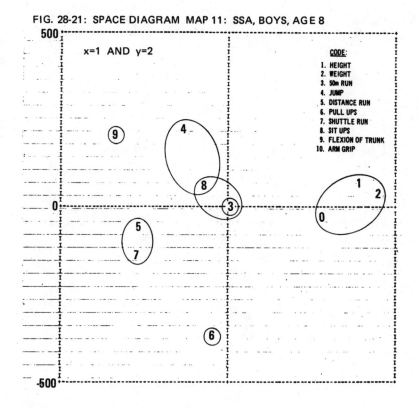

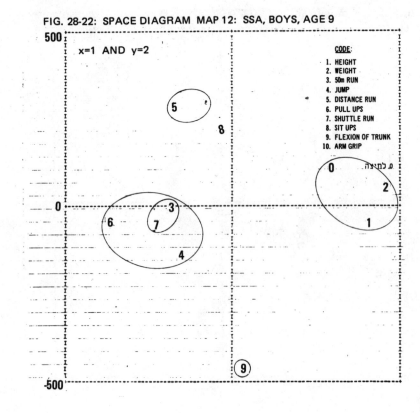

FIG. 28-22: SPACE DIAGRAM MAP 12: SSA, BOYS, AGE 9

x=1 AND y=2

CODE:
1. HEIGHT
2. WEIGHT
3. 50m RUN
4. JUMP
5. DISTANCE RUN
6. PULL UPS
7. SHUTTLE RUN
8. SIT UPS
9. FLEXION OF TRUNK
10. ARM GRIP

FIG. 28-23: SPACE DIAGRAM MAP 13: SSA, BOYS, AGE 10

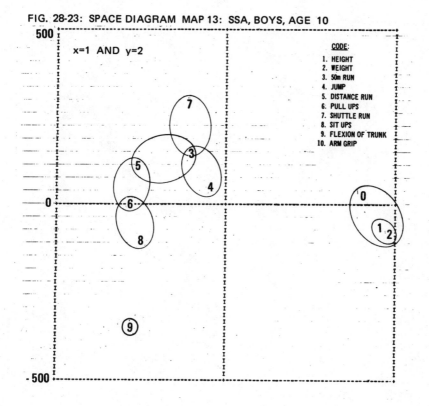

x=1 AND y=2

CODE:
1. HEIGHT
2. WEIGHT
3. 50m RUN
4. JUMP
5. DISTANCE RUN
6. PULL UPS
7. SHUTTLE RUN
8. SIT UPS
9. FLEXION OF TRUNK
10. ARM GRIP

FIG. 28-24: SPACE DIAGRAM MAP 14: SSA, BOYS, AGE 11

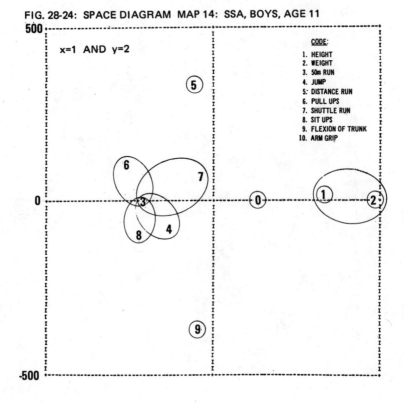

x=1 AND y=2

CODE:
1. HEIGHT
2. WEIGHT
3. 50m RUN
4. JUMP
5. DISTANCE RUN
6. PULL UPS
7. SHUTTLE RUN
8. SIT UPS
9. FLEXION OF TRUNK
10. ARM GRIP

FIG. 28-25: SPACE DIAGRAM MAP 15: SSA, BOYS, AGE 12

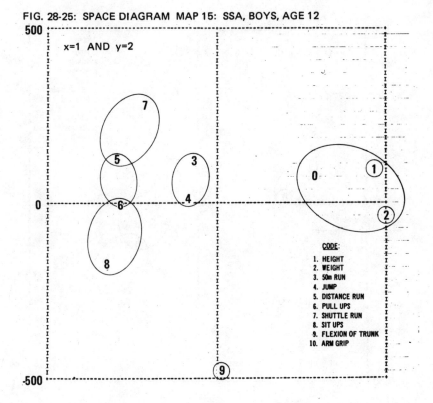

x=1 AND y=2

CODE:
1. HEIGHT
2. WEIGHT
3. 50m RUN
4. JUMP
5. DISTANCE RUN
6. PULL UPS
7. SHUTTLE RUN
8. SIT UPS
9. FLEXION OF TRUNK
10. ARM GRIP

FIG. 28-26: SPACE DIAGRAM MAP 16: SSA, BOYS, AGE 13

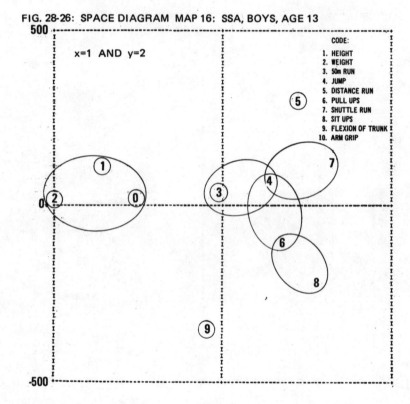

x=1 AND y=2

CODE:
1. HEIGHT
2. WEIGHT
3. 50m RUN
4. JUMP
5. DISTANCE RUN
6. PULL UPS
7. SHUTTLE RUN
8. SIT UPS
9. FLEXION OF TRUNK
10. ARM GRIP

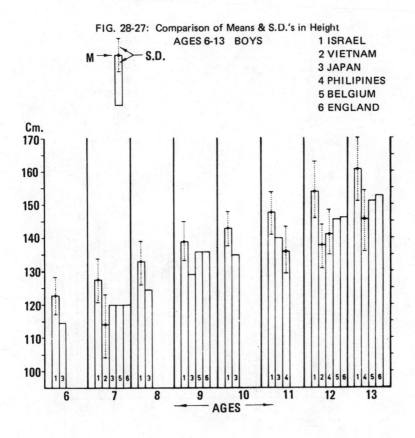

FIG. 28-27: Comparison of Means & S.D.'s in Height
AGES 6-13   BOYS
1 ISRAEL
2 VIETNAM
3 JAPAN
4 PHILIPINES
5 BELGIUM
6 ENGLAND

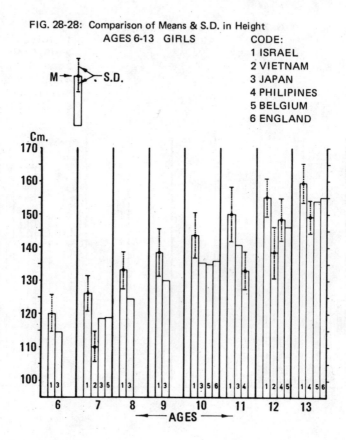

FIG. 28-28: Comparison of Means & S.D. in Height
AGES 6-13　GIRLS

CODE:
1 ISRAEL
2 VIETNAM
3 JAPAN
4 PHILIPINES
5 BELGIUM
6 ENGLAND

FIG. 28-29: Comparison of Means & S.D.'s in Weight

AGES 6-13   BOYS

1 ISRAEL
2 VIETNAM
3 JAPAN
4 PHILIPINES
5 BELGIUM
6 ENGLAND

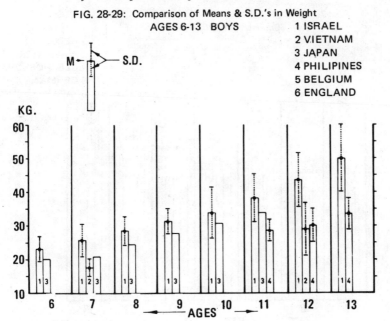

FIG. 28-30: Comparison of Means & S.D.'s in Weight

AGES 6-13   GIRLS

1 ISRAEL
2 VIETNAM
3 JAPAN
4 PHILIPINES
5 BELGIUM
6 ENGLAND

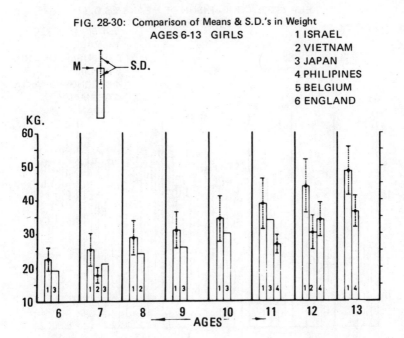

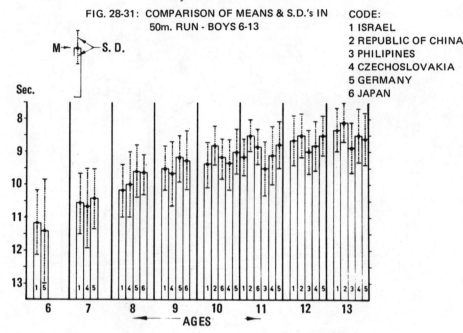

FIG. 28-31: COMPARISON OF MEANS & S.D.'s IN
50m. RUN - BOYS 6-13

CODE:
1 ISRAEL
2 REPUBLIC OF CHINA
3 PHILIPINES
4 CZECHOSLOVAKIA
5 GERMANY
6 JAPAN

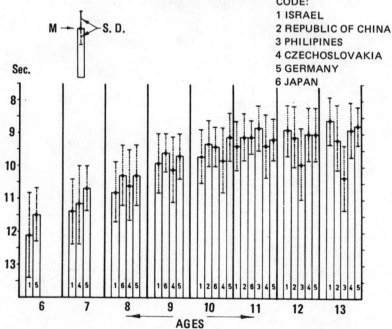

FIG. 28-32: COMPARISON OF MEANS & S.D.'s IN
50m. RUN - GIRLS 6-13

CODE:
1 ISRAEL
2 REPUBLIC OF CHINA
3 PHILIPINES
4 CZECHOSLOVAKIA
5 GERMANY
6 JAPAN

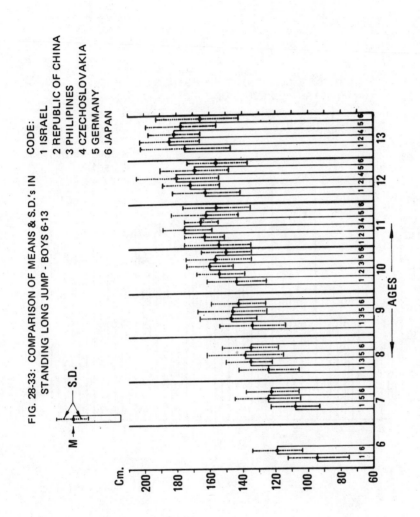

FIG. 28-33: COMPARISON OF MEANS & S.D.'s IN
STANDING LONG JUMP - BOYS 6-13

CODE:
1 ISRAEL
2 REPUBLIC OF CHINA
3 PHILIPINES
4 CZECHOSLOVAKIA
5 GERMANY
6 JAPAN

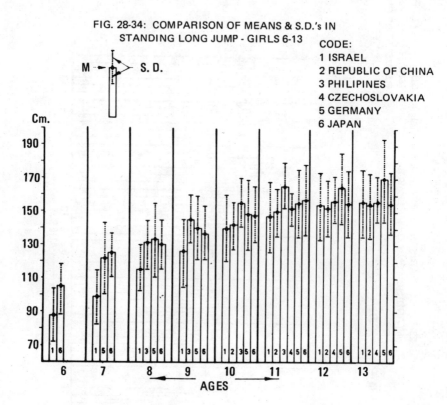

FIG. 28-34: COMPARISON OF MEANS & S.D.'s IN STANDING LONG JUMP - GIRLS 6-13

CODE:
1 ISRAEL
2 REPUBLIC OF CHINA
3 PHILIPINES
4 CZECHOSLOVAKIA
5 GERMANY
6 JAPAN

FIG. 28-35: COMPARISON OF MEANS & S.D.'s IN
LONG DISTANCE RUN - BOYS 6 13
AGES 6-11 600m.
AGES 12-13 1000m.

CODE:
1 ISRAEL
2 REPUBLIC OF CHINA
3 GERMANY

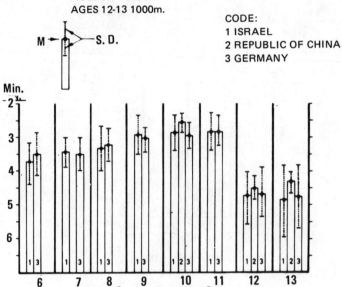

FIG. 28-36: COMPARISON OF MEANS & S.D.'s
IN LONG DISTANCE RUN - GIRLS 6-13
AGES 6-11 -600m.   CODE:
AGES 12-13 -800m.   1 ISRAEL
                         2 REPUBLIC OF CHINA
                         3 GERMANY

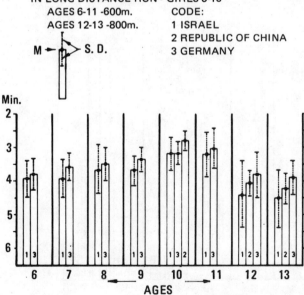

FIG. 28-37: COMPARISON OF MEANS & S.D.'s IN PULL-UPS
BOYS 11-13

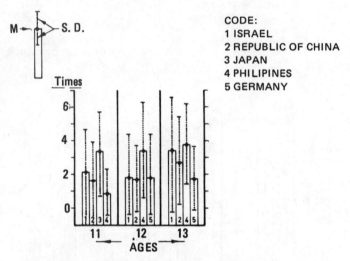

CODE:
1 ISRAEL
2 REPUBLIC OF CHINA
3 JAPAN
4 PHILIPINES
5 GERMANY

FIG. 28-38: COMPARISON OF MEANS & S.D.'s
IN FLEXED ARM HANG - GIRLS AGES 8-13

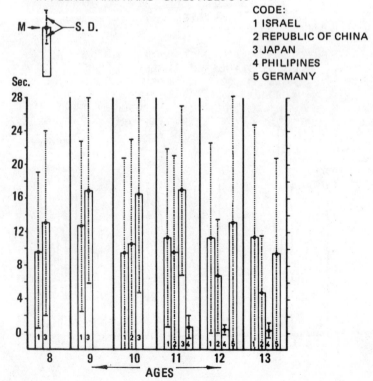

CODE:
1 ISRAEL
2 REPUBLIC OF CHINA
3 JAPAN
4 PHILIPINES
5 GERMANY

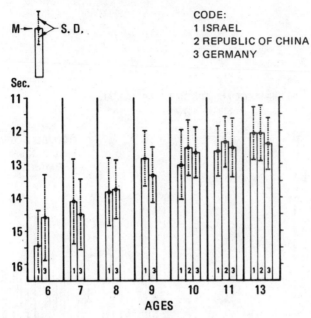

FIG. 28-39: COMPARISON OF MEANS & S.D.'s
IN SHUTTLE RUN - BOYS 6-11,13

CODE:
1 ISRAEL
2 REPUBLIC OF CHINA
3 GERMANY

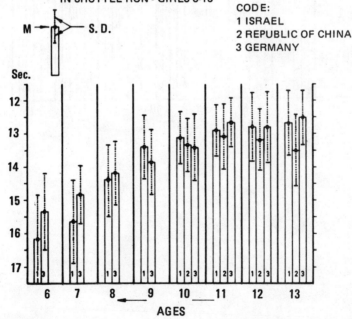

FIG. 28-40: COMPARISON OF MEANS & S.D.'s
IN SHUTTLE RUN - GIRLS 6-13

CODE:
1 ISRAEL
2 REPUBLIC OF CHINA
3 GERMANY

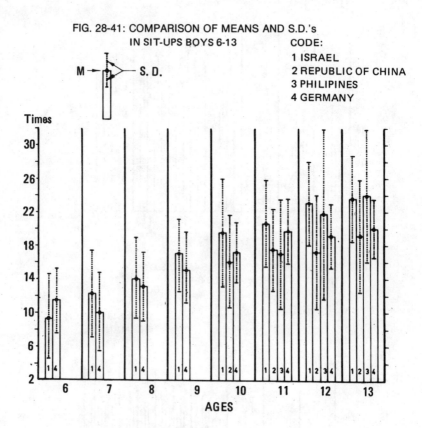

FIG. 28-41: COMPARISON OF MEANS AND S.D.'s IN SIT-UPS BOYS 6-13

CODE:
1 ISRAEL
2 REPUBLIC OF CHINA
3 PHILIPINES
4 GERMANY

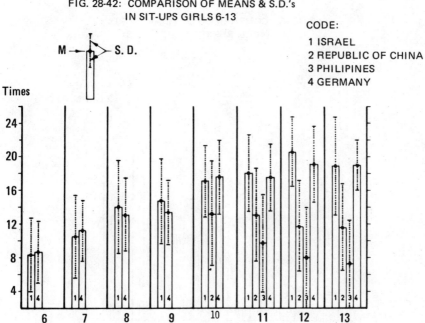

FIG. 28-42: COMPARISON OF MEANS & S.D.'s
IN SIT-UPS GIRLS 6-13

CODE:

1 ISRAEL
2 REPUBLIC OF CHINA
3 PHILIPINES
4 GERMANY

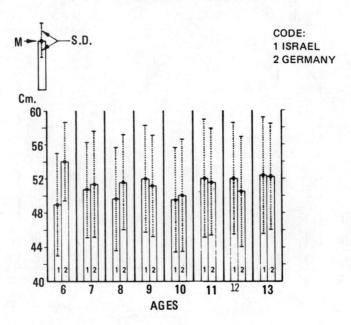

FIG. 28-43: COMPARISON OF MEANS & S.D.'s
IN FORWARD FLEXION - BOYS 6-13

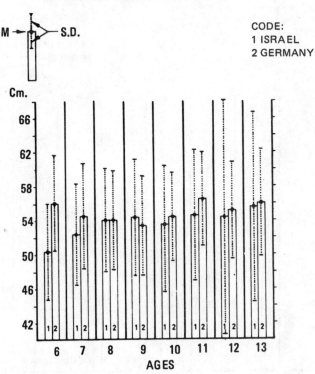

FIG. 28-44: COMPARISON OF MEANS & S.D.'s
IN FORWARD FLEXION - GIRLS 6-13

FIG. 28-45: COMPARISON OF MEANS & S.D.'s IN ARM GRIP - BOYS 7-13

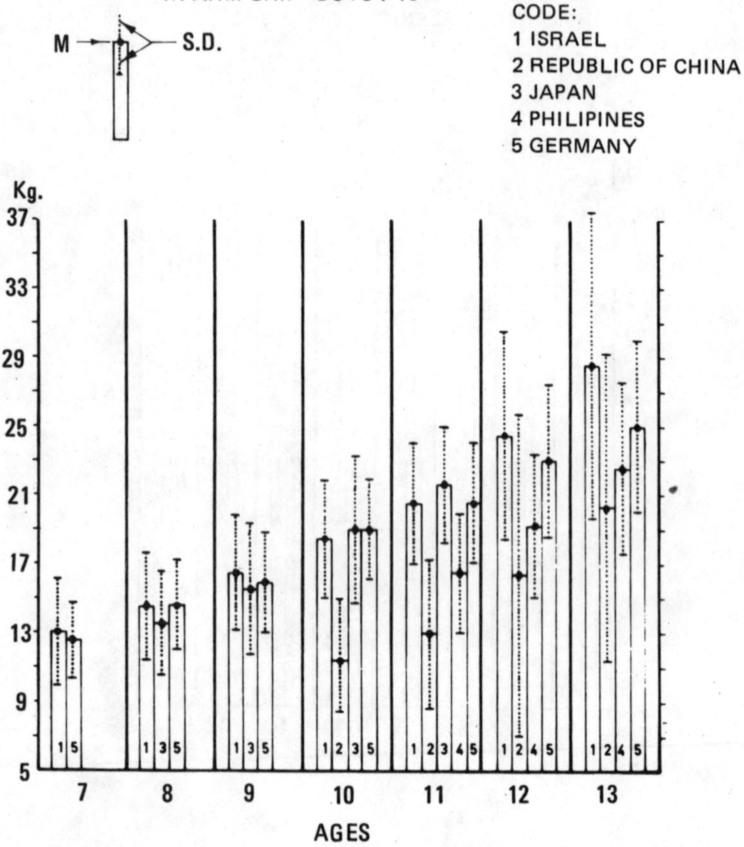
M
S.D.
CODE:
1 ISRAEL
2 REPUBLIC OF CHINA
3 JAPAN
4 PHILIPINES
5 GERMANY
Kg.
37
33
29
25
21
17
13
9
5
1 5
1 3 5
1 3 5
1 2 3 5
1 2 3 4 5
1 2 4 5
1 2 4 5
7
8
9
10
11
12
13
AGES

FIG. 28-46: COMPARISON OF MEANS & S.D.'s
IN ARM GRIP - GIRLS 7-13

CODE:
1 ISRAEL
2 REPUBLIC OF CHINA
3 JAPAN
4 PHILIPINES
5 GERMANY

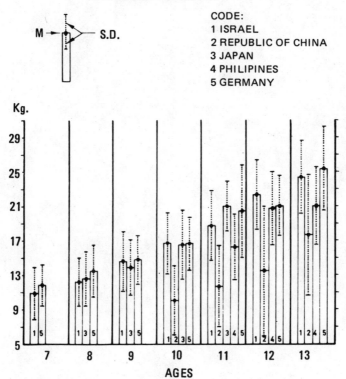

References

1. Schlesinger, Y. and Guttman L.: Smallest space analysis of intelligence and achievement tests. *Psychol Bull, 71*:95-100, 1969.
2. Ruskin, H.: Physical performance survey of pupils aged 15-18 in Israeli secondary schools, In *Standardization of Physical Fitness Test*. Basel, Birkhauser, 1974, pp. 39-48.

Chapter 29

PHYSICAL FITNESS IN YOUNG BENGALESE MALE STUDENTS*

R. N. SEN, M. R. KAR, AND D. CHAKRABARTI

Abstract

Physical fitness scores for young Bengalese male students were determined using "slow" and "rapid" Harvard step tests. The students had a very poor physical fitness compared to other groups of Indian subjects.

Introduction

O UR WORLD APPEARS headed for complete automation, but until now the process has been only partially achieved. "The advantageous use of people is still the key to success, all the machines and processes notwithstanding. Competitive advantages lie in the most efficient use of man power."[1]

Efficiency depends on individual fitness.[2] Fitness determines the safe level of occupational work, sustains alertness, and keeps away fatigue. It also increases both the quantity and the quality of production. Unfortunately, the assessment of this important variable is neither clear nor absolute. The meaning of fitness varies according to the nature of physical and mental work required of the individual. Some fitness tests demand muscular capacity, while in other tests cardiovascular and

*The authors are indebted to the students who volunteered as subjects, and to the school and college authorities. The computer service provided by Calcutta University is acknowledged with thanks. The authors also acknowledge the technical assistance of G. G. Roy, P. L. Pakrashi, and A. Dhar.

respiratory efficiency, endurance, and emotional stability are more important. No single test can assess fitness satisfactorily. Three main categories can be distinguished:[3, 4, 5]

1. tests based on anthropometric measurements,
2. tests based on cardiovascular variables such as pulse rate and blood pressure.
3. tests which measure muscle strength and endurance.

One frequently used procedure of class two is the Harvard step test. In its standard version, the subject climbs a bench, 50.8 cm high, at a uniform rate of 30 step/min for a total of five minutes (less if the subject is exhausted). After exercise, recovery pulse rates are counted in the sitting position and a fitness score is calculated as follows:

$$\text{Score} = \frac{\text{Duration of exercise in seconds} \times 100}{2 \times \text{sum of pulse counts at 1–1.5, 2–2.5, and 3–3.5 minutes of recovery}}$$

This score will subsequently be described as the "slow" method, since it requires pulse counting up to the fourth minute. In the modified Harvard step test ("rapid" method), the score is calculated from a single pulse count taken between 1 and 1.5 minutes of recovery:

$$\text{Score (rapid method)} = \frac{\text{Duration of work in seconds} \times 18}{\text{Pulse count at 1–1.5 minutes of recovery}}$$

Methods and material

In the present study, the height of the step was reduced to 40 cm and the frequency of stepping was reduced to 20/min, giving a load of 400 kg-m/min, about 50 percent of max for our subjects.[8] Many measurements of pulse rate were taken during recovery in order to get a better record of the slope òf the recovery curve. The pulse rate was also counted during exercise (counting time ten beats).

Subjects were a group of young Bengalese students aged 13 to 25 years (mean 20.7 years), drawn from middle class

TABLE 29-I
MEAN PHYSICAL CHARACTERISTICS AND RESTING PHYSIOLOGICAL VARIABLES
IN YOUNG MALE STUDENTS (N = 76)

	Mean	*SE*	*Range*
Age (yrs)	20.66	0.29	13.0 – 25.2
Height (cm)	164.89	0.69	153.7 – 181.6
Weight (kg)	47.34	0.67	28.81 – 60.45
Blood Pr. (Systolic) (mm Hg.)	116.2	1.42	85 – 150
Blood Pr. (Diastolic) (mm Hg.)	71.5	0.99	50 – 90
Vital Capacity (litres)	2.95	0.06	1.42 – 4.26
Sitting Pulse beats/min)	83.85	1.22	63 – 114
Standing Pulse beats/min)	94.75	1.20	75 – 118

TABLE 29-II
RECOVERY PULSE RATES OF YOUNG MALE BENGALESE STUDENTS (n = 76) AFTER STEP-TEST

	Pulse Rate (beats/min)	*S.E.*	*Range of count*
4' Work	145	±1.94	100-173
Recovery Time			
5"-15"	153.6	±0.33	17-33
20"-30"	144.0	±0.32	15-32.5
40"-50"	132.0	±0.31	14.5-29.6
1'-1'30"	121.6	±0.85	40-80
1'40"-1'50"	118.8	±0.29	13.5-26
2'-2'30"	112.6	±0.82	40-77
2'40"-2'50"	112.2	±0.27	13-25.5
3'-3'30"	109.6	±0.95	40-96
3'40"-3'50"	108.0	±0.26	13-24

families; ninety-one subjects were tested, but only seventy-six completed the experiments. Observations were made between 3 and 6 PM, with an interval of at least six hours after lunch. The average dry-bulb temperature, relative humidity and air velocity were 33.3°C, 62 percent and 76 cm/sec respectively.

Results

Using the rapid method of scoring, students were ranked as follows:

Above 150	=	100% Excellent
135-120	=	80% Good
105-90	=	60% Fair
85-75	=	50% Poor
70-60	=	40% Very poor

Most subjects ranked between forty percent and 60 percent, indicating poor physical fitness. The average pulse rate of young Indian industrial workers was 30 to 45 beats/min lower for an equivalent stress.[7]

The maximal physical work capacity of average healthy active Indians is about 1200 kg-m/min.[8] The average score of the students was equivalent to 400 kg-m/min, i.e. only a third of the maximal physical work capacity for average Indians. Sen et al.[6] have set the average maximal physical work capacity of sedentary Indian subjects at about 800 kg-m/min. The predicted maximum oxygen uptake was overestimated at 2.3 liters/min, even when the nomogram[9] adapted to a step test[10] was used to predict $\dot{V}O_2$ max from the body weight and the working pulse rate. In comparison, values for young western men lie between 3.0 and 5.0 l/min.[11]

Multiple correlation coefficients related score (slow method) to (a) height and standing pulse (r = 0.658), (b) height, systolic B.P., and standing pulse (r = 0.701), (c) sitting and standing pulse rates (r = 0.685), and (d) height, systolic B.P., and sitting and standing pulse rate (r = 0.728).

Regression equations were developed to predict fitness scores from resting measurements (Table 29-III).

TABLE 29-III
REGRESSION EQUATIONS FOR PREDICTING FITNESS FROM RESTING MEASUREMENTS

Regression Equations

S = (195.5 − 0.254 H − 0.6899 STP)   Stnd. Err. Estm. :11.4%

S = (159.9 − 4.214 SP − 0.3826 STP)   Stnd. Err. Estm. : 9.9%

WP = (− 6.157 + 0.636 H + 0.487 STP)   Stnd. Err. Estm. :11.8%

WP = (88.526 + 4.438 SP + 0.200 STP)   Stnd. Err. Estm. :11.9%

S = Score by Slow method,
H = Body Height
SP = Sitting Pulse
STP = Standing Pulse
WP = Working Pulse

Discussion

Limitations of the Harvard step test are discussed by Macpherson.[12] In spite of all criticism, it remains a simple, practical, and useful fitness test. The original bench height could be a handicap for short-statured Bengalese people. By reducing the height and frequency of stepping, the work load was so adjusted that average people were able to continue the exercise for the full five minutes without depending on very high motivation. In this way, all could perform the same work per unit of body mass, making comparisons more valid.

The young Bengalese students were, on the average, in extremely poor physical condition. Possible explanations include a gross absence of physical activity and bad food habits, especially with regard to the selection of food.

References

1. Walker, R. W.: An evaluation of training methods and their characteristics. *Human Factors,* 7:347, 1965.
2. Wyndham, C. H.: The effect of environmental heat on the comfort, productivity and health of workmen. *S Afr Mech Eng J 14*(10): 209-221, 1965.

3. Cureton, T. K.: Physical fitness—appraisal and guidance. St Louis, Mosby 1947.
4. American Association for Health, Physical Education and Recreation: *The A.A.H.P.E.R. Fitness Test Manual,* rev. ed. Washington, D.C., A.A.H.P.E.R. 1965.
5. Fowler, W. M., Jr. and Gardner, G. W.: The relation of cardiovascular tests to measurements of motor performance and skills. *Pediatrics, 32* (suppl):778, 1963.
6. Sen, R. N. and Sarkar, D. N.: Occupational daily work load for Indian industrial workers at three different thermal conditions. In Anand, R.L. (Ed): *Proceedings of the International Satellite Symposium on Work Physiology and Ergonomics,* Patiala, India, Netaji Subhas National Institute of Sports, Abstract No. 13. 1974, pp 32.
7. Sen, R. N., Saha, P. N., and Subramanian, A.: Assessment of work load and thermal stress in relation to physiological responses of workers in a soap factory in Bombay. *Report No. 4.* Sion, Bombay, The Industrial Physiology Division, Central Labour Institute, 1964, pp. 28.
8. Sen, R. N., Roy, B. S., and Sarkar, D. N.: *Maximal Physical Work Capacity of Indian Industrial Workers in Relation to Age and Heaviness of Job.* Read before International Conference of the Human Factors Society, Philadelphia, U.S.A., 1969.
9. Ryhming, I.: Modified Harvard step test for the evaluation of physical fitness. *Arbeitsphysiologie, 15*:235, 1953.
10. Åstrand, I.: Aerobic work capacity in men and women with special reference to age. *Acta Physiol Scand, 49* (Suppl 169): 1960.
11. Åstrand, P. O.: *Experimental Studies of Physical Working Capacity in Relation to Sex and Age.* Copenhagen, Munksgaard, 1952.
12. MacPherson, R. K.: Tropical fatigue. *University of Queensland Papers* (Department of Physiology), *I* (10):66, 1949.

Section Four

FITNESS TESTING IN PROGRAMS OF COMMUNITY HEALTH

Chapter 30

THE CANADIAN HOME FITNESS TEST IN THE HEALTH ENVIRONMENT

R. R. J. Lauzon

Abstract

The Canadian Home Fitness Test (CHFT) has been employed both as a screening procedure and as an educational-motivational tool. The author gives instances of the above uses and relates each to the role of the CHFT in an exercise program.

THE FUTURE DIRECTION of community health, public health, and occupational health in Canada should be to increase understanding of the tremendous impact that life-style has on health and well being. In the quest for appropriate health promotion techniques, the roles of exercise and physical recreation have captured the limelight and are duly recognized in the Government of Canada Working Document *A New Perspective on the Health of Canadians.*[4] The arrival of the Canadian Home Fitness Test (CHFT) coincides with this surge of interest in life-style and health.

The purpose of this chapter is to discuss the Canadian Home Fitness Test in the context of public and occupational health programs. From this point of view, two uses are envisaged for the CHFT: (1) as a screening-procedure and (2) as an educational-motivational tool.

The CHFT As A Screening Procedure

An exercise stress test is currently used as a preliminary to entering many physical activity programs. However, the most popular protocols are relatively time-consuming and perhaps unnecessarily sophisticated for the purpose. The CHFT offers a simple and efficient method of providing a submaximal exercise stress test to future program participants.

Sackett[7] has proposed that four conditions should be met before implementing any mass health screening program. His conditions are as follows:

1. Experimental results must show the reliability and validity of the test.
2. Health services must be adequate to meet the demand resulting from testing.
3. Compliance with the prescribed treatment must be high.
4. Good must exceed evil.

These principles are consistent with the W.H.O. recommendations as stated in *Principles and Practice of Screening for Disease.*[10]

Experimental results are certainly available to confirm the reliability and validity of the CHFT. Under monitored conditions, the CHFT has proven as accurate a predictor of aerobic power as other available techniques.[3, 8] However, the sensitivity of the test suffers in the self-administered situation. The question of risk to the subject is discussed below.

The second requirement is the availability of an adequate delivery system to improve the level of fitness in those individuals judged to have an undesirable or minimum personal fitness level as assessed by the CHFT. Certainly, the public health and occupational health agencies in Canada provide an as yet untapped resource for exercise testing and fitness counselling.

In the two months preceeding the Montreal Olympics the provincial public health association of Québec, l'Association de la santé publique du Québec, conducted over 70 CHFT Leader Clinics, training more than 2000 health workers, physical educators, and fitness leaders in the mechanics of group testing and providing background information for fitness counselling. One hundred and forty similar clinics have been run by the Canadian Association for Health, Physical Education and Recreation (C.A.H.P.E.R.), with the participation of over 4000 fitness leaders. Recreation Canada trained a group of federal occupational health nurses in a similar fashion; these nurses operate thirty-four health clinics, serving almost 90,000 civil servants in the National Capital Zone of Ottawa-Hull.

During 1976, the Canada Health Survey was begun. Approximately 40,000 Canadians, drawn from a multistage random sample, will be exposed to a life-style—oriented questionnaire and a physical examination. The CHFT will form one component of the physical examination.

The cost-effectiveness of the CHFT is most favorable. As a mass screening device, 100 subjects have been tested per hour in a monitored setting.[8] In terms of health risk, Shephard[8] has estimated that "if all middle aged Canadians continued to perform the test once per year without restriction, it would be 16 to 33 years before there was a death attributable to the test; exclusion of half the 'high-risk' patients by use of the 'physical activity readiness questionnaire' should lengthen the waiting period for a coronary incident to 33 to 66 years." In the evaluation of over 14000 adults, Recreation Canada has experienced no major problems.

No doubt the greatest difficulty with exercise testing and prescription is the issue of compliance with prescribed regimens of physical activity. Exercise programs in Canada, as elsewhere, are confronted with a high prevalence of program "dropouts." This is not unique to fitness programs. Similar problems occur in smoking withdrawal clinics, weight control groups, alcohol abuse programs, and so on. Nevertheless, the generality of this phenomenon does not absolve the practitioner from the responsibility of ensuring that individuals tested have access to well-structured fitness programs. If we accept that exercise compliance is low and will remain so, we must recognize the ethical dilemma of making people aware of their poor state of physical fitness, while failing to help them improve their fitness status.

Meyer and Henderson[5] have reported encouraging results from behavioral modification approaches to CHD risk-factor reduction. In an extension of the project to a community setting with the use of mass media, the encouraging results persisted.[1] Jackson's study[2] of Participation Saskatoon, a community fitness awareness program, indicated that the technology is available to improve exercise compliance.

The fourth principle of mass screening is that good must exceed evil. As just mentioned, there is an ethical issue if there is poor compliance with the prescribed regimen. There is abundant information on the physiological benefits of exercise. As yet there is no conclusive evidence that exercise will increase life expectancy, although we may accept the thesis that exercise adds "life to your years if not years to your life." Wilhelmsen et al.[9] carried out a controlled study of physical training after myocardial infarction, and they concluded that there were no significant differences of mortality between the training and the control group. However, many authors have stated on numerous occasions that the mental health benefits alone are sufficient to justify the worth of physical fitness testing and activity programs.

In summary, there is ample justification for the use of the CHFT as a screening tool. With the increasing medical emphasis upon exercise testing and prescription, it is the duty of all health workers and physical educators to take a supportive and facilitative position regarding exercise testing, recognizing that now is the time to remove barriers in order to promote a physically active lifestyle among our citizens. Thus, the CHFT is perceived by Recreation Canada as a sensible first step that a citizen should take prior to initiating his or her personal physical activity program.

The CHFT as a Motivational Tool

The CHFT was originally devised primarily as a motivational tool.[6] Although no controlled studies have been conducted to date on the motivational power of the test, Recreation Canada is encouraged by many anecdotal reports from its use.

The most popular application of the CHFT has been during special fitness weeks or fitness displays. For example, the Occupational Health Department of the Metropolitan Life Insurance Company in Ottawa used the test as a springboard for a fitness week and an employee fitness program. One initially disconcerting result was the observation that mass testing attracted employees whose scores fell in the middle and upper fitness levels. When nonparticipants were tested subsequently in private, the majority had scores in the lowest and middle categories. The lesson seems that both public and private testing should be available to the individual.

In an employee fitness program within the Department of National Health and Welfare, the CHFT is employed regularly to monitor cardiovascular progress. Accuracy is improved by using a second person to assist in pulse taking.

The test itself has inherent educational qualities, since it is based on the reaction of the cardiovascular system to a given physical workload. It facilitates the follow-up discussion with the subject concerning the need for an aerobic component in an exercise program. Moreover, the subject learns that his pulse rate can be used as a sensitive indicator of the intensity of a personal fitness program.

The CHFT is one of many items included in the life-style awareness component of a twelve-week residential middle management development program in the federal public service. Fitness testing and daily physical activity form the core of the life-style unit and are begun on entry to the program in order to demonstrate how easy it is to incorporate a physical activity program into daily living.

We have observed that participation in fitness-related activities has stimulated reductions in smoking and alcohol consumption; subjects also reported that they were much more conscientious in the selection of food during mealtimes. It has become apparent that physical activity can serve as a focal point in encouraging other changes of life-style. While the individual exercises, he does not usually continue smoking or drinking. Thus, the period that is spent exercising consumes time which might have been spent in less healthy pursuits. Furthermore, exercise may generate an interest in adopting other healthy habits. Again, anecdotal results are encouraging in this regard.

References

1. Alexander, J.: *Mass Media: The New Health Provider.* Read before the 26th Annual Meeting of the International Communication Association, Portland, Oregon, 1976.
2. Jackson, J. J.: *Diffusion of an Innovation: An Exploratory Study of the Consequences of Sport Participation Canada's Campaign at Saskatoon.* Doctoral Dissertation, University of Alberta (Edmonton, Alberta), 1975.
3. Jetté, M., Campbell, J., Mongeon, J., and Routhier, R.: The Canadian Home Fitness Test as a predictor of aerobic capacity, *Can. Med Assoc J, 114*:680-682, 1976.
4. Lalonde, M.: *A New Perspective on the Health of Canadians. A Working Document.* Ottawa, Government of Canada, 1972.
5. Meyer, A. and Henderson, J.: Multiple risk-factor reduction in the prevention of cardiovascular disease, *Prev Med, 3*:225-226, 1974.
6. *Proceedings of the National Conference on Fitness and Health,* December 1972. Ottawa, Information Canada, 1974.
7. Sackett, D. L.: *Workshop Lecture.* Halifax, Nova Scotia, Division of Family Medicine, Dalhousie University, December 1975.
8. Shephard, R. J., Bailey, D. A., and Mirwald, R. L.: Development of the Canadian Home Fitness Test, *Can Med Assoc. J, 114*:675-679, 1976.
9. Wilhelmsen, L., Sänne, H. Elmfeldt, D., Grimby, G., Tibblin, G., and Wedel, H.: A controlled trial of physical training after myocardial infarction, *Prev Med, 4*:491-508, 1975.
10. Wilson, J. L. G. and Junder, G.: *Principles and Practice of Screening for Disease.* Public Health Papers No. *34.* Geneva, World Health Organization, 1968.

Chapter 31

ON THE STAGE DURATION FOR A PROGRESSIVE EXERCISE TEST PROTOCOL

R. J. SHEPHARD AND T. KAVANAGH

Abstract

Data are presented to support the traditional view that the optimum format of a submaximal exercise test is a progressive loading, allowing three or four minutes per stage. This arrangement allows the subject to come close to steady-state values of heart rate and oxygen consumption for a given work load. Tests where the work load is increased at one-minute intervals underestimate both the steady-state heart rate and the corresponding blood pressure, while the tolerated work load and the aerobic power are overestimated by some 12 percent. In postcoronary patients, the electrocardiographic response to a given work load is also misleading. The ECG can be interpreted by relating it to heart rate, but in some patients abnormalities are more marked in the first minute than during a steady-state response. If individual stages of a progressive test are substantially extended, as when attempting steady-state measurements of cardiac output (five to eight minutes per stage), the aerobic power is underestimated by about 5 percent, and in some patients the severity of ECG changes is less than in a standard test.

SEVERAL INTERNATIONAL groups, including the International Biological Programme,[1] the World Health Organization,[2] and the International Committee for the Standardization of Physical Fitness Tests[3] have all recommended that the optimum approach to submaximal exercise testing is a progressive schedule, allowing three or even four minutes per work load. The main reason for this approach has been to allow the subjects to come close to a steady state at a given work load before proceeding to a higher intensity of effort.

Table 31-I recalls some observations of Shephard[4] on steady-state stepping. After three minutes of exercise, subjects had reached 95 to 99 percent of the heart rate to be anticipated with five minutes of effort. With the "warm-up" provided by a progressive test format, the subject is brought even closer to his steady-state value by the third minute of effort.[4] Although there remain small discrepancies of ventilatory volume, respiratory quotient, and ventilatory equivalent, the heart rate and oxygen consumption data yielded by a three-minute progressive test are extremely close to equilibrium values (Table 31-II), so that there is a close correspondence of predicted maximum oxygen intakes by steady-state and progressive test formats (Table 31-III).

One possibility raised in the W.H.O. discussions of this topic was that, whereas three minutes might allow adequate equilibration for a healthy young adult, older subjects with diseased hearts could possibly take longer to reach an equilibrium. In

TABLE 31-I

HEART RATE DURING SUCCESSIVE MINUTES OF FIVE MINUTE STEADY-STATE STEP TEST: ALL VALUES FOR A GIVEN LOADING EXPRESSED AS PERCENT OF VALUES FOR FIFTH MINUTE OF EXERCISE. DATA FOR TEN YOUNG MEN (4).

Rate of working		Heart rate at time specified (%)			
$kg\text{-}m\text{-}min^{-1}$	$kJ\text{-}min^{-1}$	1 min	2 min	3 min	4 min
320	3.14	93.1	98.2	99.3	98.8
480	4.71	88.1	94.6	96.0	98.3
640	6.28	81.1	91.6	94.3	97.0
800	7.85	75.9	90.0	95.5	97.4

TABLE 31-II

PHYSIOLOGICAL VARIABLES OBTAINED DURING A PROGRESSIVE EXERCISE TEST (3 MIN PER STAGE) EXPRESSED AS PERCENT OF VALUES OBTAINED DURING FIVE MINUTES OF EQUIVALENT STEADY STATE WORK.[4] 10 YOUNG MEN, EXERCISING ON A STEP TEST.

Rate of working		Resp min vol	Respiratory quotient	Ventilatory equivalent	Heart rate	Oxygen cons.
$kg\text{-}m\text{-}min^{-1}$	$kJ\text{-}min^{-1}$					
320	3.14	92.4%	89.0%	91.5%	101.1%	99.7%
480	4.71	93.8	83.9	95.1	101.1	100.3
640	6.28	97.8	103.4	96.2	101.3	99.6
800	7.85	96.1	105.0	102.4	99.5	96.8

TABLE 31-III

ACCURACY OF MAXIMUM OXYGEN INTAKE PREDICTION—A COMPARISON OF STEADY-STATE TESTS OF 5 MINUTES DURATION AND A STANDARD PROGRESSIVE PROTOCOL.[5]

	Predicted maximum oxygen intake $(l\text{-}min^{-1}, mM\text{-}min^{-1})$		
	Step test	*Bicycle test*	*Treadmill test*
Steady state	3.75 (167.2)	3.57 (159.2)	3.83 (170.8)
Standard progressive protocol	3.73 (166.4)	3.64 (162.3)	3.79 (169.0)
$\Delta \pm S_\Delta$	$- 0.013 \pm 0.34$	$+ 0.069 \pm 0.29$	$- 0.043 \pm 0.61$

order to test this point, we took three groups of postcoronary patients,[6] carrying out progressive tests with data recorded in the third and the fifth minute on each group. Group A comprised fifteen new entrants to our postcoronary training program, Group B were twelve patients who had been with us for a year or more but were not responding well to training, and group C were members of the program who had progressed to running a substantial distance. Table 31-IV compares data from the third and fifth minutes at each load of a progressive test. As in the previous series, the respiratory minute volumes and respiratory exchange ratios were further from equilibrium at three minutes than were the heart rate and oxygen consumption values. Heart rate and oxygen consumption figures were a little further from 100 percent than had been the case in the young normals, but nevertheless there was a good correspondence between the three-minute and the five-minute predictions of maximum oxygen intake, irrespective of the condition of the subject and his response to the training program. The one anomaly was the small drop in oxygen consumption from the third to the fifth minute at the final workload in Group C. These subjects had reached a heart rate of 154/minute, and it is likely that some of the group were at their maximum aerobic power; the decline of oxygen consumption could thus reflect a true physiological difficulty in sustaining maximum oxygen delivery for five minutes.

The data presented thus far confirms the traditional wisdom of the international organizations in advising a three– or

TABLE 31-IV

THE RATE OF ATTAINMENT OF A STEADY STATE IN POSTCORONARY PATIENTS. DATA FOR (A), 15 NEW ENTRANTS, (B) 12 PATIENTS PROGRESSING POORLY, AND (C) 9 PATIENTS PROGRESSING WELL. THREE MINUTE RESPONSES TO BICYCLE ERGOMETER EFFORT EXPRESSED AS PERCENT OF THE RESPONSE TO FIVE MINUTES AT A GIVEN LOADING.

Duration of effort and subject group		Resp Min Vol	Resp Exchange Ratio	Heart Rate	Oxygen Cons	Predicted aerobic power
5 min	A	103.9%	105.0%	100.2%	96.2%	
	B	101.7	102.2	98.4	97.7	
	C	98.8	101.7	98.7	81.2	
10 min	A	93.9	98.7	99.0	93.4	
	B	93.8	98.9	97.5	95.3	
	C	92.5	102.9	97.6	88.1	
15 min	A	94.8	100.0	98.1	97.0	97.7%
	B	88.3	100.0	96.1	89.1	96.5
	C	90.0	99.1	96.8	93.2	101.9
20 min	A	90.1	100.0	95.5	94.4	98.7
	B	93.8	102.0	98.0	98.2	101.5
	C	99.1	97.5	97.5	104.5	108.7

four-minute progressive test. However, further examination of the problem was made necessary by the commencement of a multicenter collaborative trial of exercise for the postcoronary patient.[6] Two types of test protocol were proposed for this trial. A very simple (" stage one") test was to be carried out frequently as a guide to exercise prescription. A protracted ("stage two") test would be repeated less often, with measurements of cardiac output and other variables. It quickly became apparent that neither of these new protocols was giving the same information as the traditional, internationally approved test. Accordingly, we decided to compare these procedures with the three-minute progressive test, using as our subjects two groups of fifty patients recently recruited to our exercise rehabilitation program.

The "stage one" test was carried out on a Monark bicycle ergometer. Work load, heart rate, electrocardiogram, and blood pressure response were recorded throughout. The protocol was progressive in type, but in order to reach a high work load fairly quickly, the loading was increased by 100 kg-m/min every minute.

The physiological responses (Fig. 31-1) showed a progressively developing discrepancy between the rapid, "stage one" test and the standard procedure. The "stage one" heart rate was substantially lower, about ten beats per minute at the final work load, and the blood pressure was also less, about 7 mmHg or 1 kPa in the case of the systolic reading, and 4 mmHg or 0.6 kPa in the case of the diastolic figure. This has serious implications for work prescription. The object of the test is to define a safe work load that can be sustained by the subject during his rehabilitation program. However, because a steady state has not been reached, his work potential is overestimated. If data are converted to predicted maximum oxygen intakes, using the Åstrand nomogram,[7, 8] there is a good correspondence between oxygen and work scale predictions with the standard test (Table 31-V), both showing an aerobic power of just over 2.4 liters per minute, a little under 110 mM-min^{-1}. However, the "stage one" test yields values some 12 percent higher. Rutenfranz (9) drew attention to this same problem in his evaluation of the Müller Leistungspulsindex. Accordingly, if the attained work load or the corresponding prediction of aerobic power from a "stage one" test are to be translated into an exercise prescription, they must be reduced by 12 percent to allow for failure to reach a steady state.

TABLE 31-V

A COMPARISON OF PREDICTED MAXIMUM OXYGEN INTAKES (ÅSTRAND NOMOGRAM) DERIVED FROM A STANDARD PROGRESSIVE SUBMAXIMAL TEST ON A BICYCLE ERGOMETER, AND DATA OBTAINED FROM A MORE RAPID (STAGE ONE) TEST. RESULTS FOR FIFTY POSTCORONARY PATIENTS, MEAN ± S.D.

	Predicted maximum oxygen intake (l-min^{-1} STPD, mM-min^{-1})	
	oxygen scale	*work scale*
Standard progressive test	2.46 ± 0.58 (109.7)	2.42 ± 0.59 (107.9)
Stage one test		2.72 ± 0.70 (121.3)

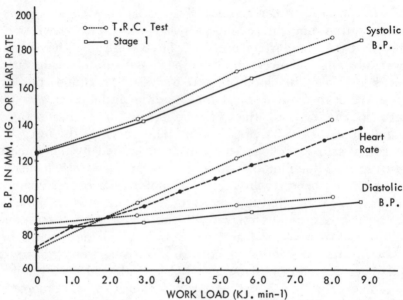

Figure 31-1. Physiological variables during a standard progressive submaximal exercise test and during a rapid (stage one) test. Data for fifty postcoronary patients.

How reliable is the ECG information from the rapid test? Again, this is an important point when prescribing exercise, since we are seeking an intensity of effort that will not cause dangerous dysrhythmias or excessive ST segmental depression. In terms of the attained work load, information from a "stage one" test can be dangerously misleading, since neither the heart rate nor the blood pressure have reached steady-state values equivalent to the apparent work load. If note is taken of the heart rate rather than the ergometer loading, the "stage one" test becomes more reliable. We found a total of twenty-three out of the fifty tests where the heart rate was roughly the same in standard and rapid tests, and in this group ST depressions were also roughly comparable for the two methods (Table 31-VI); in a few instances, depression was marginally greater with the rapid test—these presumably are individuals who can "run through their angina," with coronary vasodilatation and

TABLE 31-VI

A COMPARISON OF ST SEGMENTAL DEPRESSION IN A STANDARD PRO-
GRESSIVE SUBMAXIMAL TEST AND IN A RAPID (STAGE ONE) TEST AT
COMPARABLE HEART RATES. DATA FOR 23 POSTCORONARY PATIENTS.
MEANS ± S.D.

	Standard test	*Stage one test*
Heart rate	137.5 ± 15.1	137.0 ± 15.4
ST depression (mV)	0.115 ± 0.099	0.133 ± 0.102

an increase of systemic perfusion pressure giving a lesser ST
response to steady-state than to rapidly induced exercise.

The "stage two" tests are of unpredictable length, since each
stage is prolonged until oxygen and carbon dioxide concentrations show that a respiratory steady state has been reached and
satisfactory cardiac output determinations have been completed. As we saw above, ventilation stabilizes more slowly than
heart rate and oxygen consumption (Table 31-II), and in
different individuals the test format may require five to eight
minutes per stage.

Physiological responses to the "stage two" test and the
standard progressive test are compared in Figure 31-2. Blood
pressures were almost identical with the two protocols, but the
more prolonged work load gave a heart rate about four beats
per minute faster at each of the three work loads tested. In
consequence, the "stage two" test led to some underprediction
of maximum oxygen intake relative to the standard protocol
(Table 31-VII); however, if the oxygen consumption of the
subject was measured, the error from prolongation of the task
was not more than about 5 percent.

With regard to the electrocardiographic changes, twenty-
three of the fifty subjects in this series also had roughly
comparable heart rates (Table 31-VIII). Average ST segmental
depressions were similar for standard and "stage two" tests,
although in occasional examples depression was a little less with
the longer test.

We may conclude that the present data support use of a
progressive submaximal exercise test that allows three or four
minutes per stage. Where there are departures from this

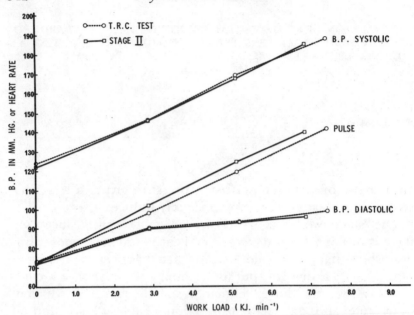

Figure 31-2. Physiological variables during a standard progressive submaximal exercise test and during a more protracted (stage two) test. Data for fifty postcoronary patients.

TABLE 31-VII

A COMPARISON OF PREDICTED MAXIMUM OXYGEN INTAKES (ÅSTRAND NOMOGRAM) DERIVED FROM A STANDARD PROGRESSIVE SUBMAXIMAL TEST ON A BICYCLE ERGOMETER, AND DATA OBTAINED FROM A MORE PROTRACTED (STAGE TWO) TEST. RESULTS FOR FIFTY POSTCORONARY PATIENTS, MEAN ± S.D.

	Predicted maximum oxygen intake $(l\text{-}min^{-1}\ STPD,\ mM\text{-}min^{-1})$	
	oxygen scale	*work scale*
Standard progressive test	2.42 ± 0.47	2.38 ± 0.50
	(107.9)	(106.1)
Stage two test	2.29 ± 0.49	2.06 ± 0.42
	(102.1)	(91.9)

TABLE 31-VIII

A COMPARISON OF ST SEGMENTAL DEPRESSION IN A STANDARD PRO-
GRESSIVE SUBMAXIMAL TEST AND IN STAGE TWO TESTING AT COMPAR-
ABLE HEART RATES. DATA FOR 23 POSTCORONARY PATIENTS,
MEAN ± S.D.

	Standard test	*Stage two test*
Heart rate	136.0 ± 14.5	138.4 ± 14.6
ST depression (mV)	0.124 ± 0.108	0.106 ± 0.085

routine, misleading impressions may be formed with respect to work tolerance and associated electrocardiographic abnormalities. If the load is increased at one minute intervals, aerobic power is underestimated by about 12 percent. ECG changes must be related to heart rate rather than the attained work load—even with this precaution, the brief test sometimes indicates a larger change than the steady-state progressive test.

If it is necessary to extend stages to longer than three minutes for such purposes as the meaurement of cardiac output, the estimate of aerobic power will be a little ($\approx$ 5%) low, and in some patients the severity of ECG changes will be less than in a standard test.

References

1. Weiner, J. S. and Lourie, J. A.: *Human Biology: A guide to field methods.* Oxford. Blackwell, 1969.
2. Anderson, K. L. et al.: *Fundamentals of Exercise Testing.* Geneva W. H. O., 1971.
3. Larson, L.: *Physical fitness measurements standards.* Final report of International Committee for the standardization of physical fitness tests, Tel Aviv, 1969.
4. Shephard, R. J.: The prediction of "maximal" oxygen consumption using a new progressive step test. *Ergonomics, 10*:1-15, 1967.
5. Shephard, R. J. et al.: Standardization of sub-maximal exercise tests. *Bull W.H.O. 38*:765-775, 1968.
6. Rechnitzer, P. A. et al.: A controlled prospective study of the effect of endurance training on the recurrence rate of myocardial infarction—a description of the experimental design. *Am J Epidemiol, 120*:358-365, 1975.

7. Åstrand, I.: Aerobic work capacity in men and women with special reference to age. *Acta Physiol Scand, 40* (Supp. 169):1-92, 1960.
8. Shephard, R. J.: Computer programmes for solution of the Åstrand nomogram. *J Sports Med Fitness 10*:206-210, 1970.
9. Rutenfranz, J.: *Entwicklung und Beurteilung der korperlichen Leistungsfahigkeit bei Kindern und Jugendlichen.* Basel, Karger, 1964.

Suggested Additional Reading

Shephard, R. J.: *Endurance Fitness,* (2nd ed.) Toronto: University of Toronto Press, 1977.

Chapter 32

FACTORS AFFECTING AN EXERCISE TOLERANCE TEST

B. LAKE

Abstract

Various conditions diagnosed from a standard medical history and examination influence scores on an exercise tolerance test. Clinical data for 300 subjects has been related to scores on a relative fitness index, adjusted for height, age, and sex (TW19R). The mean and standard deviation of scores was 0 ± 18.0 with a range from -53.7 to $+79.0$. In subjects who had >50 percent compliance with a prescribed training program, retest scores increased by an average of 9.0 units. With less than 50 percent compliance the index showed virtually no change over a three month period, and if no exercise had been undertaken, there was a decrease in score averaging 6.0 units. The degree of improvement with training depended partly on the initial fitness level of the individual. Positive influences on the TW19R score included the habit of restful and refreshing sleep, FEV_1 and FVC 10 percent above predicted values and mid and peak expiratory flows above the normal range. Adverse influences included cigarette smoking, acute alcohol intake, chronic alcoholism, manifest anxiety (largely self-directed repression), restrictive airway disorder and chronic bronchitis, ischemic heart disease, other forms of heart disease, a variety of abnormalities in the resting and the exercise ECG, a hematocrit above 51 percent, a serum uric acid level above 7.2 mg%, and the use of a variety of drugs.

THE RESIDUAL FITNESS index (Lake, 1976) is a simple fitness score based on the variance of work output after allowance for the effects of sex, age, height, and weight. The present chapter describes variations of this index encountered in the course of medical practice.

Materials and Methods

A total of 300 subjects (219 males, 81 females) aged 17 to 68 years performed a progressive bicycle ergometer test. The residual fitness index (TW19R) was calculated according to the following equations:

Men: TW19R = Total work (kpm) to level 19 on Borg scale of perceived exertion −1.41 (height in cm) +0.74 (age in years) +113.0

Women: TW19R = Total work (kpm) to level 19 on Borg scale of perceived exertion −0.60 (height in cm) −0.16 (weight in kg) +0.27 (age in years) +25.9

This index is normally distributed, the mean and standard deviation of scores being 0 ± 18.0 arbitrary units with a range of −53.7 to +78.2 units.

Reproducibility of residual fitness index

Twenty-nine subjects had at least three submaximal exercise assessments over a period of six to twelve months. All were reliable, consistent subjects who had stabilized on their exercise programs. The likely maximal daily variation, of the TW19R, calculated as $\frac{\Sigma(d^2)}{2n}$ was $\pm$ 3.76 units. Differences in residual fitness index greater than these limits were considered as due to factors other than intrapersonal daily variation. The influence of conditions noted during medical examination was subjected to analysis of variance or to student t tests where applicable.

Results

Sleep

The sleep pattern was categorized as (a) always restful and refreshing, (b) mostly restful and refreshing, (c) acutely disturbed within the past few weeks, or (d) chronically disturbed. Those in group (a) had a significantly higher TW19R than the remaining three categories.

Sleep Category	Mean TW19R	S.D.	N
a	10.9	23.9	14
b	−1.4	17.6	204
c	−3.5	15.5	10
d	−3.9	17.5	72

F= 2.74   p<0.05

Tobacco

There was a progressive deterioration in the TW19R score with a currrent tobacco usage >60 g/wk. This was unlikely to have been due to an immediate pharmacologic effect of nicotine or other constituents of cigarette smoke, as all smokers refrained for a minimum of three hours prior to ergometry.

Weekly tobacco usage	Mean TW19R	S.D.	N
No smoking	0.4	18.2	190
≤ 60g/wk	0.7	15.9	36
60 to 120 g/wk	−5.2	19.3	34
≥ 120 g/wk	−9.6	15.4	40

F= 4.22   p<0.01

The number of years of tobacco usage was also related to the loss of TW19R.

Years of tobacco usage	TW19R	S.D.	N
0	0.9	18.1	163
1 to 9	−3.3	16.6	42
≥ 10	−4.8	17.9	95

F = 3.26   p<0.05

However, TW19R was unrelated to the history of inhalation. The use of cigarettes was more injurious than cigars or pipe.

Pattern of tobacco usage	TW19R	S.D.	N
No smoking	1.1	18.2	141
Cigarettes ± other forms	−4.5	17.8	147
Cigars ± pipes only	3.3	12.8	12

$F = 4.01$ $p < 0.05$

Alcohol

Alcohol intake did not generally affect the TW19R. However, scores were low if unusual amounts of alcohol had been taken within twenty-four hours of the test. In ten such subjects, the gain of TW19R index with at least four days of abstinence from alcohol averaged 9.08 ± 2.65, more than twice the maximum expected chance variation in scores.

Anxiety/depression

Anxiety and depression were assessed separately, on a clinical basis. Anxiety was subclassified as (a) chronic frustration/suppressed aggression, (b) manifest anxiety, largely self-directed, and (c) manifest anxiety, largely environmentally directed. There was a significant difference in residual fitness index according to the presence or absence of anxiety, the greatest deviation from normal being in those with self-directed anxiety.

Anxiety	TW19R	S.D.	N
Nil	2.5	19.1	110
Type a	−2.9	17.3	60
Type b	−6.4	16.6	51
Type c	−3.0	16.8	59

$F = 3.34$ $p < 0.01$

Depression was diagnosed on the basis of significant symptoms (persistent negative feelings, flat mood, early waking, etc.), usually accompanied by a positive response to such direct questions as "Do you often feel depressed?" or "Are you depressed now?" Those with depression untreated by drugs had significantly lower residual fitness indices than a normal matched control group.

	TW19R	S.D.	N
Not depressed	−0.5	18.6	153
Depressed	−14.0	16.8	24

F = 3.14   p<0.01

Ischemic Heart Disease

Severity of ischemic heart disease was graded as nil, mild, moderate, or severe. The TW19R supported this grouping.

Severity of disease	TW19R	S.D.	N
Nil	0.7	17.3	244
Mild	−6.7	15.1	25
Moderate	−12.0	18.0	27
Severe	−36.3	13.9	4

F = 11.0   p<0.001

A more detailed classification of clinical history included the categories of no disease, history of angina without and with confirmatory clinical findings, proven myocardial infarction within three months, within three to six months, within six to twelve months, and longer than one year. Again, the relative fitness index showed significant intercategory differences.

Clinical History	TW19R	S.D.	N
No heart disease	0.4	17.2	253
Angina without clinical findings	−6.9	12.7	12
Angina with clinical findings	−12.5	17.5	18
M.I.≤ 3/12	−33.5	28.6	2
M.I. 3/12 to 6/12	−6.7	26.7	3
M.I. 6/12 to 12/12	−39.9	11.2	2
M.I. >12/12	−5.5	23.8	8
M.I. uncertain date classification	−19.1	9.4	2

F = 4.31   p<0.01

Respiratory Disorders

Respiratory disorders had a significant effect on the relative fitness index, particularly in the case of restrictive airway disease.

Type of Respiratory Disorder	TW19R	S.D.	N
Nil	0.5	17.2	201
Asthma	−0.5	21.3	14
Obstructive (other than asthma)	−2.3	16.7	14
Restrictive	−10.2	17.7	16
Restrictive & Obstructive	−10.3	19.4	22
Chronic bronchitis (with normal spirogram)	−4.0	19.0	31

$F = 2.48 \qquad p \approx 0.05$

Other conditions

All patients considered under this heading were on specific and/or symptomatic treatment at the time of ergometry and so were supposedly able to work relatively free of the limitations imposed by the basic disorder. Results are shown for categories containing five or more subjects.

Condition	TW19R	S.D.	N
Urinary tract disorder	−3.2	19.1	34
Arthritis (other than gout)	−0.2	13.9	26
Other heart disease	−9.0	16.7	15
Gout	0.7	15.5	13
Chronic alcoholism	−8.3	14.3	7

Obesity

This was assessed clinically as underweight; normal; mild, moderate, or severe obesity. Interclass differences of TW19R were not significant.

Initial Blood Pressure

In almost all instances of hypertension, treatment was instituted between the initial reading and the ergometry procedure. Only those with initial hypotension or a hypertension with systemic pressures greater than 180/120 mmHg showed significant decreases of TW19R.

Electrocardiographic Findings

Findings were classified on the basis of a resting standard twelve-lead ECG and the response to climbing fifty 22.9 cm steps as quickly as possible.

Resting ECG appearance	TW19R	S.D.	N
Normal	1.0	17.2	228
Frequent premature ventricular contractions	−6.1	19.3	3
Specific abnormalities (T_1 ST, small complexes etc . . .)	−8.3	16.1	39
Previous Myocardial Infarction	−18.7	25.4	11
Left ventricular hypertrophy	0.6	19.3	8
L.V.S./B.B.B./Other/combinations	−8.9	13.6	11

$F = 3.80$ $p < 0.01$

ECG appearance after step test	TW19R	S.D.	N
No significant change from resting trace	−0.1	17.7	244
ST <2mm depression	−14.9	16.3	18
ST ≥2mm depression	−8.0	16.6	14
Premature ventricular beat only after effort	10.5	17.1	9
ST ≥2mm + P.V.B.	−12.5	10.3	2
Other (flat T or inverted T or conduction defect)	−10.6	16.4	13

$F = 4.45$ $p < 0.01$

Spirometric Findings

These were quite sensitive with respect to the relative fitness index. Individual measurements were classified as being below, above, or within normal range for age, height, and sex.

Spirometric Findings	TW19R	S.D.	N	
FEV₁				
≥ + 10% expected	5.5	16.9	78	F = 14.73
as predicted	−1.4	17.2	154	p<0.001
≤ −10% expected	−10.1	17.5	58	
FVC				
≥ +10% expected	5.3	17.0	73	F = 10.05
as predicted	−1.9	17.1	153	p<<0.001
≤ −10% expected	−7.5	18.6	74	
Mid expiratory flow				
above normal range	7.6	9.7	10	F = 3.41
within normal range	−0.6	18.3	218	p≈0.01
below normal range	−5.6	17.5	71	
Peak expiratory flow				
above normal range	5.6	14.2	10	F = 4.74
within normal range	0.1	17.5	219	p <0.01
below normal range	7.5	18.8	71	

Laboratory Tests

There was no significant relationship between TW19R and hemoglobin over the Hb range 10.0 to 18.0 g/100 ml, nor was there any relationship between TW19R and hematocrit, except that with a HCt>51 percent the relative fitness index was substantially reduced. Blood glucose, serum total lipids, cholesterol, S.G.O.T., and S.G.P.T. were unrelated to TW19R. Serum uric acid readings >7.2 mg/100 ml were associated with a low TW19R.

Drugs

The effects of drugs likely to affect work output were as follows:

Drugs	TW19R	S.D.	N
Nil	0.7	16.3	208
β adrenergic blockers	−6.2	21.5	34
Sympathomimetics/anticholinergics	−9.8	10.5	7
Other cardiac drugs	−18.6	12.5	8
Other antihypertensives	−6.6	13.6	5
Other drugs relevant to work response	−8.0	17.8	18
Other drugs	−1.5	26.6	20

F = 2.61   p<0.05

Exercise Program Response

One hundred and thirty-nine subjects were assessed approximately three months after exercise had been prescribed (91 cycle ergometer / 36 running / 2 swimming / 10 mixed exercise). Compliance with the prescribed training was classed as (1) 100 percent, (2) almost 100 percent, (3) more than 50 percent, (4) less than 50 percent, and (5) nil:

Compliance	N	Change in TW19R (Mean ± S.E.)
100%	6	+ 5.6 ± 2.9
< 100	46	+ 9.6 ± 2.3
> 50	36	+ 9.8 ± 1.6
< 50	40	− 2.3 ± 2.3
Nil	11	− 6.1 ± 3.3

If compliance was better than 50 percent, a substantial increase of fitness occurred, but if compliance was poor or no exercise had been taken, the trend was downward. There were no significant differences of compliance or fitness gains between cycle ergometer and running programs. However, gains were related to the initial fitness of the individual.

$$\text{Change in TW19R} = 4.87 - 0.22 \text{ (original fitness index)}$$
$$(p<0.001, r = -0.42)$$

Discussion

The use of the relative fitness index permitted the immediate comparison of all subjects, whatever their age, sex, or body dimensions.

This seems the first occasion when many of the routine facts collected in a medical history have been related to work performance. Effects identified included gains from restful sleep and negative effects of cigarettes (>60 g/week), whether or not the smoke was inhaled. The acute effect of alcohol intake in the preceding twenty-four hours was dramatic, masking gains from three months' training.

The effects of mood on performance were also striking, particularly for self-directed anxiety and depression not requiring psychiatric supervision. The depressed group's results were uninfluenced by drug treatment. Many depressed people seem to be physically unfit and thus should benefit from an appropriate exercise program. Psychological well-being is probably the most consistent reward from an exercise program, but it is also hard to quantitate.

The findings in ischemic disease were the most predictable in terms of their negative effect. However, angina without an infarct reduced work output almost as much as was found postinfarction. Almost as serious was the diagnosis of restrictive, or a combination of restrictive and obstructive, airway disease.

As might be expected, electrocardiographic abnormalities led to a diminution of fitness index, the exception being left ventricular hypertrophy. The association of resting but not exercise premature ventricular beats with a poor work tolerance seems worth further study. ST depression irrespective of its depth, also influenced TW19R, as did other changes in T waves. However, there was a much larger yield of electrocardiographic abnormalities with the ergometer procedure. Abnormal findings in the resting ECG and/or the 50-step test were indicative of advanced cardiac disease. Some 18 percent of those with major obstruction of all three coronary vessels had a normal resting ECG.

If a second exercise tolerance test is undertaken a week or so after the first, a somewhat "better" result is usually obtained (Åstrand and Rodahl, 1970). This could influence our training assessments, although there seems no previous information on how long such "improvement" lasts. The present findings indicated that in those maintaining a consistent exercise program, the maximum variation in fitness over periods of up to a year was less than 5 percent. The fitness index improved by 10 percent or more in the great majority of those who had better than 50 percent compliance with a thirteen-week exercise prescription. The kind of program that was followed did not appear to matter. With the bicycle ergometer it was possible to quantitate an effective training dose. On average, this amounted to 80 percent of the original work output, repeated in seven sessions every fourteen days for at least seven weeks.

References

Åstrand, P. O. and Rodahl, K.: *Textbook of Work Physiology*, New York, McGraw-Hill, 1970.

Kasselbaum, D. S., Sutherland, K. I., and Judkins, M. P.: A Comparison of hypoxaemia and exercise electrocardiography in coronary artery disease. Diagnostic precision of the methods correlated with coronary angiography. *Am Heart J, 75*:759-766, 1968.

Lake, B.: Definition of an Exercise Tolerance Test. *Med J Austral, 63*(1): 189-192, 1976.

Chapter 33

CORRELATIONS AMONG AEROBIC FITNESS TESTS AND V̇o₂ MAX IN MEN WHO VARY IN AEROBIC POWER

O. Bar-Or, D. Zwiren, and R. Dotan

Abstract

On the hypothesis that the correlation between $\dot{V}o_2$ max and other fitness criteria is lower among less fit people than among those who are more fit, forty-three men (20.3 ± 2.8 years) underwent a battery of tests related to aerobic power. Subjects were divided into those with a directly measured $\dot{V}o_2$ max of less than 52 ml/kg-min ("less fit," n = 25) and those having a $\dot{V}o_2$ max of >52 ml/kg-min ("more fit," n = 18). Correlation coefficients for the "less fit" and the "more fit" were as follows: W_{170}, 0.23 versus 0.50; 2000 m all-out run, −0.65 versus −0.71; Harvard step test fitness index, 0.11 versus 0.46; predicted $\dot{V}o_2$ max (Åstrand), 0.61 versus 0.66; work rate at which exercise perception is rated 17, 0.15 versus 0.76. Higher values among the more fit subjects suggest that their achievements in the all-out and submaximal tests reflect their aerobic power more closely than is the case for the "less fit." The former also perceive exertion in a more "accurate" manner.

A MAJOR SHORTCOMING of both field and laboratory procedures for the indirect assessment of maximal O_2 uptake ($\dot{V}o_2$ max) is the inconsistent nature of reports regarding their validity relative to direct determinations of $\dot{V}o_2$ max. Laboratory indirect tests that include various protocols of step, treadmill, and bicycle ergometer testing have yielded correlations ranging from 0.4 to 0.9 [6, 8, 10, 14] Field tests have the advantage of being generally simpler to administer than their laboratory counterparts but, as a class, they show an even wider range of validity

356

coefficients of 0.2 to 0.9.[3, 4, 5, 7, 8, 11, 12, 14] Among the various field tests, the best correlations have been reported for the two-mile or twelve-minute runs as compared with tests conducted over shorter or longer distances.[4, 5, 12, 14] This can be explained on the grounds that, although the role of the aerobic component increases with the distance run, motivation becomes an increasingly important factor over longer distances. Other factors such as training, skill, experience, range of running abilities, age, sex, general physical fitness, and climatic conditions, all of which can influence the validity of a running test, are normally not sufficiently controlled. They seem to warrant closer attention, in order to either explain or prevent the large inconsistencies found within the same or similar tests.

Byrnes and Kearney moved in that direction, finding different r values between running times and $\dot{V}o_2$ max for groups who differed in activity and/or maximal aerobic power.[3] Their groups, however, were rather small and not sufficiently different from each other to allow generalizations. The question whether fitness level could affect the relationship between measured and predicted $\dot{V}o_2$ max was also raised by Rasch,[11] although he made no further analysis of such a possibility.

In the present study, an attempt is made to relate the level of maximal aerobic power to the strength of the correlation between $\dot{V}o_2$ max and running performance.

Subjects

Our forty-three healthy young male subjects were a random sample from a population of some 350 college-age individuals who participated in a project to determine the reliability and validity of some field tests. They ranged in physical activity from sedentary to regularly participating athletes, and for the purpose of this study they were divided into two groups according to aerobic power—those with a $\dot{V}o_2$ max <52 ml/kg-min ("less fit," n = 25) and those with a $\dot{V}o_2$ max >52 ml/kg-min ("more fit," n = 18). Although of similar age, height, and lean body mass, the "more fit" subjects weighed less and were significantly leaner (Table 33-I).

TABLE 33-I

PHYSICAL CHARACTERISTICS OF SUBJECTS, CLASSIFIED BY FITNESS

		Age yrs	Height cm	Weight kg	% fat*	Lean Body mass kg
Less Fit	$\overline{X}$	20.3	172.8	71.3	14.0	60.7
n = 25	S.D.	2.8	6.4	12.8	8.7	7.3
More Fit	$\overline{X}$	20.3	170.2	63.6	5.9	59.8
n = 18	S.D	2.7	5.4	6.0	2.7	6.1
All Subjects	$\overline{X}$	20.3	171.7	68.6	10.7	60.3
n = 43	S.D	2.7	6.1	11.4	7.9	6.8

*Using the Allen equation[1] from 10 skinfolds

Methods

Among other field measurements, a 2000 m run was performed in triplicate, the best result being taken for this analysis. Laboratory tests were as follows:

a. *An all-out continuous progressive treadmill run* to determine $\dot{V}O_2$ max, using the Douglas bag, microScholander method. The initial load was based on previously observed submaximal heart rate (f_h) values, so that the overall test would last six to eight minutes. The slope was increased 2.5 percent every two minutes.

b. *A three-stage continuous progressive bicycle test* (300,600,900 kpm/min, three minutes each). The f_h was determined at the end of each load, using a bipolar chest ECG lead. W_{170} was calculated, and the Åstrand method was used to predict $\dot{V}O_2$ max. In the latter test, a mean value was calculated for subjects who had a f_h of 120 to 170 beat/min in more than one load. The power at which each subject perceived his effort as "very hard" (WR_{17}) was rated by the Borg scale.[2]

c. *The abbreviated Harvard step test* (50.8 cm) took one measurement of f_h from 1 to 1.5 minutes of recovery.

Results

The two groups of subjects differed distinctly in all measures of aerobic power except the WR_{17}.

TABLE 33-II

CORRELATIONS BETWEEN INDICATORS OF AEROBIC POWER AND DI-
RECTLY MEASURED $\dot{V}_{O_2}$ MAX (ML/KG-MIN)
SUBJECTS CLASSIFIED BY FITNESS

	Predicted $\dot{V}_{O_2}$ max, ml/kg-min	$\dot{W}_{170}$ kpm/kg.min	$\dot{W}R_{17}$ kpm/kg.min	Step Fitness Index	2000m Time (sec)
Less Fit	.61	.23	.15	0.11	−.63
More Fit	.66	.50	.76	0.46	−.71
All Subjects	.69	.45	.30	0.55	−.72

Correlation coefficients relating the measured $\dot{V}_{O_2}$ max with other indicators were somewhat higher for the "more fit" subjects (Table 33-II), both on maximal and submaximal tests.

Discussion

The indirect tests that were used proved sensitive enough to distinguish two groups of individuals who differed markedly in aerobic power. However, individual tests varied in terms of their predictive usefulness (Table 3-II), the 2000 m run and Åstrand's predicted $\dot{V}_{O_2}$ max showing the closest correlation with the directly measured $\dot{V}_{O_2}$ max. Irrespective of fitness level, Åstrand's method underestimated "real" aerobic power by some 16 to 17 percent, a finding previously observed by others.[13]

Of special interest to the authors was the predictive strength of 2000 m running *speed*. It seems that the spread of data about the least square regression line is not uniform over the entire fitness range (Fig. 33-1). Correlations for the "fittest" fifteen subjects ($\dot{V}_{O_2}$ max of 62.3 ± 6.9 ml/kg-min) and the twelve "least fit" subjects ($\dot{V}_{O_2}$ max of 43.8 ± 4.1 ml/kg-min) were 0.80 and 0.39, respectively.

Data from the literature are inconclusive as to whether fitness affects the correlation between direct and indirect determination of $\dot{V}_{O_2}$ max. Cooper took data for 115 young and middle aged men and reported an r of 0.897. By projecting his graph on a screen and using a digitizer (Numonics), we have

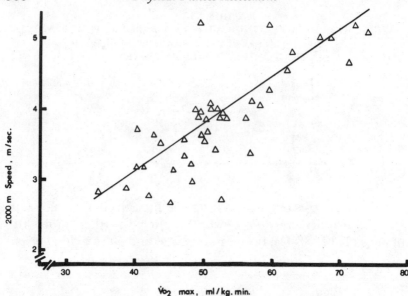

Figure 33-1. Relationship between 2000 meter running speed and measured $\dot{V}O_2$ max. Individual data for forty-three young men and line of best fit.

calculated correlation coefficients for two fitness subgroups, taking a $\dot{V}O_2$ max of 48 ml/kg-min as the dividing line. The "fitter" subjects then had an r value of 0.76 versus 0.65 for the less fit.

Ribisl[12] related two-mile running time to measured $\dot{V}O_2$ max in twenty-four fit middle-aged men. Again dividing his subjects into two fitness groups (dividing line = 48.5 ml/kg-min) we obtained an r of 0.88 for the less fit versus 0.37 for the fitter subjects. We cannot offer any explanation of the discrepancy between this finding and ours.* The range of aerobic power in Ribisl's sample was distinctly smaller than in the present report.

In a study by Byrnes and Kearney,[3] thirty-three subjects were

---

*The magnitude of the respective correlation coefficients would be influenced by the dispersion of data in "fit" and "unfit" subsamples. In the usual heterogenous collections of data, such dispersions are not necessarily equal. See Table 33-III—Ed.

TABLE 33-III
AEROBIC POWER INDICATORS
SUBJECTS CLASSIFIED BY FITNESS

		Measured $\dot{V}o_2$ max ml/kg-min	Predicted $\dot{V}o_2$ max ml/kg-min	$\dot{W}_{170}$ kpm/min	WR_{17} kpm/min	Step Fitness Index	2000m Time (sec)
Less Fit	$\overline{X}$	46.4	39.8	1,056	1,165	47.7	576.5
	S.D	4.6	7.6	266	331	26.2	81.1
More Fit	$\overline{X}$	60.6	52.3	1,362	1,317	74.6	474.0
	S.D	7.4	10.0	521	387	22.8	87.8
t		7.8	4.3	2.53	1.38	3.50	3.95

divided into three activity groups: trained runners, P.E. majors and non-P.E. majors. The respective r values relating $\dot{V}o_2$ max and one-mile running time were -0.72, -0.25, and -0.51. However, when we reclassified the subjects into two or three groups according to their $\dot{V}o_2$ max, no intergroup differences of r were evident. Generalization of these findings cannot be made, because their "trained" runners and P.E. majors had surprisingly low mean $\dot{V}o_2$ max readings (50.5 and 41.2 ml/kg-min, respectively) with a marked overlap between the latter and non-P.E. majors (41.1 ml/kg-min).

A specific design to assess the role of fitness as a determinant of validity for indirect tests would call for a priori selection of two or more groups differing distinctly in fitness but not in other variables. Such was not the case either in this report or in the other quoted studies. One cannot exclude the possibility that the above findings are an artifact of the data, highly dependent on the characteristics of the specific samples measured.

Bearing this reservation in mind, and based on our data, one may suggest that in highly fit individuals measured $\dot{V}o_2$ max is better correlated with indirect determinations of aerobic power (all-out running ability) than is the case for unfit individuals. Such a difference could be the result of lower motivation and lack of running experience among the less fit, long distance performance failing to reflect their "real" aerobic power.

References

1. Allen, T. H. et al.: Prediction of total adiposity from skinfolds and the curvilinear relationship between external and internal adiposity. *Metabolism, 5*:346-352, 1956.
2. Borg, G.: *Physical Performance and Perceived Exertion.* Lund, Gleerup, 1962.
3. Byrnes, W. C. and Kearney, J. T.: Measures of max $\dot{V}o_2$ and their relationship to running performance among three subject groups. *Am Corr Ther J, 28*:145-150, 1974.
4. Cooper, K. H.: A means of assessing maximal oxygen intake. *J.A.M.A. 203*:135-138. 1968.
5. Doolittle, T. L. and Rigbie, R.: The 12 min. run-walk: A test of Cardiorespiratory fitness of adolescent boys. *Res Quart, 39*:491-495, 1968.
6. Glassford, R. G. et al.: Comparison of maximal oxygen uptake values determined by predicted and actual methods. *J Appl Physiol, 20*:509-513, 1965.
7. Katch, V. L.: *The Role of Maximal Oxygen Intake in Endurance Performance.* Paper presented at the A.A.H.P.E.R. National Convention, Seattle, Washington, 1970.
8. Kurucz, R. L., Fox, E. L. and Mathews, D. K.: Construction of a submaximal cardiovascular step test. *Res Quart, 40*:115-121, 1969.
9. Maksud, M. G. and Coutts, V. D.: Application of the Cooper 12' run-walk test to young males. *Res Quart, 42*:54-59, 1971.
10. McArdle, D. et al.: Reliability and inter-relationships between maximal oxygen intake, physical work capacity and step-test scores in college women. *Med Sci Sports, 4*:182-186, 1972.
11. Rasch, P. J.: Maximal oxygen intake as a predictor of performance in running events. *MMFRL Report (US Navy), 22* (16): 1972.
12. Ribisl, P. M. and Kachadorian, W.: Maximal oxygen intake prediction in young and middle-aged males. *J Sports Med Phys Fit, 9*:17-22, 1969.
13. Shephard, R. J. (Ed.): *Frontiers of Fitness.* Springfield, Thomas, 1971, pp. 233-264.
14. Wiley, J. F. and Shaver, L. G.: Prediction of maximal oxygen intake from running performance of untrained young men. *Res Quart, 43*:89-93, 1972.

Chapter 34

EVALUATION OF WORK CAPACITY IN "HEALTHY" OLDER PEOPLE AND PATIENTS WITH CORONARY HEART DISEASE

R. ROST AND W. HOLLMANN

Abstract

This chapter reports results on 120 men, 50 to 70 years old, who thought themselves in good health. The exploration consisted of a clinical investigation, ECG, radiographic evaluation of cardiac volume, examination of risk factors in blood, and spiroergometric tests. More than 40 percent of the sample showed cardiac damage of varying severity. We also investigated 127 patients suffering from myocardial infarction who wanted to take part in a special training program. These men cannot be considered representative of all infarction patients but may indicate the status of those who want to train; 30 percent of this group were unable to exercise at 75 watts without severe disturbances of cardiac rhythm or signs of myocardial or coronary insufficiency. Nevertheless, the response to training was very good. Our results demonstrate the necessity of an exercise test for all older people before training is commenced.

PHYSICAL TRAINING is ever more frequently recommended for the prevention and rehabilitation of coronary heart disease. However, since many of the subjects concerned are quite elderly, the recommendation is not without problems. On the one hand, the benefits of training for such a purpose remain scientifically unproven, and, on the other hand, exercise will be advised for people who are either potentially endangered by diseases of the circulation or are already suffering from coronary arterial disease. Therefore, it is hardly surprising that fatal accidents have been reported during training. The present study was conducted to form an impression of both the degree of danger and the possibility of recognizing endangered individuals by means of an exercise test.

"Healthy" older subjects

The group investigated were 120 men who thought that they were healthy and wished to take part in an experimental training program for the 50 to 70 year age group. Their average age was 63 years. The initial investigation included a general physical examination, ECG, measurement of cardiac volume, and a bicycle ergometer test conducted according to the schedule of Hollmann and Venrath (40 watt increments of load every three minutes up to exhaustion, with measurements of oxygen uptake, heart rate, ECG, and arterial pressure).

We found that 41 percent of the subjects had disturbances of health which restricted performance in varying degrees, many subjects having more than one pathology. Arterial pressure was elevated in 22 percent and a pathological ECG was seen in 23 percent, 7 percent of the latter having a normal ECG at rest. The most common alterations of ECG were changes in repolarization, extra beats, and left or right bundle branch block either present at rest or appearing only during exercise. In one case, a large and previously unrecognized myocardial infarction was demonstrated. Other reasons, especially orthopedic problems, restricted performance in a further 8 percent; because they were not as dangerous to life as the circulatory problems, the exercise limitations imposed on these cases were less severe.

Measurement of cardiac volume did not result in further restrictions, since cardiac enlargement was seen only in subjects already showing striking abnormalities by other test methods. The same was true of an elevation of serum cholesterol; the latter was not considered a contraindication to training if there was no overt arterial disease.

The total of problems was even greater than 41 percent if we include those subjects who developed pathologies during training. Some had to stop training. It thus seems mandatory to demand a thorough examination, including an exercise test, before embarking upon the training of "healthy" men in the age group 50 to 70 years.

"Postcoronary" patients

In the patient who has already suffered a myocardial infarction, the aim of an exercise test is not to discover disease but rather to judge the possibility of taking part in a training program, to determine performance capacity and therefore to prescribe an optimal exercise load. In infarction patients, it seems unnecessary and risky to perform maximal tests. We thus limited the laboratory exercise to 125 watts, approached in steps of 25 watts. Other parts of the investigation were the same as for the "healthy" subjects.

We tested 127 patients who wanted to take part in a training program after myocardial infarction. The group was positively selected, patients thinking themselves capable of physical activity, but the results may be representative of patients coming to a "postcoronary" sports program. The average age of the group was 52.3 years and twenty-four of the subjects were female.

Some 27 percent of patients were judged as unable to participate in the training program. In three cases the family doctor did not agree as a matter of principle. In another three patients there was suspicion of an aneurysm. Two patients demonstrated signs of myocardial insufficiency at rest. Four patients were older than 65 years, a relative contraindication for our team. The remaining twenty-three patients did not fulfill the minimum criterion for commencing rehabilitation (a performance capacity of 75 watts), due to chest pain, severe disturbances of repolarization, abnormalities of cardiac rhythm (especially extra beats), and in three cases the appearance of left bundle branch block during exercise. Extra systoles were considered a reason for exclusion only if their number increased during work, if they showed a short interval, if they were polyfocal, or if they came in couplets. Before excluding the patient, we tried to suppress such disturbances by pharmacological means. In no case was high arterial pressure a contraindication to training, since pharmacological control of systemic pressures was always successful.

Our results with this group again demonstrated the need for an exercise test prior to physical activity prescription. With the "postcoronary" patient there may even be virtue in measuring pulmonary-arterial pressures during exercise in order to pick out patients with insipient myocardial insufficiency. In some cases, even the ergometer test was insufficient to demonstrate a hazardous response, since occasional patients showed an ectopic rhythm only during certain forms of gymnasium exercise. Telemetric supervision is therefore desirable at the beginning of training.

Chapter 35

PROLONGED EFFECTS OF A CAUTIOUS EXERCISE PRESCRIPTION*

C. W. POOLE, B. J. CREPIN, AND N. J. RICK

Abstract

Data is reported from a large urban fitness center. A total of 664 subjects, aged 16 to 64, were stress tested during 1974. Body fat percentage, anthropometric measures, and vital capacity were determined prior to exercise. Subjects were monitored by electrocardiograph, and blood pressures were determined throughout multistage, continuous bicycle exercise. Aerobic power ($\dot{V}O_2$ max) was predicted from work performed. Seventy subjects were retested after periods of physical training ranging from two to seventeen months. Linear regression analysis related significant ($p<.01$) physiologic and anthropometric adaptations to the duration of training. The gain of $\dot{V}O_2$ max was time dependent ($p<.001$), amounting to 27 percent after seventeen months. Multiple regression analysis demonstrated that the relationship was linear ($p<.001$). The increase of $\dot{V}O_2$ max continuing beyond twelve months of training was unusual and may reflect the gentle progression of the exercise prescribed at our fitness center.

CENTERS FOR PHYSICAL FITNESS testing have become quite common in recent years in major urban centers across Canada. However, little data from private centers has yet been published. There are also few longitudinal studies concerning the effects of prolonged physical training;[5, 8, 11] interpretation of all existing reports is limited by small sample size. The purpose of this chapter is to describe the effects of gradual and long-term physical training on 70 of the 664 subjects tested at

*The authors thank Ms. Eleanor Thomas for work on the statistical analysis and Ms. Carolyn Monsour for preparation of the manuscript.

Carleton University's Fitness Centre during 1974. Such data may be useful in evaluating the feasiblity and effectiveness of long-term exercise in achieving and maintaining recommended fitness levels.

Methods

The Fitness Centre at Carleton University provides a stress test and an appropriate exercise prescription to any applicant for a moderate fee. The purposes of the stress test are to (1) provide a basic screening procedure for a beginner in a fitness program, (2) determine the present level of cardiorespiratory fitness and body composition for educational and motivational reasons, and (3) prescribe appropriate exercise.

PRETEST SCREENING. Each subject completes a health questionnaire and has a physical examination by a physician prior to the stress test. Subjects classified as having a high risk of coronary disease and those with detected cardiovascular disease are scheduled to be tested with a physician present. Subjects classified as "low-risk" are tested by experienced laboratory technicians, medical assistance from Carleton's Sports Medicine Clinic being available within seconds.

TEST PROTOCOL. Each "high-risk" subject is given a resting twelve-lead electrocardiogram (ECG) which is evaluated by the physician prior to the stress test. Height, weight, and ten selected skinfolds are taken in order to estimate the percentage of body fat.[3] Selected girths and bone diameters are taken and the subject is somatotyped by the Heath-Carter method.[9] Vital capacity is measured by a modified Parkinson Cowan dry gas meter.

The stress test is carried out on a Von Döbeln bicycle ergometer. The subject warms up by pedalling at 50 rpm (no load) for two minutes. This is followed by a continuous, multistage exercise test, each work rate lasting four minutes. The test is terminated at 90 percent of the subject's age-predicted maximal heart rate or when standard objective or subjective clinical criteria are met.[6]

A single bipolar chest lead, CM_5 is used for ECG monitoring and analysis.[4, 6] Heart rates are displayed digitally by a Quinton 609 Cardiotachometer. The ECG is observed continuously on an oscilloscope associated with the cardiotachometer and recorded on a Cambridge VS$_4$ electrocardiograph for subsequent analysis by the physician. Blood pressures are measured at rest, during exercise, and during recovery by the cuff method. Maximal oxygen uptake ($\dot{V}O_2$ max) is predicted by standard methods,[2] with two modifications: (1) only heart rates exceeding 70 percent of age-predicted maximum are used for calculations, and (2) the age correction factor is based on recent reviews of maximal heart rates,[6, 18] higher than suggested by Åstrand[2] but lower than reported by Cumming.[4]

The subject returns for an evaluation of his results and an exercise prescription within seven days. A one-hour weekly group presentation explains the significance of the test results and describes the principles of the exercise prescription. Subjects with heart disease or those having abnormal cardiovascular responses to exertion (positive ECG, exercise hypertension, etc.) are advised individually by the exercise physiologist in consultation with the testing physician.

EXERCISE PRESCRIPTION. A person with a normal exercise test is given a standard aerobic exercise program. The warm-up period consists of ten to fifteen minutes of static stretching and abdominal, hip, and leg strengthening exercises. The cardiorespiratory exercise which follows the warm-up meets three criteria: (1) a minimum *frequency* of three sessions per week, (2) a *duration* of fifteen to thirty minutes of continuous exercise, and (3) an *intensity* eliciting 65 to 90 percent of age-predicted maximal heart rates (50 to 80 percent $\dot{V}O_2$ max) as monitored by ten-second pulse counts taken immediately after exercise.[10]

A beginner is advised to jog, swim, etc. for no longer than three minutes to avoid muscle or joint soreness. This minimal duration is increased gradually, never more than one to two minutes per training session. If muscle or joint tenderness occurs, the duration of exercise is held constant until the symptoms disappear. A typical middle-aged beginner takes four to eight weeks to reach fifteen to thirty minutes of continuous jogging.

A postexercise warm-down of five to six minutes utilizes

more static stretching in the supine position to promote effective circulatory recovery.

SUBJECTS. In the first eleven months of operation of the Carleton University Fitness Centre, 664 subjects were tested. They were 80 percent male, mean data being age 34.7 years (SD ± 10.8), weight 74.5 kg (± 13.2), body fat percent 20.1 percent (± 4.8), and $\dot{V}O_2$ max 34.5 ml/kg-min (± 8.6). Seventy of those subjects were retested on their own initiative after the elapse of two to seventeen months (mean 6.9). The pretraining

TABLE 35-I

EFFECT OF 6.9 MONTHS (RANGE 2 TO 17) OF PHYSICAL TRAINING ON ANTHROPOMETRIC VARIABLES (56 MALES, 14 FEMALES, AGED 40.2 ± 10.1 YEARS).

	Weight (kg)	Body Fat %	Somatotype* I	II	III
Pretraining	74.7	20.0	4.4	5.0	1.9
± SD	±12.1	±5.2	±1.6	±1.3	±1.2
Post training	72.9	18.0	3.9	5.0	2.2
± SD	±11.6	±5.1	±1.4	±1.3	±1.1
Difference	−1.8	−2.0	−0.5	−0.0	+0.3
± SD	±3.5	±2.6	±0.9	±0.9	±1.1
p	.001	.001	.05	ns	ns
n†	67	55	39	36	31

†n = number of paired pre– and posttraining observations available for comparison.
*Somatotype I = endomorphy; II = mesomorphy; III = ectomorphy. ns = not statistically significant.

TABLE 35-II

EFFECT OF 6.9 MONTHS (RANGE 2 TO 17) OF PHYSICAL TRAINING ON SELECTED CARDIORESPIRATORY VARIABLES (56 MALES, 14 FEMALES, AGED 40.2 ± 10.1 YEARS).

	Resting Heart Rate	$\dot{V}O_2$ max (ml/kg-min)	Vital Capacity (l)
Pretraining	76	32.2	4.4
± SD	±13	±8.1	±0.9
Post training	71	39.5	4.5
± SD	±12	±10.0	±0.9
Difference	−5	+7.3	+0.1
± SD	±12	±6.4	±0.4
p	.001	.001	.01
n	65	70	46

characteristics of the retested group were very similar to the entire group of 664 subjects (Tables 35-I and 35-II). The retested subjects were not grouped according to sex, since females respond to training in the same manner and degree as men.[13]

STATISTICAL ANALYSIS. A one-tailed *t*-test compared pretraining and posttraining data, ignoring differences in the duration of training in months (DT).

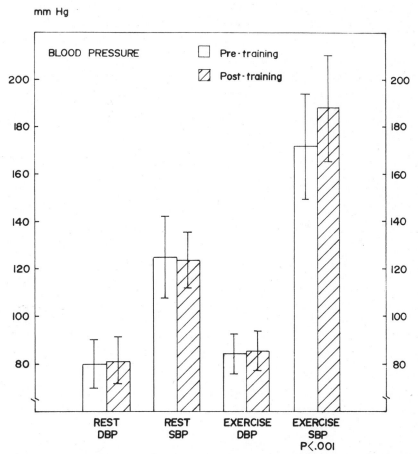

Figure 35-1. Effect of 6.9 months (range 2 to 17 months) of training on resting and standard submaximal exercise blood pressures of seventy subjects.

Significant (p<0.05) training adaptations were related to DT by linear regression analysis.

Results

The effects of physical training on anthropometric and cardiorespiratory measures are shown in Table 35-I and 35-II. The increase in $\dot{V}o_2$ max averaged 23 percent. There was also an unexpected increase of the systolic blood pressure (SBP) for a standard submaximal work rate (Fig. 35-1), but there were no significant changes of resting blood pressure or exercise diastolic blood pressure (DBP).

Linear regression analysis suggested that the increased in $\dot{V}o_2$ max was significantly (p<.001) related to DT (Fig 35-2). The equation $y = 2.96 + 0.60 (\pm 0.14) x$ (where y is the gain in $\dot{V}o_2$ max in ml/kg-min and x is DT) illustrates the slow but

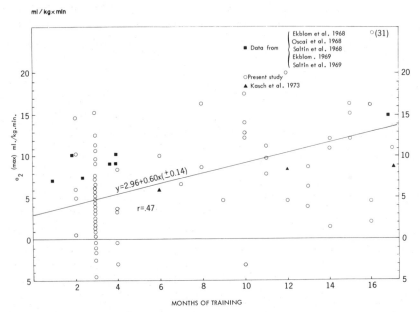

Figure 35.-2. Gain in $\dot{V}o_2$ max related to the duration of training in months (DT), where y = $\dot{V}o_2$ max gain in ml/kg.min and x= DT.

seemingly linear increase in Vo_2 max with training periods as long as seventeen months. Multiple regression analysis did not reveal any quadratic component[16] to this relatinoship, although the variability was quite large (Fig. 35-2). The magnitude of other training adaptations was independent on DT.

Discussion

LIMITATIONS OF THE STUDY. Analysis of data from a community stress-testing center has inherent limitations. The population studied is selected, being mainly white-collar, sedentary, adult males. Little control can be exercised over the intensity, frequency, and duration of training once the exercise prescription has been given, unless the subject is a participant in a group exercise program at the center. The time interval between pretraining and repeat tests varies widely (two to seventeen months), making group analysis and interpretation of training changes more difficult. Also, submaximal predictions of Vo_2 max have known limitations. Habituation may account for some of the observed "training effect."[21] Underestimation of Vo_2 max may occur with young[4] and middle-aged populations.[1] However, such data may provide valuable information of the effects of prolonged training on large populations.

EFFECTS OF PHYSICAL TRAINING. The observed adaptations in body weight, body fat percentage, resting heart rate, and Vo_2 max have been reported by many investigators.[2, 18] Increases in vital capacity with training are less consistently reported.[2] Pollock,[18] in his review of endurance training studies, indicates that resting blood pressures are typically reduced or show no change. Submaximal exercise blood pressure for a standard work rate typically does not change with training in healthy men.[2, 18] However, in the present study, the exercise SBP rose from a pretraining mean value of 172 (± 22) mmHg to 188 (± 23) mmHg (p<.001) following training (Fig. 35-1). Ekblom[5] also noted a rise in mean arterial pressures at a standard submaximal task. No mechanism can be suggested to explain this observation. However, it is unlikely to be an artifact, given the sample size (n = 32) and high degree of significance of the change (p<.001). More longitudinal data on the effects of training on the hemodynamics of the circulation of healthy adults is needed.

EFFECT OF PROLONGED TRAINING ON AEROBIC POWER. The effects of endurance training on the oxygen transport system are well known. In mature adults, gains of $\dot{V}o_2$ max occur without an enlarged heart volume.[5] The increased stroke volume of the heart results from an improved contractility of the myocardium. However, there is a lack of detailed data on the influence of prolonged training. Ekblom[5] has published data on two subjects who were followed over eighteen months of intensive (80 to 100 % $\dot{V}o_2$ max) training. This data, along with other shorter Scandinavian studies using similar high intensities of training, is compared to the present study in Figure 35-2. Kasch et al.[11] have recently published the effects of a two-year training program on seven middle-aged men. However, the intensity and duration of exercise that they used was lower than in Scandinavia. The intensity was initially 50 to 60 % $\dot{V}o_2$ max and progressed to 75 to 80 %; the mileage run was only 7.4 miles per week after eighteen months of training.

The time course of the $\dot{V}o_2$ max increments from the San Diego study is remarkably similar to that seen here. However, increases of $\dot{V}o_2$ max ceased after twelve months in the San Diego study.

Gains in aerobic power tend to increase with the length of training.[18] Training for ten weeks or less results in gains of 4 to 14 percent, whereas training in excess of twenty weeks results in 14 to 43 percent gains in aerobic power. The limited data of Ekblom[5] and Kasch et al[11] (Fig. 35-2) support the belief that gains of aerobic power "plateau" after six months to one year of training. Recent studies by Hanson and Nedde[8] on eight females and Fox et al.[7] verify this theory. However, this may simply be a function of the degree of the training stimulus and how gradually it is applied.

From Figure 35-2, it appears that intense training (>80% $\dot{V}o_2$ max) produces large gains in the initial weeks. Much smaller gains result from the light to moderate regimens (50 to

80% $\dot{V}o_2$ max) of the San Diego study and the present material. However, the rapid response to intense training results in a "plateauing" of $\dot{V}o_2$ max sooner than with the more cautious training methods. The San Diego subjects also stopped increasing in training mileage after eight months. It may be that the very slow progression of intensity and duration of training in the present study resulted in the training stimulus increasing throughout the seventeen-month study.

The philosophy of exercise training at Carleton University is in part derived from the San Diego workers.[10] The extremely cautious approach in the initial weeks of training (50% $\dot{V}o_2$ max for up to three minutes and slowly increasing the intensity and duration) has merit in a long-term approach to physical fitness and health. It also reduces the frequency of orthopedic complications. Intense training methods result in a 50 percent incidence of orthopedic injury.[12, 14] Such injuries are detrimental to adherence to an exercise program.

The advantages of cautious exercise prescription may be (1) greater safety, (2) better adherence rates due to less overexertion, (3) a longer duration of positive reinforcement from the slow training gains made over a long period of time, and (4) a form of training which is easier to tolerate over many years. The disadvantage of cautious exercise prescription is that the high levels of $\dot{V}o_2$ max attained through intense training are not achieved (Fig. 35-2). However, for improvement of subjective well-being and possibly preventing coronary heart disease such very high levels of aerobic power may not be important.[15]

References

1. Åstrand, I. et al.: Reduction in maximal oxygen uptake with age. *J Appl Physiol, 35*:649-654, 1973.
2. Astrand, P. O. and Rodahl, K.: *A Textbook of Work Physiology.* New York, McGraw-Hill, 1970.
3. Buskirk, E. R.: *Determination of Lean Body Mass and Its Relationship to Fitness.* Paper presented at American Academy of Orthopaedic Surgeons Symposium on Physical Fitness, Atlanta, Georgia, 1974.

4. Cumming, G. R. Put graded exercise testing in your medical office. *Can Family Physician,* 102-113, March, 1975.
5. Ekblom, B.: Effect of physical training on the oxygen transport system in man. *Acta Physiol Scand, 77* (Suppl. 328): 1969.
6. Ellestad, M. H.: *Stress Testing: Principles and Practices.* Philadelphia, F. A. Davis Co., 1975.
7. Fox, R. et al.: Frequency and duration of interval training programs and changes in aerobic power. *J Appl Physiol, 38*:481-484, 1975.
8. Hanson, J. S. and Nedde, W. S.: Long-term physical training effect in sedentary females. *J Appl Physiol, 37*:113-116, 1974.
9. Heath, B. and Carter, J. E. L.: A comparison of somatotype methodology. *Am J Phys Anthropol 24*:87-99, 1966.
10. Kasch, F. W. and Boyer, J. L.: *Adult Fitness.* San Diego. American International Press, 1969.
11. Kasch, F. W. et al.: Cardiovascular changes in middle-aged men during two years of training. *J Appl Physiol, 34*:53-57, 1973.
12. Kilbom, A. et al.: Physical training in sedentary middle aged and older men. I. Medical evaluation. *Scand J Clin Lab Invest, 24*:315-323, 1969.
13. Kilbom, A.: Physical training in women. *Scand J Clin Lab Invest, 28* Suppl. 119:1-34, 1971.
14. Mann, G. V. et al.: Exercise to prevent coronary heart disease. *Am J Med, 46*:46-49, 1969.
15. Morris, J. N. and Crawford, M. D.: Coronary heart disease and physical activity of work. *Br Med J, 12*:1485-1490, 1958.
16. Oscai, L. B., Williams, B. T. and Hertig, B. A.: Effect of exercise on blood volume. *J Appl Physiol, 24*:622-624, 1968.
17. Pollock, M. L.: The quantification of endurance training programs. *Exer Sports Sci Rev, 1*:155-188, 1973.
18. Saltin, B. et al.: Response to exercise after bed rest and after training. *Circulation, 38* (Suppl. 7): 1-78, 1968.
19. Saltin, B. et al.: Physical training in sedentary middle-aged and older men. II oxygen uptake, heart rate and blood lactate concentration at submaximal and maximal exercise. *Scand J Clin Lab Invest, 24*:323-334, 1969.
20. Shephard, R. J. and McClure, R. L.: The prediction of cardiorespiratory fitness. *Arbeitsphysiologie, 21*:212-223, 1965.

Chapter 36

VARIABILITY OF HEART RATE, BLOOD PRESSURE, AND RATE-PRESSURE PRODUCT DURING BICYCLE ERGOMETER EXERCISE IN MIDDLE-AGED MEN

W. E. SIME, I. T. WHIPPLE, J. STAMLER, AND D.M. BERKSON

Abstract

The variability of the heart rate (HR), systolic blood pressure (SBP), diastolic blood pressure (DBP), and heart rate times systolic pressure (rate-pressure) product responses to a standardized bicycle ergometer exercise were evaluated by test repetition. Two submaximal exercise tests were carried out on forty-four sedentary, middle-aged men with an intertest interval of one week. Values for SBP and DBP were taken simultaneously by auscultatory and phonoarteriographic methods. All comparisons except one showed a reduction of scores from the first to the second test; however, the mean decreases were significant only for HR at 300 and 600 kpm/min. Coefficients correlating HR, SBP, and DBP data for the two tests were high, ranging from 0.69 to 0.89. The standard error of the measurement was 5.2 to 5.7 beats/min for HR, 4.2 to 4.5 mmHg for DBP and 8.0 to 16.3 mmHg for SBP. When tests were repeated, the rate-pressure product showed a small mean decrease both at rest and during exercise. Auscultatory SBP and DBP readings were 3 to 8 mmHg lower than phonoarteriographic values. The results suggest that exercise HR, SBP, and rate-pressure product are sufficiently stable measurements to be used in long-term assessments of myocardial oxygen consumption in middle-aged men. However, the small but consistent decrease of these variables over a short intertest interval must be considered when evaluating the significance of apparent training responses.

Introduction

THE VARIABILITY OF physiological responses to exercise testing is of concern when evaluating the effects of physical activity on cardiovascular function either in normal subjects (Froelicher et al., 1974) or in rehabilitation after myocardial infarction (Fabian et al., 1975). Heart rate (HR), systolic (SBP) and diastolic (DBP) blood pressure are monitored routinely as estimates of cardiovascular function. In addition, the heart rate times systolic pressure (rate pressure) product is calculated as an index of myocardial oxygen consumption (Jorgensen et al., 1973). It is more practical to use auscultatory than intraarterial pressure measurements. However, the reliability and validity of auscultatory SBP as an estimate of central aortic pressure requires analysis. One possible validation criterion is the phonoarteriographic method of blood pressure measurement; this is also noninvasive and has been demonstrated previously to correlate well with intraarterial readings (Mastropaolo et al., 1964). The present investigation was undertaken to determine the reliability of HR, SBP, DBP, and rate-pressure product responses to standardized bicycle ergometer tests in middle-aged men.

Methods

The subjects were forty-four healthy, sedentary male volunteers aged 40 to 57 years. Medical eligibility, i.e. freedom from signs and symptoms of disease (including cardiovascular disease), was established by a thorough medical evaluation, including a complete history, physical examination, resting twelve-lead electrocardiogram, 14 by 17 inch teleroentgenogram of the chest, and extensive laboratory tests. Men exhibiting ST segment depression equal to or greater than 1 mm (0.1 millivolt) during or after the standard exercise were excluded from the analysis. Medical supervision and personnel trained in cardiopulmonary resuscitation were available for all tests. No incidents occurred.

Two submaximal exercise tests were performed with an intertest interval of one week. All participants reported to the laboratory in the afternoon, at least two hours after eating and six hours after ingesting any coffee, tea, cocoa, or alcohol. Smokers were asked to refrain from smoking for at least one hour preceding the test. A Monark® bicycle ergometer was pedalled at 50 rpm. The initial work load of 300 kilopond meters per minute (kpm/min) was sustained for six minutes and after a three-minute rest there was a further six minutes of exercise at 600 kpm/min. The laboratory was air conditioned, with a humidity ranging from 18 to 59 percent, and a temperature of 22.2 to 24.5°C.

Heart rates were determined from a bipolar ECG, transmitted by a Parks radiotelemetry system and recorded on a Sanborn® recorder. Phonoarteriographic blood pressures were obtained from recordings of cuff pressures with superimposed Korotkov sound markings (Mastropaolo et al., 1964). Auscultatory blood pressures were determined using the electronically amplified Korotkov sounds and a mercury manometer.

Statistical significance of group mean differences was assessed using correlated *t*-tests. Pearson coefficients of correlation (r) between repeat tests and standard errors of a single measurement (SEM = SD$\sqrt{1-r}$) were also calculated.

Results

Table 36-I shows the variability* of HR, SBP, and DBP responses to a bicycle ergometer test at 300 kpm/min. When the test was repeated, small mean decreases were observed for all three variables, although only HR was significantly lower. The intertest correlation coefficients ranged from 0.80 to 0.85. Table 36-II shows the variability of the same variables at a workload of 600 kpm/min. Again, HR was the only measurement which was significantly reduced at the second examination. The SBP was slightly higher on retesting and showed a correlation of only 0.65 with the initial set of data; correlation coefficients for HR and DBP were considerably higher (each 0.89).

Table 36-III shows the intertest variability of the rate-

---

*A portion of the following data has been published previously in separate reports discussing heart rate reproducibility (Sime et al., 1972) and blood pressure reproducibility (Sime et al., 1975).

TABLE 36-I

VARIABILITY OF HEART RATE, SYSTOLIC AND DIASTOLIC BLOOD
PRESSURE RESPONSES TO BICYCLE ERGOMETER TEST (300 KPM/MIN)

	Test		Mean		
Variable	*I*	*II†*	*Diff*	*r*	*S.E.m*
Heart Rate (bts/min)	105	102†	3	.85	5.2
Systolic BP (mmHg)†	145	141	4	.85	8.0
Diastolic BP (mmHg)†	90	88	2	.80	4.5

*Inter-test interval one week

†p < 0.05

†Auscultatory measurements of systolic and diastolic blood pressure

TABLE 36-II

VARIABILITY OF HEART RATE, SYSTOLIC AND DIASTOLIC BLOOD
PRESSURE RESPONSES TO BICYCLE ERGOMETER TEST (600 KPM/MIN)

	Test		Mean		
Variable	*I*	*II**	*Diff*	*r*	*S.E.m*
Heart Rate (bts/min)	138	135†	3	.89	5.7
Systolic BP (mmHg)†	174	176	−2	.65	16.3
Diastolic BP (mmHg)†	92	92	0	.89	4.2

*Inter-test interval one week

†p < 0.05

†Auscultatory measurements of systolic and diastolic blood pressure

TABLE 36-III

VARIABILITY OF HEART RATE X SYSTOLIC BLOOD PRESSURE PRODUCT
AT REST AND IN RESPONSE TO BICYCLE ERGOMETER TEST.

			Mean
Variable	*Test I*	*Test II**	*Diff*
HR × SBP†	89	84	5
At Rest			
Ergometer Test	152	144	8
At 300 kpm			
Ergometer Test	240	238	2
At 600 kpm			

*Inter-test interval one week

†Heart rate (N = 44) × systolic blood pressure (N = 31) × 10^{-2}; auscultatory
observations of SBP

TABLE 36-IV

COMPARISON OF AUSCULTATORY AND PHONOARTERIOGRAPHIC MEA-
SURES OF SYSTOLIC AND DIASTOLIC BLOOD PRESSURE AT REST AND IN
RESPONSE TO BICYCLE ERGOMETER TEST.

Variable	Auscul*	Phono**	Mean Diff
Systolic BP			
At Rest	126	123	3
300 kpm	143	149	−6
600 kpm	175	183	−8
Diastolic BP			
At Rest	86	88	−2
300 kpm	89	92	−3
600 kpm	92	99	−7

*Auscultatory values were obtained using a Maico electronic stethoscope and a mercury manometer.

**Phonoarteriographic values were obtained by measuring the cuff pressure tracing at the time the microphone signal of the first Korotkov sound appeared (Mastropaolo et al., 1964).

pressure product. On retesting, there was a mean decrease ranging from 2 to 8 units (bts/min $\times$ mmHg $\times$ 10^{-2}), the largest decrease occurring at the 300 kpm/min workload. These results indicate that HR and auscultatory SBP are reliable measures which can be used to calculate rate-pressure product as an estimate of myocardial oxygen consumption.

Auscultatory blood pressure readings were consistently lower than phonoarteriographic values in all comparisons except SBP at rest (Table 36-IV). The intertest correlation coefficients were lower for the auscultatory values, and the SEM was lower for the phonoarteriographic values.

Discussion

These findings agree with several other reports that the heart rate response to bicycle ergometer exercise is a reliable measurement which nevertheless shows a small and consistent decrease when testing is repeated after a short interval (Blair and Vincent, 1971; Borg and Dahlstrom, 1962; Durnin et al., 1960; Hellstrom and Holmgren, 1966). Treadmill exercise apparently has a slightly more reproducible HR response than bicycle exercise (Sime et al., 1972). Froelicher et al. (1974) found much larger decreases of treadmill HR when tests were repeated. However, their experiment included three repetitions of three different treadmill protocols, which in itself may have induced significant cardiovascular training.

There has been some controversy over the reliability (Blair and Vincent, 1971) and validity (Karlefors et al., 1966; Nagle et al., 1966) of noninvasive blood pressure measurements. In the present study, SBP and DBP were found to be reliable measurements, with a tendency towards a small decrease at the second testing. Jorgensen et al. (1973) found that the HR × SBP product correlated well with myocardial oxygen consumption. We may, therefore, further conclude that the rate-pressure product is a reliable estimate of myocardial oxygen consumption. In one comparable study, Fabian et al. (1975) demonstrated that the maximal rate-pressure product of ischemic heart disease patients was reproducible with a three-month intertest interval. The auscultatory blood pressure values were nearly as reliable as the phonoarteriographic values but were slightly lower. Mastropaolo et al. (1964) previously concluded that the phonoarteriographic SBP gave a more accurate estimate of intraarterial pressure than auscultatory SBP. It is thus probable that the auscultatory rate-pressure product underestimates myocardial oxygen consumption.

Consideration should be given to systematic intertest differences when making comparisons of HR, SBP, DBP, and rate-pressure product for evaluation of exercise training.

References

Blair, S. N. and Vincent, M.: Variability of heart rate and blood pressure measurements on consecutive days. *Res Quart, 42*:7-13, 1971.

Borg, G. and Dahlstrom, H.: The reliability and validity of a physical work test. *Acta Physiol Scand, 55*:353-361, 1962.

Durnin, J. V. G. A., Brockway, J. M., and Whitcher, H. W.: Effects of a short period of training of varying severity on some measurements of physical fitness. *J Appl Physiol, 15*:161-165, 1960.

Fabian, J. et al.: Reproducibility of exercise tests in patients with symptomatic ischemic heart disease. *Br Heart J, 37*:785-789, 1975.

Froelicher, V. F., Jr. et al.:A comparison of the reproducibility and physiological response to three maximal treadmill exercise protocols *Chest, 65*:512-517, 1974.

Hellstrom, R. and Holmgren, A.: On the repeatability of submaximal work tests and the influence of body position on heart rate during exercise at submaximal workloads. *Scand J Clin Lab Invest, 18*:479-485, 1966.

Jorgensen, C. R. et al.; Effect of propranolol on myocardial oxygen consumption and its hemodynamic correlates during upright exercise. *Circulation, 48*:1173-1182, 1973.

Karlefors, T., Nilsen, R., and Westling, H.: On the accuracy of indirect auscultatory blood pressure measurements during exercise. *Acta Med Scand 180* Suppl 449:81-87, 1966.

Mastropaolo, J. A. et al.: Validity of phonoarteriographic blood pressures during rest and exercise. *J Appl Physiol, 19*:1219-1233, 1964.

Nagle, F. J., Naughton, J., and Balke, B.: Comparison of direct and indirect blood pressure with pressure-flow dynamics during exercise. *J Appl Physiol, 21*:317-320, 1966.

Sime, W. E. et al.: Reproducibility of heart rate at rest and in response to submaximal treadmill and bicycle ergometer test in middle-aged men. *Med Sci Sports, 4*:14-17, 1972.

Sime, W. E. et al.: Reproducibility of systolic and diastolic pressure at rest and in response to submaximal bicycle ergometer tests in middle-aged men. *Human Biol, 47*:483-492, 1975.

Chapter 37

RELATIONSHIP BETWEEN SEGMENTAL AND WHOLE BODY WEIGHTS OF SOME INDIAN SUBJECTS*

R. N. SEN, G. G. RAY, AND P. K. NAG

Abstract

Information regarding relationships between segmental and whole body weights, volumes, and centers of mass is important in biomechanics, sports, and industrial technology. For the present report, five Indian adult male cadavers were weighed by a servoindicator. The whole body was dissected into fourteen segments, severing each of the primary joints across its approximate center of rotation and weighing the resultant segment on a baby-weighing platform balance. The segmental volume (water displacement technique) and the center of mass (plumb-line technique) were also determined. The relative weight of the limbs (total arm 4.3 percent and total leg 12.9 percent of body weight) were much lower in Indians than values reported for Western and Japanese subjects. On the other hand, the relative weight of the trunk (58.2 percent) was much higher in Indian cadavers. The segmental volumes of the trunk and the limbs represent 59.4 and 32.4 percent of the total body volume respectively. The center of mass of the upper arm and of the thigh both lie some 48.9 percent of the total segmental length from the proximal end of the part. Simple regression equations are derived for the prediction of segmental weights; these may be used at least until further cadavers have been studied.

INDIAN PEOPLE DIFFER from Westerners with respect to body weight, body height and other dimensions, body surface area,

---

*The authors acknowledge their gratitude to the staff of the Calcutta Corporation, Calcutta, for facilities provided at Mysore Crematorium. Thanks are also due to Dr. D. Chakroborti for his assistance and to the Indian Council of Medical Research for partial financial support.

384

basal metabolic rate, physical fitness, efficiency, and working capacity. Predictions of weight, volume, and center of mass for individual body segments are useful when analyzing biomechanical aspects of both sports and other activities including industrial work. However, no information on such variables has yet been reported for the Indian population. The present report thus describes a direct determination of segmental body composition in Indian cadavers. Comparative data for Western populations have been reported by Borelli,[2] the Weber brothers,[12] Harless,[9] Braune and Fischer[3] Dempster,[5] Williams and Lissner,[13] and Clauser et al.,[4] while information on the Japanese population has been presented by Mori and Yamamoto[10] and Fujikawa.[8]

Methods

Five unclaimed Indian adult male cadavers were selected for the present study, which was made during the cooler months of January and February. The selection of the cadavers was based on such considerations as the date of death, nutritional status, and the absence of wasting or debilitating disease. The sample was with one exception somewhat undernourished, and bodies had been preserved for approximately twenty-four hours in the hospital morgue.

After selection, the cadavers were placed inside a polythene bag, to avoid collection or evaporation of moisture. The experimental procedures were undertaken during the night, when the average room temperature was about 22°C. Each body was cleaned and swabbed with a solution containing equal proportions of phenol, glycerine, and water. The whole body weight was recorded with the help of a sensitive (± 0.05 kg) servoindicator calibrated by standard weights. Dissection of the various body segments used a method similar to that of Braune and Fischer[3] and Dempster.[5] Parts were severed at each of the primary joints, about the approximate center of rotation. Localized freezing during dissection was unfortunately impracticable. The joints severed were as follows:

HIP JOINT: The leg was abducted by about 30°. The plane of segmentation passed across the groin from the lower level of the iliac crest along the external shaft of the ilium, cutting the rim of the acetabulum across the ball and socket joint to sever the ischial tuberosity.

KNEE JOINT: The knee joint was bissected in an extended position. The plane of separation began near the lower part of the patella and bissected the maximum protrusion of the medial and lateral epicondyles of the femur. The patella was included with the lower leg.

ANKLE JOINT: The feet were plantar extended. The line of cutting began at the anterior superior edge of the neck of the talus and passed across the superior edge of the calcaneum.

SHOULDER JOINT: The shaft of the humerus was rotated laterally by about 15° to ensure that the cut passed from the tip of the acromion to the anatomical neck of the humerus and into the axilla without touching the shaft of the humerus or the medial surface of the upper arm.

ELBOW JOINT: Separation was begun by bissecting the olecranon process, crossing the greatest projection of the medial epicondyles of the humerus to end at the skin crease on the superior aspect of the elbow.

WRIST JOINT: The line of severance passed through the palpable groove between the lunate and capitate bones, bissecting the volar surface of the pisiform to end at the wrist crease.

NECK JOINT: The trunk was beheaded along the neck-chin intersection, commencing just above the hyoid bone and proceeding between the second and third cervical vertebrae.

In total, the body was thus dissected into fourteen segments. As soon as each segment had been detached from the body it was weighed on a calibrated baby-weighing platform balance. The beheaded trunk was reweighed with the servoindicator.

The center of mass of each limb segment was obtained by the plumb-line technique,[4] while volumes were determined by water displacement.

Results and Discussion

The cadavers included in the present study were of lower economic status. With one exception they were suffering from undernutrition. Their average age was 49 years. The average body weight was 37.3 kg, much lower than the fiftieth percentile value (45.9 kg)[11] for the Indian population.

The total arm and the total leg (including the thigh) represented an average of 4.3 and 12.9 percent of body weight respectively (Table 37-I). The weights of both limbs were relatively lower in Indian cadavers than in Westerners, a possible advantage in rapid unloaded movements in sports or assembly work. In consequence, the trunk (58.2 percent of body weight) was relatively heavier than in Western and Japanese studies. The relative values for individual limb segments (forearm, palm, total right leg and lower leg) are similar to those found in Japanese cadavers.[10] The relative weight of the head was similar to the values reported by Fujikawa[8] and Fischer.[7] The weight of the right arm of the Indians was greater than that of the left, but the weights of both legs were almost equal.

The sum of percentages for all segments was 94.4 percent, rather than 100 percent, the discrepancy reflecting loss of fluid and tissue during segmentation. The weight of the fluid and tissue collected during segmentation was thus added to the segmental weights in equal proportions to give the corrected values of Table 37-I. Dempster[5] and Clauser et al.[4] noted 6.4 and 1.4 percent loss of body weight respectively during dissection. The smaller losses of Clauser et al. were possibly due to use of the dry ice localized cooling technique.

The mean total body volume was 33.86 liters (Table 37-II). The volume of the trunk was 20.07 liters (59.39 percent of body volume), while that of the limbs (total arm and total leg, including thigh) represented only 32.4 percent of the body volume. Relative to Western studies,[6] the percentile distribution of most segmental volumes except the hands and feet were lower for the Indians.

Segmental centers of mass (right upper arm, forearm, thigh, and calf) could be determined in only two cadavers (Table 37-III). Centers for the upper arm and thigh both lay at some 48.9 percent of the total length from the proximal end of the segment, much as reported by Dempster.[5]

Simple linear regression equations for the prediction of

TABLE 37-I

AVERAGE WEIGHTS OF BODY SEGMENTS EXPRESSED AS PERCENTAGES OF TOTAL BODY WEIGHT.

Cadaver	Sen, Ray, and Nag (1976)	Clauser et al. (1969)	Fujikawa (1963)	Mori and Yamamoto (1959)	Dempster (1955)	Fischer (1906)	Braune and Fischer (1889)	Harless (1860)
Sample Size (n)	5	13	6	6	8	1	3	2
Segments:								
Head	9.0	7.3	8.2	11.7	7.1	8.8	6.9	7.6
Trunk	58.2	50.7	53.6	53.5	45.4	45.2	46.1	44.2
Total Right Arm	4.3	4.9	4.8	4.7	4.9	5.4	6.3	5.8
Upper arm	2.1	2.6	2.6	2.7	2.7	2.8	3.3	3.2
Forearm & Palm	2.2	2.3	2.2	2.0	2.2	2.5	3.0	2.6
Forearm	1.4	1.6	1.4	1.3	1.6	—	2.1	1.8
Palm	0.8	0.7	0.8	0.6	0.6	—	0.9	0.8
Total Left Arm	3.9	4.9	4.6	4.6	4.8	5.6	6.1	5.4
Total Right Leg including Thigh	12.2	16.1	14.4	12.6	15.7	17.8	17.3	18.5
Thigh	6.8	10.3	9.4	7.2	9.6	11.0	10.7	11.9
Leg and Foot	5.4	5.8	5.0	5.1	6.0	6.8	6.5	6.5
Leg	3.5	4.3	3.3	3.5	4.5	4.7	4.8	4.6
Foot	1.9	1.5	1.7	1.6	1.4	2.1	1.7	1.9
Total Left Leg including Thigh	12.2	16.1	14.5	12.6	15.7	17.3	17.3	19.3
Total	100.0	100.0	100.1	9.7	93.6	100.1	100.0	100.8

TABLE 37-II

AVERAGE SEGMENTAL VOLUMES, EXPRESSED AS PERCENTAGES OF WHOLE BODY VOLUME.

Segments	Sen et al. (1976) n = 5		Drillis and Contini (1966) n = 12	
	Mean (l.)	% of TB	Mean (l.)	% of TB
Total Body (TB)	33.855	100.00	—	100.00
Head	2.775	8.226	—	—
Neck & Trunk	20.071	59.395	—	—
Total Arm	2.933	8.630	3.971	5.730
Upper Arm	0.731*	2.158*	2.412	3.495
Forearm & Hand	0.763*	2.255*	—	—
Forearm	0.489*	1.455*	1.175	1.702
Hand	0.271*	0.800*	0.384	0.566
Total Leg	8.078	23.810	10.091	14.620
Thigh	2.133*	6.299*	6.378	9.241
Calf & Foot	1.861*	5.496*	—	—
Calf	1.173*	3.464*	2.818	4.083
Foot	0.688*	2.023*	0.895	1.297

*Values for right side of the body only.

TABLE 37-III

RATIO OF CENTER OF MASS OF SEGMENT LENGTH.

Source	This Study Sen et al. 1976	Clauser et al. 1969	Dempster 1955	Fischer 1889	Braune and Fischer 1889	Harless 1860
Total Body		41.2%				41.4%
Head		46.6	43.3%			36.2%
Trunk		38.0*				44.8
Total Arm		41.3		44.6%		
Upper Arm	48.9%	51.3	43.6	45.0	47.0	
Forearm & Hand		62.6*	67.7*	46.2	47.2	
Forearm	44.0	39.0	43.0		42.1	42.0
Hand		18.0*	49.4			39.7
Total Leg		38.2*	43.3	41.2		
Thigh	48.9	37.2*	43.3	43.6	44.0	48.9
Calf & Foot		47.5	43.7	53.7	52.4	
Calf	42.3	37.1	43.3	43.3	42.0	43.3
Foot		44.9	42.9		44.4	44.4

*These values are not directly comparable due to variations in the definition of segment length used by the different investigators.

TABLE 37-IV

REGRESSION EQUATIONS FOR PREDICTING SEGMENTAL WEIGHTS (Kg)
FROM WHOLE BODY WEIGHT (INDIAN SUBJECTS)

Weight of Head	= 0.04 × Body Wt. + 1.47 ± 0.22*
Weight of Trunk	= 0.63 × Body Wt. − 2.88 ± 0.54
Weight of Total Right Arm	= 0.06 × Body Wt. − 0.67 ± 0.15
Weight of Right Upper Arm	= 0.03 × Body Wt. − 0.48 ± 0.06
Weight of Right Forearm	= 0.03 × Body Wt. − 0.43 ± 0.06
Weight of Right Palm	= 0.02 × Body Wt. − 0.26 ± 0.05
Weight of Total Left Arm	= 0.05 × Body Wt. − 0.31 ± 0.11
Weight of Total Right Leg Including Thigh	= 0.14 × Body Wt. − 1.0 ± 0.23
Weight of Right Thigh	= 0.09 × Body Wt. − 1.0 ± 0.21
Weight of Right Calf	= 0.03 × Body Wt. 0.0 ± 0.06
Weight of Right Foot	= 0.02 × Body Wt. − 0.01 ± 0.09
Weight of Total Left Leg including Thigh	= 0.14 × Body Wt. − 0.67 ± 0.20

*Standard Error of Estimate.

segmental weights from the whole body weight are given in
Table 37-IV. The total number of cadavers studied was very
small, as in other studies,[1,4] but the equations developed may
be useful at least for the people of eastern India until a larger
sample has been studied.

References

1. Barter, J. T.: Estimation of the mass of body segments. *Wright Air Development Center, Report TR-57-260.* Dayton, Ohio, Wright Patterson Air Force Base, 1957.
2. Borelli, G. A.: *De motu Animalium lugduni Betavorum.* 1680-1681.
3. Broune, W. and Fischer, O.: *The Center of Gravity of the Human Body as Related to German Infantrymen.* Leipzig, 1889.
4. Clauser, C. E., McConville, J. T., and Young, J. W.: Weight, volume and center of mass of segments of the human body. *Wright Air Development Center, Report AMRL-TR-69-70.* Dayton, Ohio, Wright Patterson Air Force Base, 1969.
5. Dempster, W. T.: Space requirements of the seated operator. *Wright Air Development Center, Report TR-55-159.* Dayton, Ohio, Wright Patterson Air Force Base, 1955.

6. Drillis, R. and Contini, R.: *Body Segment Parameters*. Washington, D.C. U.S. Office of Vocational Rehabilitation, Dept. of Health, Education and Welfare, Rep. 1166-03, 1966.
7. Fischer, O.: *Theoretical Fundamentals for the Mechanics of Living Bodies with Special Applications to Man as Well as to Some Processes of Motion in Machines*. Berlin, B. G. Teubner, 1906.
8. Fujikawa, K.: The center of gravity in the parts of the human body. *Okajimos Folia Anat Jap, 39*(3):117-123, 1963.
9. Harless, E.: The static moments of the component masses of the human body. *Trans of Math Phys Royal Bavarian-Academy of Sci, 8*(1, 2):69-96, 257-294, Unpublished English Translation, Wright Patterson Air Force Base, Ohio, 1860.
10. Mori, M. and Yamamoto, T. Die Massenanteile der einzelnen Körperabschnitte der Japaner. *Acta Anat, 37*(4):385-388, 1959.
11. Nag, P. K.: Thesis submitted for Ph.D. degree, Calcutta University, 1976.
12. Weber, W. and Weber, E.: *Mechnik der menschlichen Gehwerkzeuge*. Göttingen, 1856.
13. Williams, M. and Lissner, H. R.: *Biomechanics of Human Motion*. Philadelphia, Saunders & Co., 1962.

INDEX

A

A.A.H.P.E.R. tests, 14, 163-171, 184-185
Acceleration, 117 (*see also* Speed)
Acclimatization, heat, 99, 103, 105-107 (*see also* Heat; Humidity)
Acid/base balance, 96 (*see also* Lactate)
Acromiale, 47
Activity, daily, 52-53, 206-208, 271, 333
Aerobic power (*see* Maximum oxygen intake)
Age effects, 90, 165, 168, 172-176, 199-205, 214-216, 222-225, 229-236, 273-320 (*see also* Growth; Maturation; Puberty; Skeletal age)
Agility, 131-132 (*see also* Skill)
Akropodion, 49
Alcohol and test results, 353
Alcoholism, 333
Altitude, 57-58, 94-96
Anaerobic capacity, 118, 120-123, 124-127, 142-147, 177
Anaerobic power, 10, 118, 142-147
Anaerobic threshold (turnpoint), 156-162
Androgens, 235
Angina, 354
Antero-posterior plane, 45
Anthropometric measures, 219, 251-252, 257-262 (*see also* Body form; Circumferences; Girth)
Anthropometric rating, 258
Anxiety, 83, 119, 138-140, 353
Arm ergometry, 124
grip (*see* Handgrip)
Arousal, 114-115
Åstrand nomogram, (*see* Predicted maximum oxygen intake)
Athletic performance, 113-141, 172-176, 251-252 (*see also* Performance predictions)
Atmospheric pollution, 100
pressure, 96 (*see also* Altitude)
Attitudes, 184
Axes, anatomical, 45-46

B

Balance, 132, 134
Ball-control, 134 (*see also* Skill)

Ballistic movements, 115-116
Bantu subjects, 53
Basketball players, 33-38, 261
Behavioral modification, 331
Belgian students, 305-320 (*see also* Leuven boys' growth study)
Bengalese students, 321-326
Bicycle ergometry, 19-20, 39-43, 75-84, 142-147, 154, 173, 338-344, 344-355, 358, 368, 378-379 (*see also* PWC $_{170}$)
Biorhythms, 208
Birth order, 255
Blood glucose, 126
Blood pressure, 102-110, 323, 339-344, 351, 364, 372, 377-383
Blood volume, 109
Body build (*see* Body form)
Body composition, 13-14, 15
Body fat, 14, 15, 26, 120, 124, 129, 132, 166, 206, 244, 252, 259-262, 263-272, 368, 370
Body form, 115-116, 120-123, 132, 138-140, 167-168, 186, 240, 242-244, 251-252, 263-272, 384-391
Body segments, 384-391
Body size, 18-31, 32-38, 56-57, 62-73, 115-116, 384-391 (*see also* Height; Weight; Body form)
Body temperature, 100, 119
Body volume, 384-391
Body weight, 19-31, 39-43, 62-73, 132, 158, 168, 206, 214, 231, 239, 259-262, 274, 281, 283, 307, 370
Borg scale, 346
Bruce test, 21-24
Bundle branch block, 364
Buoyancy, 120, 122
Bushmen, 53

C

C.A.H.P.E.R. survey, 67
tests, 85-93, 169, 186
Calf width, 169
Canada Health Survey, 331
Canadian Home Fitness Test, 329-334
Canoeing, 123-126
Car exhaust, 100

Cardiac output, 96, 107-108
  volume, 364, 374
Cardiovascular factors, 169-170 (*see also*
  Angina; Cardiac output; Muscle
  blood flow; Post-coronary patients)
Cell number, 235
Cellular factors, 116
Center of gravity, 116, 244, 384-391
Central inhibition, 114
Central processing, 116, 236
Cervicale, 49
Children-testing, 22-23, 142-147, 164,
  172-176, 184-190, 273-320 (*see also*
  Performance testing)
Circuit training, 129-130
Circumferences, 239, 243, 244, 259-262
  (*see also* Girths; Muscle bulk)
Clothing, 97, 119 (*see also* Heat)
Coach's rating, 120-123, 124-128, 211
Cold, 96-97, 138-140
Collapse, cardiovascular, 102-110
Community programs, 331
Compliance, 330, 331, 353, 354 (*see also*
  Motivation)
Contact sports, 115, 119
Control, 248
Cooper test, (*see* Twelve min. run)
Coordination, 115, 132, 135, 217, 218,
  233, 236 (*see also* Motor ability)
Coronal plane, 45
Coronary patients (*see* Post-coronary pa-
  tients)
Cost effectiveness, 331
Crampton index, 103, 109
Curriculum research, 182-183
Cycling, 208
Cyclists, 119 (*see also* Bicycle ergometry)
Czechoslovakian students, 186, 308-320

D

Dactylion, 47
Danish students, 195
Data synthesis, 136-138
Deceleration, 117
Decision time, 131
Depression, 353
Dexterity, manual, 97 (*see also* Motor
  ability; Skill)
Dinghy sailors, 117, 119, 126-127
Distribution, data, 62-63

Divers, 117
Drugs (*see* Medication)
Dry-land training, 129-130
Duration, test (*see also* Stage duration)
  training, 369, 374
Dynamic strength, 118 (*see also* Strength)
Dynamometry, 17

E

Economic factors, 239, 246 (*see also*
  Socio-cultural factors)
Ectomorphy, 257-262 (*see also* An-
  thropometry; Body form)
Education, 181-193, 251
Efficiency, 19-22, 83, 150, 321 (*see also*
  Agility; Coordination; Learning;
  Skill)
Electrocardiogram, 340-343, 351, 364,
  368
Electromyogram, 148-155
Employee fitness programs, 333
Endomorphy, 257-262 (*see also* An-
  thropometry; Body form)
Endurance, 131, 135-136, 225
English Canadian children, 64-73
English children, 305-320
Environmental variables, 94-101
Epigastrale, 46
Eskimo subjects, 54, 64-66
Ethnic groups, 53-54, 56-57, 72-73, 282,
  305-320 (*see also* individual nations)
Excess weight, 124, 126 (*see also* Body fat)
Exercise prescription, 331, 338, 366,
  367-376
Experience, 124 (*see also* Learning)
Explosive force, 118, 131, 134, 233-234,
  253 (*see also* Jump and reach test)
Extrasystoles, 364

F

Factor analyses, 170, 186
Fading, 156-162
Fainting, 107 (*see also* Collapse)
Family size, 240, 255
Fat mobilization, 119
Fatigue, 96, 138-140, 156-162, 321
Fiber type, 118, 143, 167
Field tests, 127-136 (*see also* Performance
  tests)
Figure skating, 208
Filipino subjects, 305-320

Film analysis, 117
Fitness centers, 367-376
  counselling, 330
  dimensions, 183, 185, 321-322
  and performance tests, 356-362
Flexed arm hang, 164, 286, 312 (*see also*
  Performance tests)
Flexibility, 117-118, 132-134, 212, 214,
  217, 219, 225 (*see also* Sit and reach
  test)
Fluid needs, 119
Flume, swimming, 120
Footballers, North American, 119 (*see also*
  Soccer)
Force, explosive, 117
Force platform, 117
French Canadian children, 64-73, 85-93
  (*see also* Trois Rivières study)
Frequency, exercise, 369
Friction, ground, 117
Frontal plane, 45

G

Gaussian distribution, 62-63
General social action system, 248
Genetic factors, 54-56, 72-73, 245
Genitalia (age assessment), 222-224 (*see
  also* Puberty; Skeletal age)
German students, 305-320
Girths, 214-215, 259 (*see also* Circumfer-
  ences)
Glucose drinks, 119
Gluteale, 49
Glycogen, 119, 135
Glycolysis, 177 (*see also* Acid/base; Blood
  lactate)
Gnathion, 45
Golf, 115
Goniometry, 118, 133-134 (*see also* Flexi-
  bility)
Ground conditions, 138-140, 207
Group objectives, 114
Growth, 168, 175, 184, 186, 215-216,
  222-226, 229-236, 244 (*see also* Age
  effects; Maturation; Performance
  tests; Puberty)
Growth hormone, 235
Gymnastic ability, 164 (*see also* Motor
  ability)
Gymnasts, 116, 117

H

Habituation, 75-84, 195, 373, 381-382
Hair (axillary, facial, pubic), 224
Handball, 211-221
Handgrip, 288, 318-319
Harvard step test, 14, 165, 321-326, 358
Health, general, 138-140 (*see also* Injury;
  Medical examination; Safety)
Health promotion, 329-334
  screening, 330
Heart rate, 77-84, 99, 105-107, 158, 244,
  323-326, 336, 377-383
  maximum, 96, 159
Heart rate-blood pressure product, 377-
  383
Heart volume (*see* Cardiac volume)
Heartometer, 166
Heat, 98-100, 102-110, 131, 138, 146
Heat loss, 56-57, 119
Heath-Carter somatotype, 258
Height, 62-73, 116, 124, 132, 166, 168,
  206, 214, 223-224, 231-232, 234-235,
  239, 259-262, 274, 281, 283, 306, 325
Height² standardization, 24-25, 32-38,
  206
Height/weight ratios, 259-262, 263-272
Hemoglobin, 169
Heritability estimate, 55-56
Hop, step and jump test, 134
Humidity, 98-100, 1146
Hypertension 351, 364
Hypoxia, 57, 95

I

I.B.P. tests, 7-17, 335
Ice-hockey, 208
I.C.P.F.R. tests, 7-17, 98, 189, 273-320,
  335
"Ideal" weight, 124
Iliocristale, 48
Iliospinale, 48
Indian subjects, 321-326, 384-391
Indices, 214
Industrial workers (Indian), 324
Inhibition (neural), 236
Injury, 164, 369, 375
Integration (neural), 236
Intensity (training), 369, 374 (*see also*
  Exercise prescription)
Interests, 184

International comparisons, 282, 305-320
  (*see also* Ethnic groups)
  competition, 122, 125-126, 129
  cooperation, 140, 189
Interpretation of data, 138-140
Israeli students, 273-320

J

Japanese students, 186, 263-272
Jump and reach test, 134, 231-233, 235, 255
Jumpers, 118, 134, 245

K

Kayak paddling, 123-126
Kicking, 131, 134
Kolmogorov-Smirnov test, 62-63
Kraus-Weber test, 184-185
Kurdish Jews, 54

L

Laboratory data, 9
  and fitness, 352
Lactate, blood, 120-127, 135, 143, 156-162, 177 (*see also* Anaerobic capacity)
Lateral axis, 46
Lean body mass, 26-27, 124, 208, 244, 271
Learning, motor activities, 236 test, 75-84, 118, 119, 138-140, 185, 195, 354
Leistungspulsindex, 339
Leuven boys' growth study, 187-188, 213, 229-237, 248-256
Life expectancy, 332
  style awareness, 333
Linearity, 253, 257 (*see also* Body form)
Ling's philosophy, 183
Longitudinal axis, 46
  studies, 186-193
Lung volumes, 10, 122, 124, 129, 323, 351-352, 370

M

Malayan subjects, 51-54
Marathon runners, 119
Margaria's two step test, 146
Maturity, 15, 138-140, 175, 222-228, 229-237 (*see also* Puberty; Skeletal age)
Maximum oxygen intake, 10-14, 24-28,

33-41, 51-55, 78-82, 96, 99, 103-107, 118-119, 120-123,124-127, 129, 135, 137, 156-162, 165-169, 172-176, 196, 198-200, 225, 357-362
Maximum testing, 173
Maximum voluntary force, 119 (*see also* Strength)
McCloy "drop-off" test, 165
Meals, 138-140
Medford growth study, 185-186
Medical examination, 8-9, 138-140, 172, 368 (*see also* Health; Injury; Post-coronary patients; Safety)
Medication and fitness, 352
Menarche, 224 (*see also* Maturity)
Mental fatigue, 126
Mental health, 332, 354
Mesomorphy, 252, 257-262 (*see also* Body form)
Mesosternale, 46
Metacarpale radiale, 47
Metacarpale ulnare, 47
Metatarsale fibulare, 49
Metatarsale tibiale, 49
Mood and test results, 353
Morphology, 258 (*see also* Anthropometry; Body form; Somatotype)
Motivation, 114, 138-140, 146, 173, 184, 332, 357
Motor ability, 168, 218, 235-236, 244, 252 (*see also* Agility; Coordination; Skill)
Motor development, 188
Motor vehicle registrations, 271
Movement patterns, 117
  time, 131
Multicenter exercise heart trial, 338
Muscle biopsy, 119, 135
  blood flow, 119, 135
  bulk, 115, 122, 149, 154, 167, 239
Muscle soreness, 369
  tone, 115
Myocardial infarction, 332, 368, 375 (*see also* Post-coronary patients)
Myocardial oxygen consumption, 378 (*see also* Heart rate-blood pressure product)

N

National comparisons, 64-73, 183-190, 305-320 (*see also* Ethnic groups)

Negro subjects, 53
Netherlands, 188-189
Neuromuscular factors, 116-118, 153, 170, 235
Nomograms, Åstrand (*see also* Predicted maximum oxygen intake)
  Silverman-Anderson, 22-23
  Workman, 20-22
Normal tables, 136-138
Normality, data, 62-63, 137, 268

O

Obesity, 19-20, 122, 245, 263-272, 350-351 (*see also* Body fat)
Objective ratings, 127-129
Omphalion, 46
One-leg ergometry, 75-84
Open-close hands test, 239, 245
Orthostatism, 102-110
Oxygen debt, 119, 124, 143, 146, 148-155 (*see also* Anaerobic capacity, lactate)
Oxygen dissociation curve, 57
Oxygen partial pressure, 94-96

P

Pace, 161
Parental education, 253
  participation, 255
Path analysis, 166-167, 170
Peer ratings, 126
Perceived exertion, 346
Percentile scores, 136-138
Performance predictions, 120-127, 136-140, 177, 218, 251-252
Performance tests, 14-17, 24, 85-93, 96, 98, 127-136, 163-171, 181-193, 225, 230-236, 239, 245, 250-255, 273-320, 356-362
Peripheral factors, 83-84
Personality, 184, 187
Peruvian Indians 57
Phenotypes, 257
Phonoarteriography, 378
Phosphagen stores, 117, 118
Photo cells (sprint speed), 149 (throwing speed), 212
Photoscopy, 257-262
Physical activity readiness questionnaire (PAR-Q), 331

Physical education, additional, 64-73, 181-193, 194-210, 238-247
Physical examination, 9 (*see also* Medical examination)
Physiological tests, 10-14 (*see also* Individual tests)
Physique, 13-14, 15 (*see also* Body form)
Pistol shooting, 115
Planes, anatomical, 45-46
Plate-tapping test, 233
Playing position, 137
Polish subjects, 186
Ponderal Index, 263-272
Pooling, venous, 102-110
Post-coronary patients, 332, 336-343, 354, 363-366
Posture, 102-110, 244, 324-325
Predicted maximum oxygen intake, 25-28, 79-82, 98-99, 119, 135, 325, 330, 336-344, 359, 369, 370-371
Pre-school children, 238-247
President's Council for Physical Fitness, 185
Probit scores, 136-138
Program assessment, 129-130
Progressive pulse ratio, 165
Progressive test schedules, 335-344
Psychological factors, 114-15, 122, 126
Psychomotor development, 183-184 (*see also* Motor ability)
Pternion, 49
Pubertal rating, 15 (*see also* Genitalia; Maturity; Skeletal age)
Puberty, 175, 217-218, 225, 235
Pull-ups, 286, 312 (*see also* Performance tests)
PWC$_{170}$, 28, 197, 201-205 (*see also* Bicycle ergometry)
Pyramidal system, 235

R

Racial factors, 51-59, 62-73 (*see also* Ethnic groups; National comparisons)
Radiale, 47
Reaction time, 114, 116-117, 131
Recovery curves, 323-326
Rehabilitation, 130
Reliability, 186, 330, 331, 346, 356, 377-383
Residential fitness programs, 333

Residual fitness index, 345-355
Respiratory disorders, 350
quotient, 336
Rowers, 115, 129-130, 156-162
Run, *(see also* Performance tests)
50 yard, 134, 135, 142-147, 284,
600 yard, 135, 142-147, 166, 285, 311
twelve min, 135, 163-171, 356-362
Running, 19-24, 39-43, 116, 148-155,
225, 253
Running ability, 170, 356-362
Rural life, 64-73, 194-210, 223

S

Safety, 173, 331, 363-365, 368
Sagittal plane, 45
Sample selection, 186-193
size, 186-193, 195
Saskatchewan growth and development
study, 187
Schlesinger-Guttman, 281-282
School programs, 181-193 *(see also* Physi-
cal education; Sports schools)
Screening test, 330
Seasonal factors, 85-93, 194-210
Secular trend, 263-272
Self-concept, 187
Sensorimotor skills, 245 *(see also* Motor
ability)
Sex differences, 64-73, 169, 175, 199,
239, 273-274, 305-320
Sheldon somatotype, 257-258
Shivering, 97
Shortening velocity, 153
Shuttle-run, 287, 313 *(see also* Perfor-
mance tests)
Sit and reach test, 134, 288, 316-317 *(see
also* Performance tests)
Sit-ups, 134, 164, 287, 314 *(see also*
Performance tests)
Size, 18-31 *(see also* Body form; Body size;
Height)
Skaters, 116
Skeletal age, 187, 222-225, 229-237, 251
(see also Maturity; Puberty)
Skeletal development, 243-244
Skiers, 258-262
Skill, 120-127, 131-132, 168, 213, 236,
239

Skilled sports, 115, 117, 120-127, 131-
132, 211-221 *(see also* individual
sports)
Skinfold readings, 197, 252, 259 *(see also*
Body fat; Obesity)
Sleep and fitness, 346-347
Smallest space analysis, 281-282
Smokers, 95, 333, 347-348
Snow, 207
Soccer players, 117, 127-140
Socio-cultural factors, 184, 187, 239,
248-256
Softball throw, 164
Somatotype, 15, 186, 187, 257-262, 368,
370 *(see also* Anthropometry; Body
form)
Specificity, 120, 132, 164
Speed, 116-117, 131, 135, 150, 167, 177,
212-218, 225, 233, 253
Sphyrion, 48-49
Spirometry, 351-352 *(see also* Lung vol-
umes)
Sports participation, 252
schools, 222-226
Sprinters, 117, 118, 142-147, 148-155
ST segmental depression (ecg), 340-343,
351, 354 364, 368
Stabilometer, 134
Stage duration, test, 335-344
Staircase sprint, 117, 143
Standardization, test, 7-17
Standing, 102-110
Standing broad jump, 89-92, 284, 310
Static effort, 43, 119, 124, 134, 214, 216,
219, 235
stretching, 370
Statistical tests, 61-62, 197-198 *(see also*
Factor analysis; Normality of data)
Steady state, 335-344
Step height, 325
Stepping, 19-20, 51-52, 104, 143, 146,
242, 253, 322, 329-334, 336-337, 354
(see also Staircase sprint)
Stork-stand, 117, 134
Strength, 118-119, 120-123, 124-127,
129, 131, 134, 167, 197, 206, 212,
214-218, 225, 235, 245, 252
Stride, 150
Stroke rate, 161
volume (heart), 96, 109, 169

Student evaluation, 183-190
Stylion, 47
Summer (*see* Seasonal factors)
Suprasternale, 46
Swedish students, 195
Swimmers, 33-38, 115, 120-123, 254
Symphysion, 46

T

Taiwanese students, 305-320
Technique (*see* Skill)
Telemeter (emg), 149
Temiars, 51-54
Temperature (*see* Heat; Cold)
   room, 119
Tennis players, 254
Tensiometry, 134, 166, 212
Terminology, kinanthropometric, 44-50
Test selection, 184-193
Thelion, 46
Thermoregulation, 119
Throwers, 118, 211-221, 225, 245 (*see also* Handball; Softball)
Tibiale, 48
Tilt-tests, 102-110
Track and field results, 28-29 (*see also* Running)
Training, 83-84, 118, 129-130, 138-140, 156-162, 168, 172-176, 177, 271, 332, 353, 363-366, 367-376
Transverse plane, 46
Treadmill tests, 19-24, 39-43, 104, 120, 124, 158, 196, 358, 381
Trochanterion, 48
Trois Rivières regional study, 64-73, 85-93, 188, 194-210
Twelve minute run, 26-28, 356-362 (*see also* Running)
Twin studies, 54-56

U

United States students, 185-186
Urban life, 64-73, 194-210, 223, 246

V

Validity, 330, 331, 356, 377-383
Vanves experiment, 183
Variance analyses, 197-198
Velocity, shortening, 153
   throwing, 214-218
Ventilation, 77-84, 95-96, 100, 158, 169, 336-344
Ventilatory equivalent, 336
Venous pump, 108
Venous reservoirs (*see* Pooling)
Vertex, 46
Vietnamese students, 305-320
Viscosity, tissue, 97, 117
Vital capacity (*see* Lung volumes)
Volleyball, 254
Volumes, segmental, 384-391

W

Walking, 19-24, 207
Warm-down, 370
Warm-up, 97, 158, 336
Water intake, 99
Weather, 207 (*see also* Heat; Cold)
Weight (*see* Body weight)
   segmental, 384-391
Weight $^{0.67}$ standardization, 33-38
Weight-supported sports, 122, 124
Wet-bulb temperature, 98-99 (*see also* Heat; Cold)
Whitewater paddlers, 123-126
W.H.O. tests, 7-17, 335
Wind resistance, 96, 117
Winter (*see* Seasonal factors; Cold)
   training, 129-130
Wrist breadth, 122

Y

Yemenite Jews, 54